W9-AQE-021

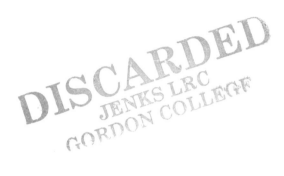

PERCEIVED EXERTION

Bruce J. Noble, PhD
Purdue University

Robert J. Robertson, PhD
University of Pittsburgh

Human Kinetics

Library of Congress Cataloging-in-Publication Data

Noble, Bruce J., 1934-
    Perceived exertion / Bruce J. Noble, Robert J. Robertson.
        p.   cm.
    Includes bibliographical references and index.
    ISBN 0-88011-508-4
    1. Kinesiology.   2. Muscle contraction--Regulation.   3. Muscular
sense.   I. Robertson, Robert J., 1943-   . II. Title.
    QP303.N55   1996   96-374
    612'.044'019--dc20   CIP

ISBN: 0-88011-508-4

Permission notices for material reprinted in this book from other sources can be found on page(s) 305-308.

Acquisitions Editor: Rik Washburn; **Developmental Editor**: Kirby Mittelmeier; **Assistant Editors**: Chad Johnson, Jackie Blakley, and John Wentworth; **Editorial Assistant:** Amy Carnes; **Copyeditor**: Karen Bojda; **Proofreaders**: Erin Cler and Bob Replinger; **Indexer**: Norman Duren, Jr.; **Typesetting and Text Layout**: Yvonne Winsor; **Text Designer**: Judy Henderson; **Cover Designer**: Jack Davis; **Illustrators:** Tom Janowski, Tara Welsch, Craig Ronto, and Jennifer Delmotte; **Printer**: Braun-Brumfield

Human Kinetics books are available at special discounts for bulk purchase. Special editions or book excerpts can also be created to specification. For details, contact the Special Sales Manager at Human Kinetics.

Printed in the United States of America   10   9   8   7   6   5   4   3   2   1

Human Kinetics
Web site: http://www.humankinetics.com

United States: Human Kinetics
P.O. Box 5076
Champaign, IL 61825-5076
1-800-747-4457
e-mail: humank@hkusa.com

Canada: Human Kinetics, Box 24040
Windsor, ON N8Y 4Y9
1-800-465-7301 (in Canada only)
e-mail: humank@hkcanada.com

Europe: Human Kinetics, P.O. Box IW14
Leeds LS16 6TR, United Kingdom
(44) 1132 781708
e-mail: humank@hkeurope.com

Australia: Human Kinetics
57A Price Avenue
Lower Mitcham, South Australia 5062
(08) 277 1555
e-mail: humank@hkaustralia.com

New Zealand: Human Kinetics
P.O. Box 105-231, Auckland 1
(09) 523 3462
e-mail: humank@hknewz.com

We dedicate this text:

To my wife, Amy, and my children Andrew, Bruce, John, and Marjorie

    BJN

To my wife, Margaret, and son, Ian

    RJR

To Gunnar A.V. Borg in honor of his retirement and to acknowledge a great intellectual debt

    BJN and RJR

Contents

Foreword

It is very pleasing that a book on perceived exertion has been written. There has been a great need for a long time for a compilation of facts and theories in this growing field. This is true with regard both to scientific and laboratory investigations and to clinical applications in various fields.

The authors, Bruce J. Noble and Robert J. Robertson, are both prominent professors in the field of exercise science. They have not only an extraordinary knowledge and general view of their science but also a very special insight in the field of perceived exertion. This is due to the fact that, for a quarter of a century or more, they have been doing research on fundamental problems in the area of perceived exertion. As a matter of fact, Bruce Noble was the one who contributed most to the introduction of perceived exertion in the United States.

In 1967, I received a generous invitation from Bruce Noble to visit Pittsburgh to do research with him and his colleagues at the University of Pittsburgh. Five years before that, in 1962, I had published a monograph in Sweden entitled *Physical Performance and Perceived Exertion*. In this book, I introduced the concept of perceived exertion along with some methods to measure it, presented laboratory studies on perceived exertion and physiological correlates, and offered some examples of clinical applicatons. Noble read this book along with some preceding articles that I—as a psychologist interested in perception and psychophysics with a background in sports—had done earlier with Hans Dahlstrom, a medical doctor and head of a laboratory for clinical physiology. Bruce Noble was very interested in this work and invited me to his laboratory. A long and fruitful collaboration thus started.

During the spring semester of 1968, I visited with Ellsworth Buskirk and James Skinner at Pennsylvania State University. Oded Bar-Or also worked there at that time, and we all got to know each other very well and have collaborated during the intervening years. In 1973, I returned to Pittsburgh to continue my collaboration with Bruce Noble. During that visit I was also invited to the University of Wisconsin by William P. Morgan. Morgan specifically wanted to stress the emotional/motivational and personality aspects of perceived exertion.

Bruce Noble got several students (e.g., Robert Robertson, Kent Pandolf, and Enzo Cafarelli) interested in the study of perceived exertion. Robertson took over leadership in the exercise lab at Pittsburgh when Noble left for Wyoming in the middle 1970s. Robertson, in an excellent way, continued the work that Noble started.

The field of perceived exertion—as Noble and Robertson point out—is a complex, interdisciplinary field with its origins mainly in psychology and physiology. There are, however, also some influences and contributions from such diverse disciplines as philosophy, sociology, and chemistry. Properly placed, perceived exertion is a subfield within perception and psychophysics. Subjective ratings depend not only upon sensory cues but also upon cognitive and emotional factors, personality traits, and so on. Many psychological and physiological factors vary in specific ways and interact with each other during exercise. This interaction gives us a basis to understand and explain the variation of perceived exertion, depending upon the kind of performance and its duration, the environment and performance situation, the person doing the exercise, and so on. Theories that will help us understand the factors during exercise that cause a certain perception of exertion, therefore, have to be rather complex with ingredients from many subfields.

Psychophysical scaling came to flourish especially during the 1960s, thanks to the development of the ratio scaling methods of S.S. Stevens and colleagues at Harvard. Before Stevens no good methods existed for direct scaling of sensory attributes. The new methods made it possible to describe perceptual growth functions mathematically, most often with power functions. Also in the 1960s, ergometers, such as bicycles and treadmills, started to become very popular in exercise laboratories for both scientific and clinical use. The time was just right for scientific studies of perceived exertion. I was glad to get a letter from Stevens in which he congratulated me for having opened up a new field for psychophysical research.

The Stevens methodology did, however, have an inherent drawback. It was possible to get growth functions for intermodal comparisons with results based on groups of subjects. However, when individual functions were the main interest and the purpose was to make direct intra- or interindividual comparisons of an "absolute" character, then the methods were not suitable. The main drawback in the ratio scaling methodology may be elucidated by a simple example. If one percept (e.g., the subjective weight of an object) is estimated to be twice as intense as another percept, this does not say if it is strong (e.g., heavy) or not. Special methods therefore had to be developed that not only could give a reasonably valid growth function for different performances but also could provide information about the individual's perceived intensity level.

The main reason for the development of these level-directed methods was the great need for simple procedures to determine perceived exertion that included perceptions from the working muscles and joints and from the central cardiopulmonary system. It should also be possible to distinguish between normal healthy symptoms and pathological signs, such as angina pain. Outside of Stevens' group of psychophysicists at Harvard, there was no great interest in psychophysical scaling in the United States. Scientists and practioners in medicine and physiology were not acquainted with the methods that facilitated the introduction of the new level-anchored scaling methods, such as my RPE scale. The lack of specific knowledge in scaling and related application among these people made acceptance of the RPE scale easier because they did not have any prejudices or biases against the methodology.

I have often said, "Two things make my heart beat: walking up stairs and watching pretty girls. But only one thing makes me perceive exertion." Although this statement is, of course, not entirely true, the point is that heart rate is sensitive not only to physical exercise but also to emotional sensations and anxiety. As there are more than two things that make the heart rate increase, there are also many things underlying the variations in perceived exertion. The human brain integrates many peripheral and central signals and cues into a kind of gestalt. Physiological variables are often more specific than the overall perception made by the brain. For example, psychological defense mechanisms may make us suppress the subjective intensity of exercise, whereas anxiety may make us overreact and overestimate exertion. In pathological cases, the situation becomes very complex with several physiological signs and symptoms needed for a precise clinical determination. Many factors that influence perceived exertion need to be theoretically anchored in a psychobiological frame of reference.

It has been a great pleasure for me to read this book. It covers most of the important areas of research and clinical application in the area of perceived exertion. It deals with perception of exertion as it arises from physiological cues coming from both cardiopulmonary sources and musculoskeletal functions and from psychological factors of a conscious or unconscious kind, as well as the use of perceived exertion during exercise testing and during training and rehabilitation.

Perceived Exertion by Bruce Noble and Bob Robertson is warmly recommended to everyone who wants to know the background and development of the field, to penetrate ideas and theories, and to obtain descriptive facts about many different kinds of exercises, situations, and groups of subjects. It not only helps in understanding the advantages of using perceived exertion in clinical diagnostics, rehabilitation, and sports, but it also gives the reader an insight into the difficulties and pitfalls of the scaling methodology.

Gunnar A.V. Borg
Stockholm, Sweden

Preface

Interest in human perceptual response goes back to the very roots of modern psychology. Pioneering in a new branch of philosophy, William James at Harvard University and Wilhelm Wundt at the University of Leipzig are jointly credited as the founders of experimental psychology. Wundt is regarded as the seminal figure in the field we now call psychophysics. Psychophysics attempts to discover the orderly relation between physical stimuli and human sensation, what we might call subjective reality. It is interesting that James thought attempts to measure subjective reality were not possible and took experimental psychology in a different direction. As fate would have it, the torch of classical psychophysics, lit by Wundt, was eventually passed to a latterday Harvard psychologist, S.S. Stevens, who not only believed that humans could make meaningful evaluations of their sensory experience but explicated a new law stating that human sensation is a power function of the stimulus applied.

Emil Kraepelin, a psychiatrist and director of a famous clinic in Munich who trained with Wundt, adapted the new experimental techniques to psychiatry. Psychiatry, of course, has long been concerned with the disparity between subjective and objective reality. Sigmund Freud built his entire psychoanalytic theory based upon the knowledge that perception of the objective world could be altered by early caretaking experiences lodged as unconscious psychic contents.

To those of us working in the burgeoning field of sports medicine in the 1960s, several things became abundantly clear:

1. As we attempted to understand human exercise experience, physiological measurements were at once quintessentially important and, at the same time, incomplete.
2. How we *feel* about exercise, as with love and work, can affect its outcome.
3. Humans perceive muscular effort, as Stevens and Freud could have told us, not as absolute physical reality, but relative to a multitude of factors that color our response.

Swedish psychologist Gunnar Borg was the first to take up these questions in a rigorous scientific manner. He adapted Steven's power law to perceptions made during exercise and developed a practical method for measuring perceptual effort that is used today throughout the world (the Borg scale).

Interest in perception of muscular effort in the United States can be traced to the visit of Gunnar Borg to the University of Pittsburgh and Pennsylvania State University in 1967-68. A psychological Johnny Appleseed, Borg spread his perceptual seeds throughout the United States and subsequently the world. Those of us who remember that period continue to be amazed at the rapidity with which the Borg scale took hold and became an accepted tool in both research and clinical settings. The scale added a dimension to the study of the exercising human that was needed, but, more important, it was simple to use and had an easily understood construct validity.

Although research interest and productivity has increased exponentially since the late 1960s, the lack of a comprehensive text in the area of perceived exertion is notable. The current bibliography comprises over 450 published articles.[1] Although several important edited symposia reports and review papers have been published, none have attempted an all-embracing synthesis of this most important field of inquiry.

This collection of chapters has taken on a life of its own, with eight years of manuscripts written, revised, and rewritten, but the work has been consistent and the goal unchanging. While we have tried to be theoretically provocative for the researchers, the concerns of those who monitor subjective effort in testing and field environments have not been forgotten.

We begin with a historical review of the field of study. Historical perspective and scientific geneology, we believe, provide a grounding that serves as the genesis for further consideration of the body of knowledge on perceived exertion.

One of our concerns has been that the Borg scale is so easy to use and understand that its acceptance and proliferation occurred without much appreciation for the basics of perceptual measurement. Therefore, we have reviewed, in moderate detail, the psychophysical measurement of what might be called the ''effort sense.''

The study and practical use of perceived exertion has become so identified with a single technique of measurement, the category scale variously known as the Borg scale or rating of perceived exertion (RPE) scale, that we have devoted an entire chapter to its development, administration, and experimental use. It is our view, despite our continued commitment to the Borg scale, that the study of human perception during movement should not be linked to a single measurement tool. As is always the case, measurement must be linked to the demands of the research or clinical goal.

For a field of study to mature it must move from description to theoretical explanation. The study of perceived exertion has grown to the point where fourth

---

[1]The use of ratings of perceived exertion as a supplemental or descriptive measure has become standard in many research protocols. Often such data is reported with interesting comments. However, when we speak of the perceived exertion bibliography, we have chosen to include only those articles that study the exercise perception process per se.

generation models are being adapted and refined. Several chapters have been devoted to the discussion of theoretical models developed over the years to explicate the manner in which sensory signals mediate the intensity of exertional ratings. Respiratory-metabolic mediators and peripheral mediators are discussed in separate chapters. One chapter is devoted to the development of a global model that attempts a broad explanation of not only physiological but also psychological inputs to the effort sense. This latter chapter also includes a discussion of the future directions of perceived exertion research.

We recognize a number of exercise psychologists, especially William Morgan, Jack Rejeski, and the team of Bob Kinsman and Phil Weiser, for their valuable contributions to our understanding of the role of psychological factors to the setting of exertional ratings. Their work, and that of many other authors, serves as the foundation for our chapter dealing with this subject.

In keeping with our goal to be complete we have even delved into the topic of the unconscious as a mediator of perceptual ratings. Certainly a construct such as personality may play a role in how we perceive physical effort, but we do not consciously monitor such an input. Nor are we consciously aware of many physiological correlates to the effort sense, such as oxygen consumption.

Last, two chapters have been written that address the topics of graded exercise testing and exercise prescription. Specifically, we discuss the research that has examined the role of perceived exertion ratings in each of these activities. Borg scale ratings serve as a valuable subjective supplement to physiological data recorded during an exercise test. How one is feeling can be as valuable as how one is responding physiologically to exercise graded according to intensity. Likewise, ratings of perceived exertion have been found to be useful to the exercise client as well as the exercise leader in the control of prescriptive dosage.

It is our hope that this book will provide a practical and theoretically complete resource for those interested in using perceived exertion in either clinical or research settings. We have passed the 25-year mark, using 1967-68 as a starting point, in our search for answers to the mechanisms by which humans perceive their effort during physical exercise. The next 25 years will be the responsibility of those who read this book.

We owe a huge debt of gratitude to our many colleagues and graduate students who have in so many ways, directly and indirectly, contributed to the writing of this book. At the risk of slighting someone, we would like to single out Enzo Cafarelli, Ken Metz, Kent Pandolf, and Fredric Goss. Special appreciation is extended to Donna Farrell and many wonderful graduate students for their support, encouragement, and clerical assistance in preparing this book. These pages serve as the conduit for the work of many. We thank all of you!

I

PART

Background and Development

Most exercise scientists associate the study of perceived exertion with its founder, Swedish psychologist Gunnar Borg. Less known are the circumstances under which the construct was first developed, and the sequence of events that led to its rapid popularity. Although Borg first published his seminal studies in 1961, rapid growth of the construct is usually attributed to the introduction of his category scale during a sabbatical visit to the United States in 1967-68. Since that time over 450 articles have appeared about perceived exertion. Chapter 1 addresses where we have been in our collective search for answers to questions related to perception of effort during physical activity.

The study of perception is the central concern of the science of psychophysics. Chapter 2 attempts to establish a link between 19th century studies by E.H. Weber and G.T. Fechner, both classical psychophysicists who pioneered in the discovery of perceptual laws, and 20th century scientists such as S.S. Stevens and Borg. Stevens, considered by many to be the father of modern psychophysics, established a power law using a ratio method known as magnitude estimation which states that sensation grows with the power of the stimulus. Borg, making a conceptual and methodological leap from earlier psychophysicists, was concerned with methods that enabled clinical studies to emphasize interindividual subjective differences—a feat not possible using conventional ratio scaling methods.

Chapter 3 outlines the development of the so-called Borg scale, often referred to as the RPE scale (rating of perceived exertion). A major feature of this chapter is the detailing of the empirical steps required to justify the Borg scale as a legitimate interval scale. The scale was designed so that subjective intensity paralleled physiological intensity, i.e., heart rate. Verbal expressions on the scale

1

were progressively ordered according to subjective intensity and intervals between expressions were subjectively equal. The simplicity and "common sense" character of the Borg scale has often led to a more or less casual approach to its administration. This chapter argues for rather rigorous standards when perception is measured both in research and clinical environments.

The capstone of both individual and collective scholarly inquiry is the development of theory that generalizes knowledge beyond limited description. Although the great majority of empirical reports dealing with perceived exertion have been more descriptive than theoretical, a thread of model building by various authors can be identified from the very beginning. Chapter 4 takes a look at the development of models of exertional perception whose focus on exertional symptoms can be traced to the landmark work of Phillip Weiser and Bob Kinsman. Their model defined the alpha source of symptoms to be in the "physiological substrata." "Discrete symptoms" reach the terminus after passing through several levels of processing. The Kinsman-Weiser model was modified by Pandolf to include the concept of differentiated perceptual ratings, i.e., peripheral and central inputs to the effort sense.

This classification of differentiated symptoms is an extension of Ekblom and Goldbarg's hypothesis that the effort sense is shaped by local peripheral signals reflecting feelings of muscular discomfort and central signals of cardiopulmonary exertion. Models with a "perceptual-cognitive reference filter," reflecting a broad range of psychological and cognitive processes through which physiological symptoms are screened, are also discussed.

1

Historical Development of Perceived Exertion

We all perceive exertion. Monitoring how we feel about the exercise we are performing is a minute-by-minute process for active humans. The intensity of our perception provides the major intrinsic input for making decisions about our energy output. Sensations that we perceive to be within the comfort zone do not alert us to the need for altering pace. On the contrary, sensations that we perceive as too intense for toleration require a decision to adjust pace.

Most of our perceptions associated with exertion are made so automatically that their presence and usefulness are often taken for granted. One of my former students was fond of chiding me with the statement, "But isn't perceived exertion just common sense?" Indeed, our senses and how we interact with them are used so reflexively that they are just that, common senses. Nevertheless, over the past 30 years there has been growing scientific and clinical interest in the measurement concept we have come to know as perceived exertion.

The purpose of this chapter is to provide the reader with a historical perspective of how this field of study began and developed. To provide this perspective, we have assembled here what we believe to be a reasonably complete collection of related publications. This collection of roughly 450 articles represents the body of knowledge related to perceived exertion that is located in published manuscripts. Thus, the historical perspective that we wish to share will primarily be based on the written productivity of the authors who have generated this collected body of knowledge.

Although we believe to have completed a comprehensive review of the literature, we make no claim that it is exhaustive. To be sure, it is virtually impossible to assemble every piece of literature related to a particular field of study. For example, foreign language articles are often difficult to locate and translate, and, in fact, some manuscripts often receive only very local distribution. We made the conscious decision not to include manuscripts until they had been published, with two exceptions. We elected to include Borg's unpublished reports from the

University of Stockholm because of their historical and scientific value. Also, a few unpublished but peer-reviewed abstracts have been utilized. We have consciously opted not to include articles that have used perceived exertion as a secondary dependent variable. In such articles, perceptual data is collected for descriptive purposes without the intention of studying the perceptual process per se or the interaction of perception with physiological or psychological processes. Some of these publications coincidentally have made insightful contributions; however, most are merely descriptive in nature.

Our attempts at history here are rather chronological, quantitative, and anecdotal. We offer apologies to professional historians who may read our humble attempts at recording and interpreting history. We certainly do realize that written history may better be left to those who are not living it. So, let us say that we are only trying to provide reasonably accurate data for future historians. We also admit that quantification of author research productivity may or may not be related to quality of their contributions. Nevertheless, we believe the following chronology and quantification of the literature will provide a useful perspective to the reader. Likewise, since we have been very close to those who have written in the area, our anecdotes can be considered primary sources for future historians.

Defining the Concept

There can be no doubt that Gunnar Borg, Swedish psychologist, is the father of the concept of perceived exertion. He coined the term, developed the first rating scale that measures perceptual intensity during exercise, and served as a scientific missionary, spreading knowledge of the concept throughout the world. Borg was interested in studying the way in which individuals subjectively adapt to physical exercise. The rating scale developed for this work, discussed in detail later, has come to be called the Borg scale or rating of perceived exertion (RPE) scale.

How is the concept defined? Perceived exertion can be defined as the act of detecting and interpreting sensations arising from the body during physical exercise. The term *exertion* has often been criticized as inappropriate or too specific to endurance-type activity. Some have suggested the use of terms like *perceived fatigue, perceived effort,* or *perceived force.* In fact, in one of Borg's earliest publications (1962) he suggested that *perceived force* would be preferable for short-time exercise, while *perceived fatigue* or *perceived exertion* would be more appropriate for what we now call aerobic activity. Despite such suggestions, *perceived exertion* has become the term generally accepted for use with all types of human movement.

Two other points are important relative to semantics. First, one can think of terms for describing perceived exertion as those which reflect the effort *exerted by* the person on the environment, for example, perceived effort or stress. For instance, while running up hill you can think of the effort or force necessary to overcome the grade. On the other hand, one can think of the influence the movement has on the body itself, for example, perceived discomfort or strain. An example of this would be the perception of strain *caused by* running up the hill. Such a distinction may be academic, but it emphasizes the importance of exact scaling instructions, since the perceptual response may be somewhat different in each case. The instruction should be dictated by the result desired. Usually the term *perceived exertion* has been used to refer to the latter example.

Second, we have generally found that perceived exertion can be rated independently of other competing stimuli. Cardiac patients often rate their exertion to be quite low at low exercise intensities despite the fact that angina (chest) pain is relatively intense. This is not to say that pain is consciously excluded from the internal perceptual equation providing sensory feedback that acts to adjust exercise intensity. It means that individuals can distinguish between *exertion* and non-exercise-related *pain*. The same can be said for environmental stimuli like temperature.

Publication Productivity

One method of assessing the growth of an area of study is to simply tally the frequency of published articles. In the late 1950s and early 1960s perceived exertion as a field of study gained its impetus. This period was marked by studies in the psychological discipline known as psychophysics (the study of the growth of sensation as a function of increasing physical stimuli). Psychophysics laid the methodological groundwork and provided early validation of Borg's perceptual scale. Increased use of the Borg scale, especially in the United States, began in the late 1960s. Borg visited the United States for the first time while on sabbatical leave from Sweden's Umea University in 1967-68. He spent the fall semester at the University of Pittsburgh with Bruce Noble and the spring semester at Pennsylvania State University with James Skinner and Ellsworth Buskirk. Certainly the seeds for future expansion of the concept were sowed during this period. The annual meeting of the American College of Sports Medicine (ACSM) was held in the spring of 1968 in State College, Pennsylvania. The papers delivered at this conference, with Borg, Noble, and Michael Sherman as coauthors, served as the first broad exposure of the concept of perceived exertion to an audience of exercise scientists.

The growth of the body of knowledge related to perceived exertion can be seen from the frequency of publications presented in figure 1.1. Borg's doctoral dissertation, published in 1962, as well as a few of his preliminary studies and other psychophysical investigations marked the early history of publication in this area. After a relative hiatus in the mid-1960s, the beginning of rapid growth in publication productivity seems to be coincident with Borg's visit to the United States in 1967-68. Except for two exceptional years, 1973 and 1977, publications increased linearly with time until about 1980. Shifts from linearity in 1973 ($N = 16$) and in 1982 ($N = 30$) were largely due to composite publications

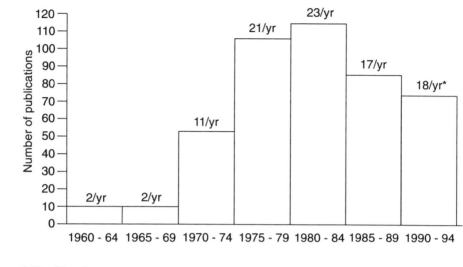

* 90 - 93 only

Figure 1.1   Publication productivity in perceived exertion research.

following perceived exertion symposia held at annual meetings of the American College of Sports Medicine. The largest output of published papers in any one year occurred in 1977 ($N = 39$). This was the year Borg published his first edited work, entitled *Physical Work and Effort*. The second largest annual output occurred in 1986 ($N = 31$) with the publication of the second Stockholm symposium, ''The Perception of Exertion in Physical Work'' (Borg and Ottoson 1986). The period between 1980 and 1984 was the apex of publication productivity for any five year period ($N = 114$). Following 1984, the publication rate seems to have plateaued at about 17 or 18 papers per year.

Author Productivity

The relatively low publication rate in the area of perceived exertion over the past 25 years compared with other subspecialties within exercise physiology or sport psychology can probably be explained by the dearth of authors with a primary interest in the topic. For example, only 10 authors have served as primary authors on five or more articles dealing with perceived exertion. Table 1.1 lists these authors. Obviously, Gunnar Borg leads the productivity list. Special mention should be made of Enzo Cafarelli, William Morgan, and Kent Pandolf, who have made major contributions to the growth of this subdiscipline.

Table 1.1   Authors With Five or More Publications

Author	Location	Publications
G.A.V. Borg	University of Stockholm, Sweden	39
R.J. Robertson	University of Pittsburgh	14
K.B. Pandolf	United States Army Institute of Environmental Medicine, Natick	11
Bruce Noble	Purdue Univeristy	10
W.P. Morgan	University of Wisconsin	9
E. Cafarelli	York University, Canada	7
K.J. Killian	McMaster University, Canada	7
R.G. Eston	University of Liverpool, UK	5
G. Ljunggren	University of Stockholm, Sweden	5
W.J. Rejeski	Wake Forest University	5

Journal Sources

Another method of identifying the proliferation of a research area is to examine the extent to which scientific journals utilize the topic in their issues. Such an analysis reveals much about the disciplinary origins of the authors as well as the clinical applications of the data. For example, the list of journals in table 1.2 indicates an interest in perceived exertion predominantly in the fields of applied physiology, applied psychology, cardiac rehabilitation, ergonomics, kinesiology, and sports medicine. The journal *Medicine and Science in Sports and Exercise* far and away leads other journals in the publication of articles about perceived exertion ($N = 61$).

Three other important sources of literature are the internally published research by Borg and his colleagues in the Department of Psychology at the University of Stockholm (Box 5602, S-11486 Stockholm, Sweden) and two books containing the proceedings of the 1976 and 1985 international symposia held in Stockholm: *Physical Work and Effort* (Borg 1977a) and *The Perception of Effort in Physical Work* (Borg and Ottoson 1986). Details of these symposia will be discussed below.

Symposia

Beginning in the early 1970s, a number of symposia were held that were entirely devoted to the topic of perceived exertion. By and large these symposia were

Table 1.2   Journals Publishing Five or More Articles

Journal	Number
Medicine and Science in Sports and Exercise	61
European Journal of Applied Physiology	33
Ergonomics	24
Perception and Motor Skills	23
Journal of Applied Physiology	14
Journal of Sport and Exercise Psychology	10
International Journal of Sports Medicine	9
Research Quarterly for Exercise and Sport	9
British Journal of Sports Medicine	7
Canadian Journal of Applied Sport Science	7
Physician and Sportsmedicine	7
Journal of Cardiopulmonary Rehabilitation	6
Journal of Sports Medicine	5
Journal of Sports Medicine and Physical Fitness	5

international in character. At the very least Gunnar Borg was a guest speaker at these symposia, and often speakers representing several countries were featured. The first such symposium organized in the United States occurred in conjunction with the annual meeting of the American College of Sports Medicine held in Philadelphia, Pennsylvania, in 1972. Presentations were given by Borg, William Morgan (University of Wisconsin), Bruce Noble (University of Pittsburgh), James Skinner (Pennsylvania State University), and William Cain (John B. Pierce Foundation, New Haven, Connecticut). These papers were published in *Medicine and Science in Sports and Exercise* in 1973 (vol. 5, no. 2). We believe that no other single event was as important to the eventual growth of perceived exertion as a viable area of research in the United States. The symposium was well attended and the subsequent publication of the proceedings reached a very large American audience. (While ice skating after a cocktail party in Philadelphia, Borg and Noble made the little known but important discovery that one could perceive exertion to be 6 or 7 on the Borg scale with a heart rate exceeding 150 beats per min. Many have subsequently confirmed the fact that RPE and heart rate are not causally related. However, not until 1990 did Borg confirm our recreational findings in a published paper.)

Two subsequent symposia were held in the United States. First, the concept of perceived exertion was initially introduced to an audience principally composed of physical educators at a symposium presented in 1977 at the annual meeting of the American Alliance of Health, Physical Education, Recreation and Dance in Seattle, Washington. Second, a symposium that represented a 10-year update of perceived exertion research was sponsored by the American College of Sports Medicine at its 1981 annual meeting held in Miami, Florida. At this symposium, in addition to Borg and Noble, what might be called the second generation of investigators interested in perceived exertion presented their work. Other speakers were Enzo Cafarelli, Kent Pandolf, and Robert Robertson. While this symposium was well attended, it was clear that the character of the audience had changed. There were many more health care specialists who had become accustomed to using the Borg scale in various clinical environments ranging from graded exercise testing to exercise training. By 1981, Borg had made several visits to the United States during which he made presentations in virtually every corner of the country and to audiences in several disciplines. In addition, many clinical exercise physiologists had advocated the use of the Borg scale for testing and training cardiac patients. For example, Michael Pollock, currently at the University of Florida, included perceived exertion as an important element in his extensive presentation schedule. As a result, it became clear to many of us in the early 1980s that the clinical use of perceived exertion far exceeded its purely scientific exposure. The Borg scale had gained acceptance as a handy instrument effective in dealing with several difficult clinical situations. For example, cardiac patients who were receiving medications that reduced their heart rate response to exercise used perceived exertion as a means of gauging their energy expenditure. Many scientists began to worry that the concept was growing beyond its substantiated value and that many were using the Borg scale with no formal training in its application. Despite this concern, the concept continued to be used and supported by a large and varied group of clinicians in sports medicine.

Perhaps the two most truly international symposia dealing with perceived exertion were organized by Gunnar Borg and held in Stockholm, Sweden. The first occurred in 1976 and resulted in the publication of the book entitled *Physical Work and Effort*. This symposium was held at the Wenner-Gren Center in Stockholm and consisted of speakers from England, Finland, Israel, Italy, Norway, Sweden, United States, West Germany, and Yugoslavia. The second, held in 1985 with an equal array of international speakers, was published in 1986.

Borg has played an active role in the International Congress of Applied Psychology for many years and as a result organized important symposia for this organization in 1971 and 1974. These symposia, held in Leige, Belgium, and Montreal, Canada, were not entirely devoted to perceived exertion per se but definitely had a strong focus in that direction. The proceedings of the Leige Congress were published in 1972 (Piret 1972).

It can be said that the presentation of symposia, especially in conjunction with important national and international conferences, has played a prominent role in the growth of the concept of perceived exertion.

Research Topics

It should be obvious, even to the casual observer, that when the body of knowledge concerned with perceived exertion reaches 450 published articles that a wide variety of topics have been explored. This is indeed the case. Categorizing these topics is a useful aid to understanding the nature of the study of perceived exertion. Table 1.3 represents such a categorization of articles. This process was definitely arbitrary since the complexity of many papers make single categorizations almost impossible.

To those of us working in the subspecialty called perceived exertion, the generation of more than 450 articles in approximately 25 years seems quite extraordinary. The truth of the matter is that, although productivity has been adequate, it has been far from maximal. There is certainly plenty of ground to

Table 1.3   Categories of Research Productivity (1957–1993)

Category	Published topics
Relationship of perceived exertion to various physiological factors or conditions (e.g., "anaerobic threshold," lactate, electromyography, heart rate, catecholamines, menstruation, sleep loss, etc.)	48
Clinical applications	41
Psychological factors	39
Psychophysics and research methodology	38
Exercise testing and prescription	29
Perceived exertion in various types of exercise (isometric, dynamics, walk, run, bike, swim, arm, leg, etc.)	28
Differentiated perceptions; local and central factors	25
Environmental factors	25
Occupational applications	24
Review articles	23
Pulmonary function	22
Physical training and fitness level	22
Ergogenic aids	15
Growth, aging, and gender	14
Pedal rate and resistance	10
Prediction and theoretical modeling	10
Sport applications	8

be plowed and replowed by future scientists. The larger specialty of psychobiology, within which the area of perceived exertion exists, has only begun to be explored.

Until the last 5 or 10 years research productivity was dominated by studies that explored the relationship between perceived exertion and various physiological factors or conditions that alter physiological response. Likewise, many papers compared perceived exertion among various modes of exercise. Some of these studies were experimental in nature, but many were purely descriptive. A preponderance of descriptive studies is predictable in a new field of study as investigators search for variables that might be fruitful for future study. The comparatively large number of studies in the area of psychophysics and research methodology also seems logical, given the need for the proper development and validation of a new measurement tool and concept.

More recent productivity originates from three pools of scientific interest. First, increasing interest has been shown over the past 10 years in various psychological factors that mediate exertional ratings. Second, more inquiry has focused on the accuracy of perceived exertion as a method of prescribing and controlling exercise intensity. The third interest area, clinical application of perceived exertion in various medical settings and conditions, continues unabated from early years.

With regard to future study, no interest area has been exhausted of potential. There is no limitation to the future investigator with innovative ideas and a passion for understanding more about the interaction of psychology and physiology in human performance. Several areas of inquiry, however, require increased effort. For example, very little has been accomplished regarding the efficacy of perceived exertion in sport environments. How can perceived exertion be used in sport to promote successful and efficient performance? Perhaps the most neglected area can be seen in theoretical conceptualization. After 25 years a great deal of descriptive data has been amassed, but few papers have attempted the difficult task of building theoretical models that help to explain human perception of effort. We hope this book will be the beginning of a new interest in theory building. Further, we look forward to greater measurement diversity in the future. As in every other field of scientific interest, choice of perceptual measurement should be dictated by the research question and not by historical precedent.

Synthesis

Table 1.4 lists the major literature reviews that consider the scientific study of perceived exertion. The earliest of these reviews represented attempts by Borg to educate the scientific community about the new concept and its psychophysical underpinnings. More recent reviews reflect the desire of investigators to synthesize an accelerating body of knowledge for a rapidly growing scientific and clinical audience. In addition to a general audience, these reviews

Table 1.4   Major Perceived Exertion Reviews

Borg, G. 1970. Perceived exertion as an indicator of somatic stress. *Scand. J. Rehab. Med.* 2-3:92-98.

Borg, G. 1971. The perception of physical performance. In *Frontiers of fitness*, ed. R. Shepherd. Springfield, IL: Charles C. Thomas.

Borg, G., and B.J. Noble. 1974. Perceived exertion. *Exer. Sport Sci. Rev.* 2:131.

Borg, G. 1978. Subjective effort in relation to physical performance and working capacity. In *Psychology: From research to practice*, ed. H.L. Pick et al. New York: Plenum Press.

Pandolf, K.B. 1978. Influence of local and central factors dominating rated perceived exertion. *Percept. Motor Skills* 46:683-98.

Rejeski, W.J. 1981. The perception of exertion: A social psychophysiological integration. *J. of Sports Psych.* 4:305-20.

Mihevic, P.M. 1981. Sensory cues for perceived exertion. A review. *Med. Sci. Sports Exerc.* 13:150-63.

Nishimura, J. 1983. Problems of perceived exertion. *Japanese Psychol. Rev.* 24(2):174-202.

Pandolf, K.B. 1983. Advances in the study and application of perceived exertion. In *Exerc. Sport Sci. Rev.* 11:118-58.

Maresh, C.M., and B.J. Noble. 1984. Utilization of perceived exertion ratings during exercise testing and training. In *Cardiac rehabilitation: Exercise testing and prescription*, ed. L.K. Hall. New York: Spectrum Books.

O'Sullivan, S.B., 1984. Perceived exertion: A review. *Phys. Ther.* 64:343-46.

Gamberale, F. 1985. The perception of exertion. *Ergonomics* 28:299-308.

Carton, R.L., and E.C. Rhodes. 1985. A critical review of the literature on ratings for perceived exertion. *Sports Med.* 2:198-222.

have been written for specialists in exercise physiology, sport psychology, sports medicine, cardiac rehabilitation and preventive exercise, physical therapy, and ergonomics.

Seminal Articles

It goes without saying that the work of Gunnar Borg provided the foundation for the development of the area that we refer to as perceived exertion. His early publications described the theoretical and psychophysical basis for the study of perception during human movement as well as potential practical applications. Borg's motivation has always been to provide a theoretical construct and technique that could be practically used to assess the subjective cost of exercise and to compare interindividual ratings of exertion. His work was definitely seminal. However, any attempt at providing a historical perspective to the growth of an area of study would be remiss if it did not pay homage to others who provided the building blocks for later creative advancement. Scientific interest in human sensation has its roots in both physiology and psychology. Physiologist C.S. Sherrington reported the results of his work on muscular sense as early as 1900. Likewise, psychologist G.T. Fechner published a volume entitled *The Elements of Psychophysics* in 1860, which explored the relationship between that which we perceive in the psychical world and stimuli arising from the physical world. It is not our purpose here to elucidate the enormous scientific base developed prior to the work of Borg but only to acknowledge its importance.

The psychophysical studies of S.S. Stevens at Harvard University probably represent the most immediate precursor to those of Borg. Others, such as J.C. Stevens, G. Bernyer, and H. Eisler, were simultaneously investigating the psychophysics of force production and muscular effort during the late 1950s and early 1960s. Borg's more practical orientation, validation of an effective perceptual scale, extraordinary efforts to inform an international audience, and sustained publication record over 35 years account for his preeminence in the field of perception of muscular effort. Publications that might be considered seminal to the study of perceived exertion are listed in table 1.5. This list should in no way be considered exhaustive but should provide the interested researcher with points of origin. The articles appear in chronological order.

Where We Have Been

We must admit to a modicum of surprise about the growth of the perceived exertion concept both as a research topic and especially as a valuable clinical tool. Both of us, along with many others, have worked diligently to promote this growth, but the result far exceeds our initial imagination. Borg's visit to the United States in 1967-68 was at least partially serendipitous. In the early 1960s, while Noble searched the literature to find material related to the way in which physical performance may be enhanced by motivating conditions, he uncovered one of Borg's earliest published articles. A letter inquiring about the details of perceived exertion resulted in correspondence, which eventually led to an invitation to collaborate in Pittsburgh during the fall semester of 1967.

The field of sports medicine during the late 1960s was gathering considerable momentum. It is fair to say that exercise physiology was, and remains today, the dominant subspecialty in sports medicine. However, ACSM has always given enthusiastic support to the efforts of investigators interested in perceived exertion. Such a statement is a tribute to the eclectic nature of the college and its willingness to bring under its collective umbrella any and all of those committed to the furtherance of sport and exercise science as an important scientific endeavor.

Perhaps the answer to the unpredictably rapid growth of the concept of perceived exertion can be found in the growth of the American College of Sports

Table 1.5   Seminal Articles Related to Perceived Exertion

Fechner, G.T. [1860] 1966. *Elemente der Psychophysik.* Leipzig: Breitkopf and Harterl. Reprint, vol. 1, ed. D.H. Howes and E.G. Boring, trans. H.E. Adler. New York: Holt, Rinehart and Winston.

Sherrington, C.S. 1900. The muscular sense. In *Textbook of physiology,* ed. E.A. Schafer. Edinburgh and London: Pentland.

Stevens, S.S. 1957. On the psychophysical law. *Psycholog. Rev.* 64:153-81.

Stevens, S.S., and E.H. Galanter. 1957. Ratio scales and category scales for a dozen perceptual continua. *J. Exp. Psych.* 54:377-411.

Stevens, J.C., and J.D. Mack. 1959. Scales of apparent force. *J. Exp. Psych.* 58:405-13.

Borg, G., and H. Dahlstrom. 1960. The perception of muscular work. *Umea Vetensk. Bibiotekskr.* 5:1-27.

Borg, G. 1961. Perceived exertion in relation to physical work load and pulse rate. *Kungliga Fysiografiska Sallskapets i Lund Forhandlingar* 31(11):105-15.

Borg, G. 1961. Interindividual scaling and perception of muscular force. *Kungliga Fysiografiska Sallskapets i Lund Forhandlingar* 31(12):117-25.

Bernyer, G. 1962. Etude sur la validite d'une echelle de sensation d'effort musculaire, *Annee Psychol.* 62:1-15.

Borg, G. 1962. *Physical performance and perceived exertion.* Lund, Sweden: Gleerup.

Eisler, H. 1962. Subjective scale of force for a large muscle group. *J. Exp. Psych.* 64:253-57.

Bernyer, G. 1963. La perception de l'effort musculaire. *Biolypologie* 24:136-55.

Borg, G., and H. Linderholm. 1967. Perceived exertion and pulse rate during graded exercise in various age groups. *Acta Med. Scand.* 472 (Suppl.):194-206.

Borg, G., H. Diamant, L. Strom, and Y. Zotterman. 1967. The relationship between neural and perceptual intensity: A comparative study on the neural and psychophysical response to taste stimuli. *J. Physiol.* 192:13-20.

Borg, G. 1970. Perceived exertion as an indicator of somatic stress. *Scand. J. Rehab. Med.* 2:92-98.

Medicine itself. Perceived exertion research grew, as was the case of many other subspecialties within the college, as ACSM grew. Borg, by synchronistic chance, had aligned himself with those who were active supporters of the college. For example, William Morgan, whom Borg visited at Madison, was to be invited to present the prestigious Joseph Wolffe Lecture in 1986 for his quintessential work in sport psychology and leadership in the college. Likewise, James Skinner, an eventual ACSM president, and Ellsworth Buskirk, an ACSM past president, worked closely with Borg during his stay at Penn State in the spring of 1968. Both Morgan and Skinner were influential in the college and unabashed supporters of perceived exertion as an area of scientific inquiry. Later, as some college members such as Michael Pollock (another ACSM president) concentrated their career efforts in the area of testing and training cardiac patients, they found that perceived exertion had a very practical usefulness in their work. As previously mentioned, Pollock included discussions of perceived exertion in his presentations and research schedule.

To a certain extent the concept of perceived exertion has had an inherent believability that seems to have caused research and application activities to take on a certain life of their own. For the same reason, the practical acceptance of the concept seems to have exceeded actual scientific support. It seems that most practitioners intuitively believed that the scale "works" and patiently awaited final scientific validation to support their views.

One might ask whether this subspecialty more correctly belongs to the discipline of psychology or of physiology. Even though such a discussion is largely academic, its resolution will undoubtedly affect the future of research and development efforts. Support can be found for both sides of the argument. However, interest in perceived exertion by both exercise physiologists and sport and exercise psychologists has mostly emanated from a psychobiological point of view; that is, both disciplines have been concerned with unraveling the interactive nature of the mind and body (perception of effort and biological function). The concept of perceived exertion probably belongs to both disciplines and to neither at the same time. Just as biochemistry can be argued to be related to both biology and chemistry, it can be defended with equal authority as an independent discipline. Most important of all is the admission by workers in the key disciplines that a complex human response such as the perception of muscular effort is a composite of many inputs—psychological, physiological, and sociological, to name only three. It does little good to argue about a disciplinary home when there is so much to be done to understand the complexities of human performance.

Where We Are Going

It is difficult to discuss the historical background of any topic without conjuring up thoughts of what the future might bring. Certainly we have no crystal ball to predict the future. Still a few comments seem appropriate. Research productivity seems to have plateaued at a rate of 15 to 20 published papers per year. It is probable that this trend in research productivity will continue. There is no sign that production of research is waning, nor do we have knowledge of any situation that would predict significant growth. The major limitation to continued growth is the number of scholars choosing to concentrate their research efforts in this area. Few, if any, scholars responsible for directing doctoral programs are exclusively devoting their scholarly careers to the study of perceived exertion. Both sport psychologists and exercise physiologists who have published in this area in the past have eclectic research interests that would preclude exclusivity in research focus and the development of great numbers of young scholars to carry the torch of this subdiscipline. Nevertheless, it appears that the theoretical and practical attractiveness of the area will sustain a growing body of knowledge in the future.

Bibliography

Following is a complete listing of the collected bibliography used in the development of this chapter. It is presented here in its entirety as an aid to future scholars and clinicians who have interest in the topic of perceived exertion.

Alekseev, V. 1989. Correlation between heart rate and subjectively perceived exertion during muscular work. *Human Physiol.* 15:39-44.

Allen, P.D., and K.B. Pandolf. 1977. Perceived exertion associated with breathing hyperoxic mixtures during submaximal work. *Med. Sci. Sports* 9:122-27.

Altose, M., A. DiMarco, and K. Strohl. 1981. The sensation of respiratory muscle force. *Am. Rev. Respir. Dis.* 126:807-11.

Arioshi, M., H. Tanaka, K. Kanamori, S. Obara, H. Yoshitake, K. Yamaji, and R.J. Shephard. 1979. Influence of running pace upon performance: Effects upon oxygen intake, blood lactate, and rating of perceived exertion. *Can. J. Appl. Sport Sci.* 4:210-13.

Arnhold, R., N. Ng, and G. Pechar. 1992. Relationship of rated perceived exertion to heart rate and workload in mentally retarded young adults. *Adapt. Phys. Act. Q.* 9:47-53.

Aronchick, J., and E.J. Burke. 1977. Psycho-physical effects of varied rest intervals following warm-up. *Res. Q.* 48:260-64.

Arstila, M., K. Antila, H. Wendelin, I. Vuori, and I. Valamaki. 1977. The effect of age and sex on the perception of exertion during an exercise test with a linear increase in heart rate. In *Physical work and effort*, 199-216. See Borg 1977a.

Arstila, M., H. Wendelin, I. Vuori, and I. Valamaki 1974. Comparison of two rating scales in the estimation of perceived exertion in a pulse-conducted exercise test. *Ergonomics* 17:577-84.

Asfour, S.S., M.M. Ayoub, A. Mital, and N.J. Bethea. 1983. Perceived exertion of physical effort for various manual handling tasks. *Am. Indust. Hyg. Asso. J.* 44:223-28.

Åstrand, P.O., and J. Nystrom. 1977. Perceived exertion during running and bicycling. In *Swedish Sports Council: A review of reports, 1971-1976*, ed. L.M. Engstroem, 43. Stockholm: Swedish Sports Research Council.

Åström, H. 1986. Rating perceived symptoms during exercise in heart disease. In *The perception of effort in physical work*, 199-206. See Borg and Ottoson 1986.

Åström, H., A. Holmgren, J. Karlsson, and E. Orinius. 1983. Rated effort angina, perceived leg fatigue and blood lactate during graded exercise. In *Biochemistry of exercise*, ed. H.G. Knuttgen, 835-39. Champaign, IL: Human Kinetics.

Attaway, R., W. Bartoli, R. Pate, and J. Davis. 1992. Physiologic and perceptual responses to exercise on a new cycle ergometer. *Can. J. Sport Sci.* 17:56-59.

Bakers, J.M., and S.M. Tenney. 1970. The perception of some sensations associated with breathing. *Respir. Ther.* 10:85-92.

Balogun, J., R. Robertson, F. Goss, and M. Edwards. 1986. Metabolic and perceptual responses while carrying external loads on the head and by yoke. *Ergonomics* 29:1623-35.

Banister, E.W. 1979a. Perceiving effort. In *Science in sports: Open papers,* ed. L. Terauds, 175-83. Del Mar, CA: Academic.

———. 1979b. The perception of effort: An inductive approach. *Eur. J. Appl. Physiol.* 41:141-50.

Bar-Or, O. 1977. Age related changes in exercise perception. In *Physical work and effort,* 255-66. *See* Borg 1977a.

Bar-Or, O., and O. Inbar. 1977. Relationship between perceptual and physiological changes during heat acclimatization in 8-10 year old boys. In *Frontiers of activity and child health,* ed. H. Lavalle and R.J. Shepard, 205-14. Quebec: Editions du Pelican.

Bar-Or, O., and S. Reed. 1986. Ratings of perceived exertion in adolescents with neuromuscular disease. In *The perception of exertion in physical work,* 137-48. *See* Borg and Ottoson 1986.

Bar-Or, O., J.S. Skinner, E.R. Buskirk, and G. Borg. 1972. Physiological and perceptual indicators of physical stress in 41 to 61 year old men who vary in conditioning level and body fatness. *Med. Sci. Sports* 4:96-100.

Bartley, S.H. 1970. The homeostatic and comfort perceptual systems. *J. Psychol.* 75:157-62.

Bayles, C., K. Metz, R. Robertson, F. Goss, J. Cosgrove, and D. McBurney. 1990. Perceptual regulation of prescribed exercise. *J. Cardiopul. Rehab.* 10:25-31.

Ben-Ari, E., and J.J. Kellerman. 1982. Physiologic and perceptual responses to low and moderate training intensities in two different groups of coronary patients. *J. Cardiac Rehab.* 2:127-32.

Bergh, V., V. Danielsson, L. Wennberg, and B. Sjodin. 1986. Blood lactate and perceived exertion during heat stress. *Acta Physiol. Scand.* 126:617-18.

Bernyer, G. 1962. Etude sur la validite d'une echelle de sensation d'effort musculaire. *Annee Psychol.* 62:1-15.

———. 1963. La perception de l'effort musculaire. *Biolypologie* 24:136-55.

———. 1967. A subjective scale of the sensation of muscular effort. *Annee Psychol.* 67:23-42.

Berry, M., A. Weyrich, R. Robergs, and K. Krause. 1989. Ratings of perceived exertion in individuals with varying fitness levels during walking or running. *Eur. J. Appl. Physiol. Occup. Physiol.* 5:494-99.

Bhambhani, Y., P. Gomes, and G. Wheeler. 1990. Physiologic and perceptual responses during treadmill running with ankle weights. *Arch. Phys. Med. Rehab.* 71:231-35.

Birk, T., and C. Birk. 1987. Use of ratings of perceived exertion for exercise prescription. *Sports Med.* 4:1-8.

Blitz, P.S., and A. Van-Moorst. 1978. Application of the theory of signal detectability to the perception of differences in load. *Percept. Motor Skills* 47:1083-88.

Bloem, P., L. Goessens, P. Zamparo, M. Sacher, R. Paviotti, and P.E. diPrampero. 1991. Effects of order of presentation of exercise intensities and of sauna baths on perceived exertion during treadmill running. *Eur. J. Appl. Physiol.* 62:204-10.

Bloomberg, R. 1980. Menstruation alters perceived exertion. (Abstract). *Physician Sportsmed.* 8:29.

Bond, V., B.D. Franks, and E.T. Howley. 1983. Effect of small and moderate doses of alcohol on submaximal cardiorespiratory function, perceived exertion and endurance in abstainers and moderate drinkers. *J. Sports Med. Phys. Fitness* 23:221-28.

Borg, G. 1961a. Interindividual scaling and perception of muscular force. *Kungliga Fysiografiska Sallskapets i Lund Forhandlingar* 31 (12): 117-25.

———. 1961b. Perceived exertion in relation to physical work load and pulse-rate. *Kungliga Fysiografiska Sallskapets i Lund Forhandlingar* 31 (11): 105-15.

———. 1962. *Physical performance and perceived exertion.* Lund, Sweden: Gleerup.

———. 1968. The three effort continua in physical work. In *Proceedings of the 16th International Congress of Applied Psychology,* 18-22. Amsterdam.

———. 1970. Perceived exertion as an indicator of somatic stress. *Scand. J. Rehab. Med.* 2:92-98.

———. 1971. The perception of physical performance. In *Frontiers of fitness,* ed. R.J. Shephard, 280-94. Springfield, IL: Charles C Thomas.

———. 1972. *The basic "noise constant" in the psycho-physical function of perceived exertion.* Reports from the Institute of Applied Psychology, no. 33. Stockholm: Univ. of Stockholm.

———. 1973a. *A note on a category scale with "ratio properties" for estimating perceived exertion.* Reports from the Institute of Applied Psychology, no. 36. Stockholm: Univ. of Stockholm.

———. 1973b. Perceived exertion: A note on "history" and methods. *Med. Sci. Sports* 5:90-93.

———. 1973c. *Perceived exertion during walking: A psycho-physical function with two additional constants.* Reports from the Institute of Applied Psychology, no. 39. Stockholm: Univ. of Stockholm.

———. 1976. *Perception of panting during ergometer work.* Reports from the Institute of Applied Psychology, no. 73. Stockholm: Univ. of Stockholm.

———. ed. 1977a. *Physical work and effort.* New York: Pergamon Press.

———. 1977b. Simple rating methods for estimation of perceived exertion. In *Physical work and effort,* 38-48. *See* Borg 1977a.

———. 1978a. Psychological assessment of physical effort. In *Proceedings of the 1978 International Symposium on Psychological Assessment in Sport,* 49-57. Netamya, Isreal.

———. 1978b. Subjective effort and physical abilities. *Scand. J. Rehab. Med.* 6:105-13.

————. 1978c. Subjective effort in relation to physical performance and working capacity. In *Psychology: From research to practice,* ed. H.L. Pick, 333-61. New York: Plenum Press.

————. 1982a. Psychophysical bases of perceived exertion. *Med. Sci. Sports Exerc.* 14:377-81.

————. 1982b. Ratings of perceived exertion and heart rates during short-term cycle exercise and their use in a cycling strength test. *Int. J. Sports Med.* 3:153-58.

————. 1984. *Some characteristics of a simple run test and its correlation with a bicycle ergometer test of physical work capacity.* Reports from the Institute of Applied Psychology, no. 625. Stockholm: Univ. of Stockholm.

————. 1990. Psychophysical scaling with applications in physical work and the perception of exertion. *Scand. J. Work Environ. Health* 16:55-58.

Borg, G., and H. Dahlstrom. 1960. The perception of muscular work. *Umea Vetensk. Bibiotekskr.* 5:1-27.

————. 1962. A pilot study of perceived exertion and physical work capacity. *Acta Soc. Med. Upsal.* 67:21-27.

Borg, G., H. Diamant, L. Strom, and Y. Zotterman. 1967. The relationship between neural and perceptual intensity: A comparative study on the neural and psychophysical response to taste stimuli. *J. Physiol.* 192:13-20.

Borg, G., B. Edgren, and G. Marklund, 1971. *A simple walk test of physical working capacity.* Reports from the Institute of Applied Psychology, no. 18. Stockholm: Univ. of Stockholm.

————. 1973. *The reliability and stability of the indicators in a simple walk test.* Reports from the Institute of Applied Psychology, no. 35. Stockholm: Univ. of Stockholm.

Borg, G., B. Edgren, and B. Noble. 1975. *A study of the effect of physical conditioning on perceived exertion and working capacity.* Reports from the Institute of Applied Psychology, no. 63. Stockholm: Univ. of Stockholm.

Borg, G., C. Edstrom, and G. Marklund. 1970. *A new method to determine the exponent for perceived force in physical work.* Reports from the Institute of Applied Psychology, no. 4. Stockholm: Univ. of Stockholm.

————. 1972. *Effects of the rate of the work load increase on terminal thresholds for physical work.* Reports from the Institute of Applied Psychology, no. 25. Stockholm: Univ. of Stockholm.

Borg, G., and E. Freeman. 1979. A study of physical performance and perceived exertion. *School of Education Report, Univ. of Pittsburgh* 4:1-25.

Borg, G., P. Hassmen, and M. Lagerstrom. 1987. Perceived exertion related to heart rate and blood lactate during arm and leg exercise. *Eur. J. Appl. Physiol.* 56:679-85.

Borg, G., A. Holmgren, and I. Lindblad. 1980. *Perception of chest pain during physical work in a group of patients with angina pectoris.* Reports from the Institute of Applied Psychology, no. 81. Stockholm: Univ. of Stockholm.

————. 1981. Quantitative evaluation of chest pain. *Acta Med. Scand.* 644 (Suppl.): 43-45.

Borg, G., J. Karlsson, and L. Ekelund. 1977. A comparison between two work tests controlled subjectively and by heart rate. In *Physical work and effort,* 239-54. *See* Borg 1977a.

Borg, G., J. Karlsson, and I. Lindblad. 1976. *Quantitative variation of subjective symptoms during ergometer work.* Reports from the Institute of Applied Psychology, no. 72. Stockholm: Univ. of Stockholm.

Borg, G., M. Komserius, and L. Kaijser. 1990. Effect of alcohol on perceived exertion in relation to heart rate and blood lactate. *Eur. J. Appl. Physiol.* 60:382-84.

Borg, G., and I. Lindblad. 1976. *The determination of subjective intensities in verbal descriptions of symptoms.* Reports from the Institute of Applied Psychology, no. 75. Stockholm: Univ. of Stockholm.

Borg, G., and H. Linderholm. 1970. Exercise performance and perceived exertion in patients with coronary insufficiency, arterial hypertension and vasoregulatory asthenia. *Acta Med. Scand.* 187:17-26.

Borg, G., G. Ljunggren, and R. Ceci. 1985. The increase of perceived exertion, aches and pains in the legs, heart rate and blood lactate during exercise on a bicycle ergometer. *Eur. J. Appl. Physiol. Occup. Physiol.* 54:343-49.

Borg, G., and B.J. Noble. 1974. Perceived exertion. *Exerc. Sport Sci. Rev.* 2:131-53.

Borg, G., and M. Ohlsson. 1975. *A study of two variants of a simple run-test for determining physical working capacity.* Reports from the Institute of Applied Psychology, no. 61. Stockholm: Univ. of Stockholm.

Borg, G., and D. Ottoson, eds. 1986. *The perception of effort in physical work.* London: Macmillan Press.

Boutcher, S., L. Fleischer-Curtian, and S. Gines. 1988. The effects of self-presentation on perceived exertion. *J. Sport Exerc. Psychol.* 10:270-80.

Boutcher, S., and M. Trenske. 1990. The effects of sensory deprivation and music on perceived exertion and affect during exercise. *J. Sport Exerc. Psychol.* 12:167-76.

Bubb, W.J., B.C. Myers, R.P. Claytor, D.L. Varnum, L. Watts, and B.D. Franks. 1985. Experimenter effects in exercise tolerance testing: The race and gender of the tester/subject relationship. *Res. Q. Exerc. Sport* 56:370-77.

Buick, F.J., N. Gledhill, A.B. Froese, L. Spriet, and E.C. Meyers. 1980. Effect of induced erythrocythemia on aerobic work capacity. *J. Appl. Physiol.* 48:636-42.

Burdon, J., K.J. Killian, and E. Campbell. 1982. Effect of ventilatory drive on the perceived magnitude of added loads to breathing. *J. Appl. Physiol.* 53:901-7.

Burgess, M., R. Robertson, J. Davis, and J. Norris. 1991. RPE, blood glucose, and carbohydrate oxidation during exercise: Effects of glucose feedings. *Med. Sci. Sports Exerc.* 23:353-59.

Burke, E.J. 1979. Individualized fitness program: Using perceived exertion for the prescription of exercise for healthy adults. *J. Phys. Ed. Recr.* 50:35-37.

————. 1986. Perceived exertion: Subjectivity and objectivity in work assessment. In *The perception of exertion in physical work,* 149-59. *See* Borg and Ottoson 1986.

Burke, E.J., and M.L. Collins. 1984. Using perceived exertion for the prescription of exercise in healthy adults. In *Clinical sports medicine,* ed. R.C. Cantu, 93-105. Toronto: Collamore Press, D.C. Health.

Burke, E.J., and T.J. Keenan. 1984. Energy cost, heart rate, and perceived exertion during the elementary backstroke. *Physician Sportsmed.* 12:75-78, 80.

Butts, N.K., and D. Crowell. 1985. Effect of caffeine ingestion on cardiorespiratory endurance in men and women. *Res. Q. Exerc. Sport* 56:301-5.

Cafarelli, E. 1977. Peripheral and central inputs to the effort sense during cycling exercise. *Eur. J. Appl. Physiol.* 37:181-89.

————. 1978. Effect of contraction frequency on effort sensations during cycling at a constant resistance. *Med. Sci. Sports* 10:270-75.

————. 1982. Peripheral contributions to the perception of effort. *Med. Sci. Sports Exerc.* 14:382-89.

Cafarelli, E., and B. Bigland-Ritchie. 1979. Sensation of static force in muscles of different length. *Exper. Neurol.* 65:511-25.

Cafarelli, E., W.S. Cain, and J.C. Stevens. 1977. Effort of dynamic exercise: Influence of load, duration and task. *Ergonomics* 20:147-58.

Cafarelli, E., and B.J. Noble. 1976. The effect of inspired carbon dioxide on subjective estimates of exertion during exercise. *Ergonomics* 19:581-89.

Cafarelli, E., and J.B. Pierce. 1976. Integrated EMG and the peripheral drive for effort sensations. (Abstract). *Med. Sci. Sports* 8:69.

Cain, W.S. 1973. Nature of perceived effort and fatigue: Roles of strength and blood flow in muscle contractions. *J. Motor Behav.* 5:33-47.

————. 1977. Versatility of the constant-effort procedure. In *Physical work and effort,* 49-60. *See* Borg 1977a.

Cain, W.S., and J.C. Stevens. 1971. Effort in sustained and phasic handgrip contractions. *Am. J. Psychol.* 84:52-65.

————. 1973. Constant effort contractions related to the electromyogram. *Med. Sci. Sports* 5:121-27.

Campbell, E.J.M., R.H. Edwards, D.K. Hill, D.H. Jones, and M.K. Sykes. 1976. Perception of effort during partial curarization. *J. Physiol.* 263:186-87.

Campbell, E.J.M., and J.L. Howell. 1963. The sensation of breathlessness. *Br. Med. Bull.* 19:36-40.

Carton, R.L., and E.C. Rhodes. 1985. A critical review of the literature on rating scales for perceived exertion. *Sports Med.* 2:198-222.

Carver, C.S., A. Coleman, and D. Glass. 1976. The coronary-prone behavior pattern and the suppression of fatigue on a treadmill test. *J. Personality Soc. Psychol.* 33:460-66.

Casal, D.C., and A.S. Leon. 1985. Failure of caffeine to affect substrate utilization during prolonged running. *Med. Sci. Sports Exerc.* 17:174-79.

Ceci, R., and P. Hassmen. 1991. Self-monitored exercise at three different RPE intensities in treadmill vs. field running. *Med. Sci. Sports Exerc.* 23:732-38.

Chidea, M., N. Inase, M. Ichioka, I. Miyazato, and F. Marumo. 1991. Ratings of perceived exertion in chronic obstructive pulmonary disease—A possible indicator for exercise training in patients with this disease. *Eur. J. Appl. Physiol.* 62:390-93.

Chow, R., and J. Wilmore. 1984. The regulation of exercise intensity by ratings of perceived exertion. *J. Cardiac Rehab.* 4:382-87.

Christensen, C.L., and R.O. Ruhling. 1983. Physiological and perceptual responses of women to equivalent power outputs on the bicycle ergometer and treadmill. *J. Sports Med. Phys. Fitness* 23:436-44.

Cooper, D.F., G. Grimby, D.A. Jones, and R.H. Edwards. 1979. Perception of effort in isometric and dynamic muscular contraction. *Eur. J. Appl. Physiol.* 41:173-80.

Copeland, B., and B. Franks. 1991. Effects of types and intensities of background music on treadmill endurance. *J. Sports Med. Phys. Fitness* 31:100-103.

Costa, G., and E. Gaffuri. 1977. Studies of perceived exertion rate on bicycle ergometer in conditions reproducing some aspect of industrial work (shift work; noise). In *Physical work and effort,* 297-306. *See* Borg 1977a.

Davies, C.T., L. Fohlin, and C. Thoren. 1980. Perception of exertion in anorexia nervosa patients. In *Children and exercise IX,* ed. K. Berg and B.O. Ericksson, 327-32. Baltimore: University Park Press.

Davies, C.T., and A.J. Sargeant. 1979. The effects of atropine and practolol on the perception of exertion during treadmill exercise. *Ergonomics* 22:1141-46.

Dehlin, O., G. Grimby, S. Berg, and G.B. Anderson. 1981. Effect of physical training and ergonomic counselling on the psychological perception of work and on the subjective assessment of low back insufficiency. *Scand. J. Rehab. Med.* 13:1-9.

Dehlin, O., and E. Jaderberg. 1982. Perceived exertion during patient lifts. An evaluation of the importance of various factors for the subjective strain during lifting and carrying patients. A study at a geriatric hospital. *Scand. J. Rehab. Med.* 14:11-20.

DeMeersman, R. 1988. Personality, effort perception and cardiovascular reactivity. *Neuropsychobiol.* 19:192-94.

DeMeersman, R., D.C. Schaefer, and W.W. Miller. 1985. Effect of diet upon ventilation and effort perception during a physical stressor. *Physiol. Behav.* 35:555-58.

DeMello, J., K. Cureton, R. Boineau, and M.M. Singh. 1987. Rating of perceived exertion at the lactate threshold in trained and untrained men and women. *Med. Sci. Sports Exerc.* 19:354-62.

Dengel, D., P. Weyand, D. Black,and K.J. Cureton. 1993. Effects of varying levels of hypohydration on ratings of perceived exertion. *Int. J. Sport Nutr.* 3:376-86.

Dishman, R.K. 1982. Contemporary sport psychology. *Exerc. Sport Sci. Rev.* 10:120-59.

Dishman, R., R. Graham, R. Holly, and J.G. Tieman. 1991. Estimates of type A behavior do not predict perceived exertion during graded exercise. *Med. Sci. Sports Exerc.* 23:1276-82.

Dishman, R., R. Patton, J. Smith, R. Weinberg, and A. Jackson. 1987. Using perceived exertion to prescribe and monitor exercise training heart rate. *Int. J. Sports Med.* 8:208-13.

Docktor, R., and B. Sharkey. 1971. Note on some physiological and subjective reactions to exercise and training. *Percept. Motor Skills* 32:233-34.

Dunbar, C. 1993. Practical use of ratings of perceived exertion in a clinical setting. *Sports Med.* 16:221-24.

Dunbar, C., R. Robertson, R. Baun, M.F. Blandin, K. Metz, R. Burdett, and F.L. Goss. 1992. The validity of regulating exercise intensity by ratings of perceived exertion. *Med. Sci. Sports Exerc.* 24:94-99.

Duthie, J.H., K. Tyler, and R. Hermiston. 1977. Relationship between fitness levels, the ability to perceive exertion and beliefs about strenuous activity in adult males aged 20-60 years. *Can. J. Appl. Sport Sci.* 2:213.

Eakin, B., K. Finta, G. Serwer, and R. Beekman. 1992. Perceived exertion and exercise intensity in children with or without structural heart defects. *J. Pediatr.* 120:90-93.

Edgren, B. 1977. A work test based on preferred settings. In *Physical work and effort,* 61-74. *See* Borg 1977a.

Edgren, B., and G. Borg. 1975. *The reliability and stability of the indicators in a simple run test.* Reports from the Institute of Applied Psychology, no. 57. Stockholm: Univ. of Stockholm.

Edwards, R.H., A. Melcher, C.M. Hesser, O. Wigerbtz, and L.G. Ekelund. 1972. Physiological correlates of perceived exertion in continuous and intermittent exercise with the same average power output. *Eur. J. Clin. Invest.* 2:108-14.

Eisler, H. 1962. Subjective scale of force for a large muscle group. *J. Exper. Psychol.* 64:253-57.

Ekblom, B., and A.N. Goldbarg. 1971. The influence of physical training and other factors on the subjective rating of perceived exertion. *Acta Physiol. Scand.* 83:399-406.

Ekelund, L., J. Blumenthal, M. Morey, and C.C. Ekelund. 1986. The effect of nonselective and selective betablockade on perceived exertion during treadmill exercise in mild hypertensive type A and B males and the interaction with aerobic training. In *The perception of exertion in physical work,* 191-98. *See* Borg and Ottoson 1986.

Eklund, B. 1977. Estimation of perceived pain during treadmill testing of patients with obliterative arterial disease of the lower limbs. In *Physical work and effort,* 315-22. *See* Borg 1977a.

El-Manshawi, A., K. Killian, E. Summers, and N. Jones. 1986. Breathlessness during exercise with and without resistive loading. *J. Appl. Physiol.* 61:896-905.

Ericksson, C., and G. Tibblin. 1976. Heart rhythms, perceived exertion, and physiological responses to physical work. *Goteborg Psychol. Rep.* 6:21.

Eston, R.G. 1984a. A discussion of the concepts: Exercise intensity and perceived exertion with reference to the secondary school. *Phys. Ed. Rev.* 7:19-25.

————. 1984b. The regular menstrual cycle and athletic performance. *Sports Med.* 1:431-45.

Eston, R., B. Davies, and J. Williams. 1987. Use of perceived effort ratings to control exercise intensity in young healthy adults. *Eur. J. Appl. Physiol.* 56:222-24.

Eston, R.G., and J.G. Williams. 1986. Exercise intensity and perceived exertion in adolescent boys. *Br. J. Sports Med.* 20:27-30.

————. 1988. Reliability of ratings of perceived effort regulation of exercise intensity. *Br. J. Sports Med.* 22:153-55.

Evans, W.O. 1966. Measurement of subjective symptomatology of acute high altitude sickness. *Psychol. Rep.* 19:815-20.

Faria, I.E., and B.J. Drummond. 1982. Circadian changes in resting heart rate and body temperature, maximal oxygen consumption and perceived exertion. *Ergonomics* 25:381-86.

Fechner, G.T. 1860. *Elemente der Psychophysik.* In D.H. Howes and E.G. Boring, eds., New York, 1966, Holt, Rinehart, and Winston.

Felts, W. 1989. Relationship between ratings of perceived exertion and exercise-induced decrease in state anxiety. *Percept. Motor Skills* 69:368-70.

Felts, W., S. Crouse, and M. Brunetz. 1988. Influence of aerobic fitness on ratings of perceived exertion during light to moderate exercise. *Percept. Motor Skills* 67:671-76.

Fillingim, R., and M. Fine. 1986. The effects of internal versus external information processing on symptom perception in an exercise setting. *Health Psychol.* 5:115-23.

Fillingim, R., D. Roth, and W. Haley. 1989. The effects of distraction on the perception of exercise-induced symptoms. *J. Psychosom. Res.* 33:241-48.

Fleishman, E.A., D.L. Gebbardt, and J.C. Hogan. 1984. The measurement of effort. *Ergonomics* 27:947-54.

Frankenhaeuser, M., B. Post, B. Nordheden, and H. Sjoeberg. 1969. Physiological and subjective reactions to different physical work loads. *Percept. Motor Skills* 28:343-49.

Franklin, B.A., L. Vander, D. Wrisley, and M. Rubenfire. 1983. Aerobic requirements of arm ergometry: Implications for exercise testing and training. *Physician Sportsmed.* 11:81-85; 89-90.

Franks, B.D., and B.C. Myers. 1984. Effects of talking on exercise tolerance. *Res. Q. Exerc. Sport* 55:237-41.

Gagge, A.P., A.J. Stolwijk, and B. Stalin. 1969. Comfort and thermal sensations and associated physiological responses during exercise at various ambient temperatures. *Environ. Res.* 2:209-29.

Gamberale, F. 1972. Perceived exertion, heart rate, oxygen uptake and blood lactate in different work operations. *Ergonomics* 15:545-54.

————. 1985. The perception of exertion. *Ergonomics* 28:299-308.

Gamberale, F., and I. Holmer. 1977. Heart rate and perceived exertion in simulated work with high heat stress. In *Physical work and effort,* 323-32. *See* Borg 1977a.

Gamberale, F., I. Holmer, A.S. Kindblom, and A. Nordstrom. 1978. Magnitude perception of added inspiratory resistance during steady-state exercise. *Ergonomics* 21:531-38.

Gandevia, S. 1982. The perception of motor commands on effort during muscular paralysis. *Brain* 105:151-59.

Gandevia, S., K. Killian, and E. Campbell. 1981. The effect of respiratory muscle fatigue on respiratory sensations. *Clin. Sci.* 60:463-66.

Gandevia, S.C., and D.I. McCloskey. 1977a. Changes in motor commands in perceived heaviness, during partial curarization and peripheral anaesthesia in man. *J. Physiol.* 272:673-89.

————. 1977b. Sensations of heaviness. *Brain* 100:345-54.

Gayle, G., R. Pohlman, R. Glaser, and G. Davis. 1990. Cardiorespiratory and perceptual responses to arm crank and wheelchair exercise using various handrims in male paraplegics. *Res. Q. Exerc. Sport* 61:224-32.

Glass, S., R. Knowlton, and M. Becque. 1992. Accuracy of RPE from graded exercise to established exercise training intensity. *Med. Sci. Sports Exerc.* 24:1303-7.

Glass, S., M. Whaley, and M. Wegner. 1991. Ratings of perceived exertion among standard treadmill protocols and steady state running. *Int. J. Sports Med.* 12:77-82.

Goldberg, L.I., D.J. White, and K.B. Pandolf. 1982. Cardiovascular and perceptual responses to isometric exercise. *Arch. Phys. Med. Rehab.* 63:211-16.

Goslin, B.R., and S.C. Rorke. 1986. The perception of exertion during load carriage. *Ergonomics* 29:677-86.

Goss, F., R. Robertson, T. Auble, D. Cassinelli, R. Spina, R. Glickman, R. Galbreath, R. Silberman, and K. Metz. 1987. Are treadmill-based exercise prescriptions generalizable to combined arm and leg exercise? *J. Cardiopul. Rehab.* 7:551-55.

Gottfried, S.B., M.D. Altose, S.G. Kelson, C.M. Fogarty, and N.S. Cherbiack. 1978. The perception of changes in airflow resistance in normal subjects and patients with chronic airways obstruction. *Chest* 73:286-88.

Gutin, B., K. Ang, and K. Torrey. 1988. Cardiorespiratory and subjective responses to incremental and constant load ergometry with arms and legs. *Arch. Phys. Med. Rehab.* 69:510-13.

Gutman, M.C., R.W. Squires, M.L. Pollock, C. Foster, and J. Anholm. 1981. Perceived exertion-heart rate relationship during exercise testing and training in cardiac patients. *J. Cardiac Rehab.* 1:52-59.

Hage, P. 1981. Perceived exertion: One measure of exercise intensity. *Physician Sportsmed.* 9:136-39; 142-43.

Hagen, K., T. Vik, N. Myhr, P.A. Opsahl, and K. Harms-Ringdahl. 1993. Physical workload, perceived exertion, and output of cut wood as related to age in motor-manual cutting. *Ergonomics* 36:479-88.

Hake, M., and E. Michael. 1977. The physiological costs of box lifting. *J. Human Ergol.* 6:167-78.

Hardy, C., E. Hall, and P. Prestholdt. 1986. The mediational role of social influence in the perception of exertion. *J. Sport Psychol.* 8:88-104.

Hardy, C., R. McMurray, and S. Roberts. 1989. A/B types and psychophysiological responses to exercise stress. *J. Sport Exerc. Psychol.* 11:141-51.

Hardy, C., and W. Rejeski. 1989. Not what, but how one feels: The measurement of affect during exercise. *J. Sport Exerc. Psychol.* 11:304-17.

Hare, T.W., A.H. Hakki, D.T. Lowenthal, A.S. Iskandrian, and B.L. Segal. 1985. Simplified scale for rating perceived exertion in patients with coronary artery disease. *Ann. Sport Med.* 2:64-68.

Haskvitz, E., R. Seip, J. Weltman, A. Rodol, and A. Weltman. 1992. The effect of training intensity on ratings of perceived exertion. *Int. J. Sports Med.* 13:377-83.

Hassmen, P. 1990. Perceptual and physiological responses to cycling and running in groups of trained and untrained subjects. *Eur. J. Appl. Physiol.* 60:445-51.

Hassmen, P., R. Ceci, and L. Backman. 1992. Exercise for older women: A training method and its influences on physical and cognitive performance. *Eur. J. Appl. Physiol.* 64:460-66.

Hassmen, P., R. Stahl, and G. Borg. 1993. Psychophysiological responses to exercise in type A/B men. *Psychosom. Med.* 55:178-84.

Hellerstein, H.K., and B.A. Franklin. 1984. Evaluating the cardiac patient for exercise therapy: Role of exercise testing. *Clinics Sports Med.* 3:371-93.

Henriksson, J., H.G. Knuttgen, and F. Bonde-Peterson. 1972. Perceived exertion during exercise with concentric and eccentric muscle contractions. *Ergonomics* 15:537-44.

Hetzler, R., R. Seip, S. Boutcher, E. Pierce, D. Snead, and A. Weltman. 1991. Effect of exercise modality on ratings of perceived exertion at various lactate concentrations. *Med. Sci. Sports Exerc.* 23:88-92.

Hickey, M., W. Franke, W. Herbert, J. Walberg-Rankin, and J. Lee. 1992. Opioid antagonism, perceived exertion and tolerance to exercise-thermal stress. *Int. J. Sports Med.* 13:326-31.

Higgs, S.L. 1980. Influence of the menstrual cycle on perception of effort. In *Female athlete: Proceedings of a national conference about women in sports,* ed. A. Popma, 94-98. Burnaby, BC: Institute for Human Behavior, Simon Fraser Univ.

Higgs, S.L., and L.A. Robertson. 1981. Cyclic variations in perceived exertion and physical work capacity in females. *Can. J. Appl. Sport Sci.* 6:191-96.

Highgenboten, C., A. Jackson, N. Meske, and J. Smith. 1991. The effects of knee brace wear on perceptual and metabolic variables during horizontal treadmill running. *Am. J. Sports Med.* 19:639-43.

Hill, D., K. Cureton, S. Grisham, M. Collins. 1987. Effect of training on the rating of perceived exertion at the ventilatory threshold. *Eur. J. Appl. Physiol.* 56:206-11.

Hobbs, S.F., and S.C. Gandevia. 1985. Cardiovascular responses and the sense of effort during attempts to contract paralyzed muscles: Role of the spinal cord. *Neurosci. Letters* 57:85-90.

Hochstetler, S.A., W.J. Rejeski, and D.L. Best. 1985. The influence of sex-role orientation on ratings of perceived exertion. *Sex Roles* 12:825-35.

Hogan, J.C., and E.A. Fleishman. 1979. An index of the physical effort required in human task performance. *J. Appl. Psychol.* 64:197- 204.

Hogan, J.C., G.D. Ogden, D.L. Gebhardt, and E.A. Fleishman. 1980. Reliability and validity of methods for evaluating perceived physical effort. *J. Appl. Psychol.* 65:672-79.

Holder, C., E. Haskvitz, and A. Weltman. 1993. The effects of assistive devices on the oxygen cost, cardiovascular stress, and perception of nonweight-bearing ambulation. *J. Orthoped. Sports Phys. Ther.* 18:537-42.

Holland, L., M. Bouffard, and D. Wagner. 1992. Rating of perceived exertion, heart rate, and oxygen consumption in adults with multiple sclerosis. *Adapt. Phys. Act. Q.* 9:64-73.

Horstman, D.H., W.P. Morgan, A. Cymerman, and J. Stokes. 1979. Perception of effort during constant work to self imposed exhaustion. *Percept. Motor Skills* 48:1111-26.

Horstman, D.H., R. Weiskopf, and S. Robinson. 1979. The nature of the perception of effort at sea level and high altitude. *Med. Sci. Sports* 11:150-54.

Hueting, J.E., and H.R. Sarphati. 1966. Measuring fatigue. *J. Appl. Psychol.* 50:535-38.

Inbar, O., A. Rotstein, R. Olin, R. Dotan, and F. Sulman. 1982. The effects of negative air ions on various physiological functions during work in a hot environment. *Int. J. Biometeor.* 26:153-63.

Jackson, A., R.K. Dishman, S. LaCroix, R. Patton, and R. Weinberg. 1981. The heart rate, perceived exertion, and pace of the 1.5 mile run. *Med. Sci. Sports Exerc.* 13:224-28.

Jacobs, I., R. Schele, and B. Sjodin. 1985. Blood lactate vs. exhaustive exercise to evaluate aerobic fitness. *Eur. J. Appl. Physiol. Occup. Physiol.* 54:151-55.

Johansson, S. 1986. Perceived exertion, heart rate and blood lactate during prolonged exercise on a bicycle ergometer. In *The perception of exertion in physical work,* 199-206. See Borg and Ottoson 1986.

Johansson, S., and G. Ljunggren. 1989. Perceived exertion during a self-imposed pace of work for a group of cleaners. *Appl. Ergonomics* 20:307-12.

Johnson, A.N., D.F. Cooper, and E.H.T. Edwards. 1977. Exertion of stair climbing in normal subjects and in patients with chronic obstructive bronchitis. *Thorax* 32:711-16.

Johnson, J., and D. Siegel. 1987. Active vs. passive attentional manipulation and multidimensional perceptions of exercise intensity. *Can. J. Sport Sci.* 12:41-45.

———. 1992. Effects of association and dissociation on effort perception. *J. Sport Behav.* 15:119-29.

Jones, L.A., and I.W. Hunter. 1982a. Relation of muscle force and EMG to perceived force in human finger flexors. *Eur. J. Appl. Physiol. Occup. Physiol.* 50:125-31.

————. 1982b. The role of centrally-generated motor commands and sensory signals in the perception of muscular force. *Soc. Neurosci. Abstr.* 8:732.

————. 1983a. Force and EMG correlates of constant effort contractions. *Eur. J. Appl. Physiol. Occup. Physiol.* 51:75-83.

————. 1983b. Perceived force in fatiguing isometric contractions. *Percept. Psychophys.* 33:369-74.

Kaiser, P. 1982. Running performance as a function of the dose-response relationship to beta-adrenoceptor blockade. *Int. J. Sports Med.* 3:29-32.

Kaiser, P., and P.A. Tesch. 1983. Perceived exertion and muscle lactate accumulation during exercise following B-adrenergic blockade. In *Biochemistry of exercise,* ed. H.G. Knuttgen, 728-32. Champaign, IL: Human Kinetics.

Kamon, E., K. Pandolf, and E. Cafarelli. 1974. The relationship between perceptual information and physiological responses to exercise in the heat. *J. Human Ergol.* 3:45-54.

Kassin, S.M., and F.X. Gibbons. 1981. Children's use of the discounting principle in their perceptions of exertion. *Child Develop.* 52:741-44.

Kilbom, A., F. Gamberale, J. Persson, and G. Annwall. 1983. Physiological and psychological indices of fatigue during static contractions. *Eur. J. Appl. Physiol.* 50:179-93.

Killian, K. 1985. The objective measurement of breathlessness. *Chest* 88 (Suppl.): 845-905.

————. 1986. Breathlessness—The sense of respiratory muscle effort. In *The perception of exertion in physical work,* 71-82. *See* Borg and Ottoson 1986.

Killian, K.J., D. Bucens, and E. Campbell. 1982. Effect of breathing patterns on the perceived magnitude of added loads to breathing. *J. Appl. Physiol.* 52:578-84.

Killian, K.J., and E.J. Campbell. 1983. Dyspnea and exercise. *Ann. Rev. Physiol.* 45:465-79.

Killian, K.J., S.C. Gandevia, E. Summers, and E. Campbell. 1984. Effect of increased lung volume on perception of breathlessness, effort, and tension. *J. Appl. Physiol.* 57:686-91.

Killian, K.J., K. Mahutte, and E. Campbell. 1981. Magnitude scaling of externally added loads to breathing. *Am. Rev. Respir. Dis.* 123:12-15.

Killian, K.J., C.K. Mahutte, J.L. Howell, and E. Campbell. 1980. Effect of timing, flow, lung volume, and threshold pressures on resistive load detection. *J. Appl. Physiol.* 49:958-63.

Kinsman, R.A., and P.C. Weiser. 1976. Subjective symptomatology during work and fatigue. In *Psychological aspects of fatigue,* ed. E. Simonson and P.C. Weiser, 336-405. Springfield, IL: Charles C Thomas.

Kinsman, R.A., P.C. Weiser, and D.A. Stamper. 1973. Multi-dimensional analysis of subjective symptomatology during prolonged strenuous exercise. *Ergonomics* 16:211-26.

Kircher, M.A. 1984. Motivation as a factor of perceived exertion in purposeful versus nonpurposeful activity. *Am. J. Occup. Ther.* 38:165-70.

Kirk, J., and D. Schneider. 1992. Physiological and perceptual responses to load-carrying in female subjects using internal and external frame backpacks. *Ergonomics* 35:445-55.

Knuttgen, H.G. 1977. Physiological factors in fatigue. In *Physical work and effort,* 13-24. *See* Borg 1977a.

Kogi, K., Y. Saito, and T. Matsuhashi. 1970. Validity of three components of subjective fatigue feelings. *J. Sci. Labour* 46:251-70.

Kohl, R., and C. Shea. 1988. Perceived exertion: Influences of locus of control and expected work intensity and duration. *J. Human Move. Stud.* 15:225-72.

Koltyn, K., and W. Morgan. 1992. Efficacy of perceptual versus heart rate monitoring in the development of endurance. *Br. J. Sports Med.* 26:132-34.

Koltyn, K., P. O'Connor, and W. Morgan. 1991. Perception of effort in female and male competitive swimmers. *Int. J. Sports Med.* 12:427-29.

Komi, P.V., and S.L. Karppi. 1977. Genetic and environmental variation in perceived exertion and heart rate during bicycle ergometer work. In *Physical work and effort,* 91-100. *See* Borg 1977a.

Kostka, C.E., and E. Cafarelli. 1982. Effect of pH on sensation and vastus lateralis electromyogram during cycling exercises. *J. Appl. Physiol.* 52:1181-85.

Kraemer, W., R. Lewis, N. Triplett, L. Koziris, S. Heyman, and B. Noble. 1992. Effects of hypnosis on plasma proenkephalin peptide F and perceptual and cardiovascular responses during submaximal exercise. *Eur. J. Appl. Physiol.* 65:573-78.

Kuipers, H., F.T. Verstappen, H.A. Keizer, P. Geurten, and G. Kranenburg. 1985. Variability of aerobic performance in the laboratory and its physiologic correlates. *Int. J. Sports Med.* 6:197-201

Kuoppasalmi, K., R. Llmarinen, J. Smolander, and M. Harkonen. 1986. Relationship between physiological responses and perceived exertion of muscular exercise under various environmental conditions. *Psychiatr. Fennica* Suppl.:69-77

Kurokawa, T., and T. Ueda. 1992. Validity of ratings of perceived exertion as an index of exercise intensity in swimming training. *Ann. Physiol. Anthropol.* 11:277-88.

Lamberty, M., and H.V. Ulmer. 1980. On the importance of a feeling for performance and speed of movement from the point of view of strategy during top level performance. *Leistungssport* 30:464-69.

Lane, L., and E. Winslow. 1987. Oxygen consumption, cardiovascular response, and perceived exertion in healthy adults during rest, occupied bedmaking, and unoccupied bedmaking activity. *Cardiovasc. Nurs.* 23:31-36.

Layman, E.M. 1974. Psychological effects of physical activity. *Exerc. Sport Sci. Rev.* 2:131-53.

Legg, S.J., and W.S. Myles. 1985. Metabolic and cardiovascular cost, and perceived effort over an 8 hour day when lifting loads selected by the psychophysical method. *Ergonomics* 28:337-43.

Lewis, S., P. Thompson, N.H. Areskog, P. Vodak, and M. Marconyak. 1980. Transfer effects of endurance training to exercise with untrained limbs. *Eur. J. Appl. Physiol.* 44:25-34.

Linderholm, H. 1986. Perceived exertion during exercise in the discrimination between circulatory and pulmonary disorders. In *The perception of exertion in physical work,* 199-206. *See* Borg and Ottoson 1986.

Ljunggren, G. 1985. Studies of perceived exertion during bicycle ergometer exercise—Some applications. *Reports from the Department of Psychology,* Stockholm: Univ. of Stockholm.

———. 1986. Observer ratings of perceived exertion in relation to self ratings and heart rate. *Appl. Ergonomics* 17:117-25.

Ljunggren, G., R. Ceci, and J. Karlsson. 1987. Prolonged exercise at a constant load on a bicycle ergometer: Ratings of perceived exertion and leg aches and pain as well as measurements of blood lactate accumulation and heart rate. *Int. J. Sports Med.* 8:109-16.

Ljunggren, G., and P. Hassmen. 1991. Perceived exertion and physiological economy of competition walking, ordinary walking and running. *J. Sports Sci.* 9:273-83.

Ljunggren, G., and S. Johansson. 1988. Use of submaximal measures of perceived exertion during bicycle ergometer exercise as predictors of maximal work capacity. *J. Sports Sci.* 6:189-203.

Lloyd, A., S. Gandevia, and J. Hales. 1991. Muscle performance, voluntary activation, twitch properties and perceived effort in normal subjects and patients with the chronic fatigue syndrome. *Brain* 114:85-98.

Löllgen, H., T. Graham, and G. Sjogaard. 1980. Muscle metabolites, force, and perceived exertion bicycling at varying pedal rates. *Med. Sci. Sports Exerc.* 12:345-51.

Löllgen, H., H.V. Ulmer, R. Gross, G. Wilbert, and G. von Nieding. 1975. Methodical aspects of perceived exertion and its relation to pedalling rate and rotating mass. *Eur. J. Appl. Physiol.* 34:205-15.

Löllgen, H., H.V. Ulmer, and G. von Nieding. 1977. Heart rate and perceptual response to exercise with different pedalling speed in normal subjects and patients. *Eur. J. Appl. Physiol.* 37:297-304.

Löllgen, H., H.V. Ulmer, G. Wilbert, and R. Gross. 1974. Correlation of pedalling frequency and perceived exertion in bicycle ergometry. In *Proceedings of the 20th World Congress in Sports Medicine,* 347-53. Melbourne, Australia.

Loverin, J. 1984. Perceived level of exertion chart used to monitor heart rates. *J. Phys. Ed. Program* 81:12-14.

Mahon, A., and M. Marsh. 1992. Reliability of the rating of perceived exertion at ventilatory threshold in children. *Int. J. Sports Med.* 13:567-71.

Mak, V., J. Bugler, C. Roberts, and S. Spiro. 1993. Effect of arterial oxygen desaturation on six minute walk distance, perceived effort and perceived breathlessness in patients with airflow limitation. *Thorax* 48:33-38.

Marcus, P., and P. Redman. 1979. Effect of exercise on thermal comfort during hypothermia. *Physiol. Behav.* 22:831-35.

Maresh, C., M. Deschenes, R. Seip, L. Armstrong, K. Robertson, and B. Noble. 1993. Perceived exertion during hypobaric hypoxia in low- and moderate-altitude natives. *Med. Sci. Sports Exerc.* 25:945-51.

Maresh, C., and B.J. Noble. 1984. Utilization of perceived exertion ratings during exercise testing and training. In *Cardiac rehabilitation: Exercise testing and prescription,* ed. L.K. Hall, 155-73. New York: Spectrum.

Marks, L.E., G. Borg, and G. Ljunggren. 1983. Individual differences in perceived exertion assessed by two new methods. *Percept. Psychophys.* 34:280-88.

Martin, B.J. 1981. Effect of sleep deprivation on tolerance of prolonged exercise. *Eur. J. Appl. Physiol. Occup. Physiol.* 47:345-54.

Martin, B.J., and G.M. Gaddis. 1981. Exercise after sleep deprivation. *Med. Sci. Sports Exerc.* 13:220-23.

Martin, B.J., and R. Haney. 1982. Self-selected exercise intensity is unchanged by sleep loss. *Eur. J. Appl. Physiol. Occup. Physiol.* 49:79-86.

Matthews, P.B.C. 1982. Where does Sherrington's muscular sense originate? Muscles, joints, corollary discharges? *Ann. Rev. Neurosci.* 5:189-218.

Maw, G., S. Boutcher, and N. Taylor. 1993. Ratings of perceived exertion and affect in hot and cool environments. *Eur. J. Appl. Physiol.* 67:174-79.

McCarthy, R.T. 1975. Heart rate, perceived exertion, and energy expenditure during range of motion of the extremities: A nursing assessment. *Milit. Med.* 140:9-16.

McCauley, E., and K. Courneya. 1992. Self-efficacy relationships with affective and exertion responses to exercise. *J. Appl. Soc. Psychol.* 22:312-26.

McCloskey, D.I. 1978. Kinesthetic sensibility. *Physiol. Rev.* 58:763-820.

McCloskey, D.I., P. Ebeling, and G.M. Goodwin. 1974. Estimation of weights and tension and apparent involvement of a "sense of effort." *Exper. Neurol.* 42:229-32.

McCloskey, D.I., S. Gandevia, E.K. Potter, and J.G. Colebatch. 1983. Muscle sense and effort: Motor commands and judgements about muscular contractions. *Adv. Neurol.* 39:151-67.

Merton, P.A. 1964. Human position sense and sense of effort. *Symp. Soc. Exper. Biol.* 18:387-400.

Michael, E.D., and L. Eckardt. 1972. The selection of hard work by trained and non-trained subjects. *Med. Sci. Sports* 4:107-10.

Michael, E.D., and P. Hackett. 1972. Physiological variables related to the selection of work effort on a treadmill and bicycle. *Res. Q.* 43:216-25.

Mihevic, P.M. 1978. Psychological influences on perceived exertion. (Abstract). *Med. Sci. Sports* 10:52.

———. 1983a. Cardiovascular fitness and the psychophysics of perceived exertion. *Res. Q. Exerc. Sport* 54:239-46.

———. 1983b. Sensory cues for perceived exertion: A review. *Med. Sci. Sports Exerc.* 13:150-63.

Mihevic, P.M., J.A. Gliner, and S.M. Horvath. 1981. Perception of effort and respiratory sensitivity during exposure to ozone. *Ergonomics* 24:365-74.

Miller, G.D., R.D. Bell, M.L. Collis, and T.B. Hoshizaki. 1985. The relationship between perceived exertion and heart rate of post 50 year-old volunteers in two different walking activities. *J. Human Move. Stud.* 11:187-95.

Miyashita, M., K. Ondodera, and I. Tabata. 1986. How Borg's RPE-scale has been applied to Japanese. In *The perception of exertion in physical work,* 27-34. See Borg and Ottoson 1986.

Moffatt, R.J., and B.A. Stamford. 1978. Effects of pedalling rate changes on maximal oxygen uptake and perceived exertion during bicycle ergometer work. *Med. Sci. Sports* 10:27-31.

Monahan, T. 1988. Perceived exertion: An old exercise tool finds new applications. *Physician Sportsmed.* 16:174-79.

Morgan, W.P. 1973. Psychological factors influencing perceived exertion. *Med. Sci. Sports* 5:97-103.

———. 1977. Perception of effort in selected samples of Olympic athletes and soldiers. In *Physical work and effort,* 267-78. See Borg 1977a.

———. 1981. 1980 C.H. McCloy research lecture: Psychophysiology of self-awareness during vigorous physical activity. *Res. Q. Exerc. Sport* 52:385-427.

———. 1983. Psychometric correlates of respiration: A review. *Am. Indust. Hyg. Asso. J.* 44:677-84.

———. 1985. Psychogenic factors and exercise metabolism: A review. *Med. Sci. Sports Exerc.* 17:309-16.

Morgan, W.P., and G. Borg. 1976. Perception of effort in the prescription of physical activity. In *Humanistic and mental health aspects of sports, exercise, and recreation,* ed. T.T. Craig, 126-29. Chicago: American Medical Association.

Morgan, W.P., K. Hirta, G.A. Weitz, and B. Balke. 1976. Hypnotic perturbation of perceived exertion: Ventilatory consequences. *Am. J. Clin. Hypn.* 18:182-90.

Morgan, W.P., and M.L. Pollock. 1977. Psychologic characterization of the elite distance runner. *Ann. N.Y. Acad. Sci.* 301:382-403.

Morgan, W.P., P. Raven, B. Drinkwater, and S. Horvath. 1973. Perceptual and metabolic responsivity to standard bicycle ergometry following various hypnotic suggestions. *Int. J. Clin. Exper. Hypn.* 21:86-101.

Muza, S.R., and F.W. Zechman. 1984. Scaling of added loads to breathing: Magnitude estimation vs. handgrip matching. *J. Appl. Physiol.* 57:888-91.

Myers, J., J. Atwood, M. Sullivan, S. Forbes, R. Friis, W. Pewen, and V. Froelicher. 1987. Perceived exertion and gas exchange after calcium and beta-blockade in atrial fibrillation. *J. Appl. Physiol.* 63:97-104.

Myles, W.S. 1985. Sleep deprivation, physical fatigue, and the perception of exercise intensity. *Med. Sci. Sports Exerc.* 17:580-84.

Myles, W., and D. Maclean. 1986. A comparison of response and production protocols for assessing perceived exertion. *Eur. J. Appl. Physiol.* 55:585-87.

Myles, W.S., and P.L. Saunders. 1979. The physiological cost of carrying light and heavy loads. *Eur. J. Appl. Physiol.* 42:125-31.

Nishi, Y., R.R. Gonzalez, and A.P. Gagge. 1976. Prediction of equivalent environments by energy exchange and assessments of physiological strain and discomfort. *Isr. J. Med. Sci.* 12:808-11.

Nishimura, J. 1981a. Problems of perceived exertion. *Japanese Psych. Rev.* 24(2):174-202.

————. 1981b. The relationship between perceived exertion of daily activities and aging of physical function. *Japanese J. Psychol.* 52:219-25.

Noble, B.J. 1979. Validity of perception during recovery from maximal exercise in men and women. *Percept. Motor Skills* 49:891-97.

————. 1982. Clinical applications of perceived exertion. *Med. Sci. Sports Exerc.* 14:406-11.

Noble, B.J., and J.G. Allen. 1984. Perceived exertion in swimming. *Swimming Technique* 21:11-15.

Noble, B.J., and G. Borg. 1972. Perceived exertion during walking and running. In *Proceedings of the 17th International Congress of Applied Psychology,* ed. R. Piret, 387-92. Brussels.

Noble, B.J., G. Borg, I. Jacobs, R. Ceci, and P. Kaiser. 1983. A category-ratio perceived exertion scale: Relationship to blood and muscle lactates and heart rate. *Med. Sci. Sports Exerc.* 15:523-28.

Noble, B., W. Kraemer, J. Allen, J. Plank, and L. Woodward. 1986. The integration of physiological cues in effort perceptions: Stimulus strength vs. relative contribution. In *The perception of exertion in physical work,* 83-96. See Borg and Ottoson 1986.

Noble, B.J., W.J. Kraemer, and M. Clark. 1982. Response of selected physiological variables and perceived exertion to high intensity weight training in highly trained and beginning weight trainers. *Nat. Strength Conditioning Asso. J.* 4:10-12.

Noble, B.J., C.M. Maresh, and M. Ritchey. 1981. Comparison of exercise sensations between females and males. In *Women and sport: An historical, biological, physiological and sports medicine approach,* ed. J. Borms, M. Hebbelinck, and A. Venerando, 175-79. Basel: Karger.

Noble, B.J., K.F. Metz, K.B. Pandolf, C.W. Bell, E. Cafarelli, and W.E. Sime. 1973. Perceived exertion during walking and running II. *Med. Sci. Sports* 5:116-20.

Noble, B.J., K.F. Metz, K.B. Pandolf, and E. Cafarelli. 1973. Perceptual responses to exercise: A multiple regression study. *Med. Sci. Sports* 5:104-9.

Noble, M.M., H.L. Frankel, W. Else, and A. Guz. 1971. The ability of man to detect added resistive loads to breathing. *Clin. Sci.* 41:285-87.

————. 1972. The sensation produced by threshold resistive loads to breathing. *Eur. J. Clin. Invest.* 2:72-77.

Nordesjo, L., L. Ekelund, and L. Sporre. 1977. Heart rate controlled ergometry and its application. In *Physical work and effort,* 223-38. See Borg 1977a.

O'Neill, M., K. Cooper, C. Mills, E. Boyles, and S. Hunyor. 1992. Accuracy of Borg's ratings of perceived exertion in the prediction of heart rates during pregnancy. *Br. J. Sports Med.* 26:121-24.

O'Sullivan, S.B. 1984. Perceived exertion: A review. *Phys. Ther.* 64:343-46.

Pandolf, K.B. 1977. Psychological and physiological factors influencing perceived exertion. In *Physical work and effort,* 371-84. See Borg 1977a.

————. 1978. Influence of local and central factors in dominating rated perceived exertion during physical work. *Percept. Motor Skills* 46:683-98.

————. 1982. Differentiated ratings of perceived exertion during physical exercise. *Med. Sci. Sports Exerc.* 14:397-405.

————. 1983. Advances in the study and application of perceived exertion. *Exerc. Sport Sci. Rev.* 11:118-58.

————. 1986. Local and central factor contributions in the perception of effort during physical exercise. In *The perception of effort in physical work,* 97-110. See Borg and Ottoson 1986.

Pandolf, K.B., D.S. Billings, L.L. Drolet, N.A. Pimetal, and M.N. Sawka. 1984. Differential ratings of perceived exertion and various physiological responses during prolonged upper and lower body exercise. *Eur. J. Appl. Physiol.* 53:5-11.

Pandolf, K.B., R.L. Burse, and R.F. Goldman. 1975. Differentiated ratings of perceived exertion during physical conditioning of older individuals using leg-weight loading. *Percept. Motor Skills* 40:563-74.

Pandolf, K.B., E. Cafarelli, B.J. Noble, and K.F. Metz. 1972. Perceptual responses during prolonged work. *Percept. Motor Skills* 35:975-85.

Pandolf, K.B., and W.S. Cain. 1974. Constant effort during static and dynamic muscular exercise. *J. Motor Behav.* 6:101-10.

Pandolf, K.B., E. Kamon, and B.J. Noble. 1978. Perceived exertion and physiological responses during negative and positive work in climbing a laddermill. *J. Sports Med. Phys. Fitness* 18:227-36.

Pandolf, K.B., and B.J. Noble. 1973. The effect of pedalling speed and resistance changes on perceived exertion for equivalent power outputs on the bicycle ergometer. *Med. Sci. Sports* 5:132-36.

Patton, J.F., W.P. Morgan, and J.A. Vogel. 1977. Perceived exertion of absolute work during a military physical training program. *Eur. J. Appl. Physiol.* 36:107-14.

Pavlina, Z., and I. Saric. 1975. *The interrelationship among three measures of physical stress: Absolute heart rate, relative heart rate and ratings of perceived effort.* Reports from the Institute of Applied Psychology, no. 56. Stockholm: Univ. of Stockholm.

Pederson, P.K., and J.R. Nielsen. 1984. Absolute or relative work load in exercise testing: Significance of individual differences in working capacity. *Scand. J. Clin. Lab. Invest.* 44:635-42.

Pederson, P.K., and H.G. Welch. 1977. Oxygen breathing, selected physiological variables and perception of effort during submaximal exercise. In *Physical work and effort,* 385-400. See Borg 1977a.

Perkins, R., J. Sexton, R. Solberg-Kassel, and L.H. Epstein. 1991. Effects of nicotine on perceived exertion during low-intensity activity. *Med. Sci. Sports Exerc.* 23:1283-88.

Perkins, R., J. Sexton, R. Solberg-Kassel, and L. Epstein. 1991. Estimates of type A behavior do not predict perceived exertion during graded exercise. *Med. Sci. Sports Exerc.* 23:1276-83.

Persson, B., and C. Thoren. 1980. Prolonged exercise in adolescent boys with juvenile diabetes mellitus. Circulatory and metabolic responses in relation to perceived exertion. *Acta Paedriatr. Scand.* 283 (Suppl.): 62-69.

Pierce, E., N. Eastman, R. McGowan, and M. Legnola. 1992. Metabolic demands and perceived exertion during cardiopulmonary resuscitation. *Percept. Motor Skills* 74:323-28.

Pimental, N., and K. Pandolf. 1979. Energy expenditure while standing or walking slowly uphill or downhill with loads. *Ergonomics* 22:963-73.

Piret, R., ed. 1972. *Proceedings of the 17th International Congress of Applied Psychology*. Brussels.

Pivarnik, J., T. Grafner, and E. Elkins. 1988. Metabolic, thermoregulatory, and psychophysiological responses during arm and leg exercise. *Med. Sci. Sports Exerc.* 20:1-5.

Pivarnik, J., W. Lee, and J. Miller. 1991. Physiological and perceptual responses to cycle and treadmill exercise during pregnancy. *Med. Sci. Sports Exerc.* 23:470-75.

Pivarnik, J., and L. Senay. 1986. Effect of endurance training and heat acclimation on perceived exertion during exercise. *J. Cardiopul. Rehab.* 6:499-504.

Pollock, M., A. Jackson, and C. Foster. 1986. The use of the perception scale for exercise prescription. In *The perception of exertion in physical work*, 161-78. *See* Borg and Ottoson 1986.

Pollock, M.L., and A.E. Pels. 1984. Exercise prescription for the cardiac patient: Update. *Clinics Sports Med.* 3:425-42.

Poulus, A.J., H.J. Docter, and H.G. Westra. 1974. Acid-base balance and subjective feelings of fatigue during physical exercise. *Eur. J. Appl. Physiol.* 33:207-13.

Prusaczyk, W., K. Cureton, R. Graham, and C. Ray. 1992. Differential effects of dietary carbohydrate on RPE at the lactate and ventilatory thresholds. *Med. Sci. Sports Exerc.* 24:568-75.

Purvis, J.W., and K.J. Cureton. 1981. Ratings of perceived exertion at the anaerobic threshold. *Ergonomics* 24:295-300.

Randle, I.P.M., and S.J. Legg. 1985. A comparison of the effect of mixed static and dynamic work with mainly dynamic work in hot conditions. *Eur. J. Appl. Physiol. Occup. Physiol.* 54:201-6.

Reilly, T., and D. Ball. 1984. The net physiological cost of dribbling a soccer ball. *Res. Q. Exerc. Sport* 55:267-71.

Reilly, T., G. Robinson, and D.S. Minors. 1984. Some circulatory responses to exercise at different times of day. *Med. Sci. Sports Exerc.* 16:477-82.

Rejeski, W.J. 1981. Perception of exertion: A social psychophysiological integration. *J. Sport Psychol.* 3:305-20.

———. 1985. Perceived exertion: An active or passive process? *J. Sport Psychol.* 7:371-78.

Rejeski, W.J., G. Brodwicz, D. King, and P. Ribisl. 1982. Salience of perceptual cues during cycling: Do training and instrumentation moderate rating of perceived exertion? *Percept. Motor Skills* 54:823-29.

Rejeski, W.J., and P.M. Ribisl. 1980. Expected task duration and perceived effort: An attributional analysis. *J. Sport Psychol.* 2:227-36.

Rejeski, W.J., and B. Sanford. 1984. Feminine-typed females: The role of affective schema in the perception of exercise intensity. *Sport Psychol.* 6:197-207.

Robertson, R.J. 1982. Central signals of perceived exertion during dynamic exercise. *Med. Sci. Sports Exerc.* 14:390-96.

Robertson, R.J., C.J. Caspersen, T.G. Allison, G.S. Skrinar, R.A. Abbott, and K.F. Metz. 1982. Differentiated perceptions of exertion and energy cost of young women while carrying loads. *Eur. J. Appl. Physiol.* 49:69-78.

Robertson, R.J., J.E. Falkel, A.L. Drash, A.M. Swank, K.F. Metz, S.A. Sprungen, and J.R. LeBoeuf. 1986. Effect of blood pH on peripheral and central signals of perceived exertion. *Med. Sci. Sports Exerc.* 18:114-22.

Robertson, R., R. Gilcher, K. Metz, H. Bahnson, and T. Allison. 1978. Effect of red blood cell reinfusion on physical working capacity and perceived exertion at normal and reduced oxygen pressure. (Abstract). *Med. Sci. Sports* 10:49.

Robertson, R., R. Gilcher, K. Metz, G. Skrinar, T. Allison, H. Bahnson, R. Abbott, R. Becker, and J. Falkel. 1982. Effect of induced erythrocythemia on hypoxia tolerance during physical exercise. *J. Appl. Physiol. Respir. Environ. Exerc. Physiol.* 53:490-95.

Robertson, R., R. Gilcher, K. Metz, C. Casperson, T. Allison, R. Abbott, G. Skrinar, J. Krause, and P. Nixon. 1988. Effect of simulated altitude erythrocythemia in women on hemoglobin flow rate during exercise. *J. Appl. Physiol.* 64:1674-79.

Robertson, R.J., R.L. Gillespie, E. Hiatt, and K.D. Rose. 1977. Perceived exertion and stimulus intensity modulation. *Percept. Motor Skills* 45:211-18.

Robertson, R.J., R.L. Gillespie, J. McCarthy, et al. 1978. Perceived exertion and the field-independence-dependence dimension. *Percept. Motor Skills* 46:495-500.

Robertson, R.J., R.L. Gillespie, J. McCarthy, and K.D. Rose. 1979a. Differentiated perceptions of exertion: Part I. Mode of integration of regional signals. *Percept. Motor Skills* 49:683-89.

———. 1979b. Differentiated perceptions of exertion: Part II. Relationship to local and central physiological responses. *Percept. Motor Skills* 49:691-97.

Robertson, R., R. Goss, T. Auble, D. Cassinelli, R. Spina, E. Glickman, R. Galbreath, R. Silberman, and K. Metz. 1990. Cross-modal exercise prescription at absolute and relative oxygen uptake using perceived exertion. *Med. Sci. Sports Exerc.* 22:653-59.

Robertson, R., J. McCarthy, and R. Gillespie. 1976. Contribution of regional to overall perceived exertion during cycle ergometer exercise. *Med. Sci. Sports* 8:64-65.

Robertson, R., P. Nixon, C. Caspersen, K. Metz, R. Abbott, and F. Goss. 1992. Abatement of exertional perceptions following dynamic exercise: Physiological mediators. *Med. Sci. Sports Exerc.* 24:346-53.

Robertson, R., R. Stanko, F. Goss, R. Spina, J. Reilly, and K. Greenawalt. 1990. Blood glucose extraction as a mediator of perceived exertion during prolonged exercise. *Eur. J. Appl. Physiol.* 61:100-105.

Rodrigues, L., A. Russo, A. Silva, I. Picarro, F. Silva, P. Zogaib, and D. Soares. 1990. Effects of caffeine on the rate of perceived exertion. *Braz. J. Med. Biol. Res.* 23:965-68.

Rodriquez, A., and J. Agre. 1991. Physiologic parameters and perceived exertion with local muscle fatigue in postpolio subjects. *Arch. Phys. Med. Rehab.* 72:305-8.

Roland, P.E. 1978. Sensory feedback to the cerebral cortex during voluntary movement in man. *Behav. Brain Sci.* 1:129-71.

Roland, P.E., and H. Ladegaard-Pederson. 1977. A quantitative analysis of sensations of tension and of kinaesthesia in man. *Brain* 100:671-92.

Rosentswieg, J., D. Williams, C. Sandburg, K. Kolten, L. Engler, and G. Norman. 1979. Perceived exertion of professional hockey players. *Percept. Motor Skills* 48:992-94.

Ross, M.A., W.P. Morgan, and H. Leventhal. 1978. Perceived exertion in adults males possessing either the type A or type B behavior pattern. (Abstract). *Med. Sci. Sports* 10:51.

Ryman, D., P. Naitoh, and C. Englund. 1989. Perceived exertion under conditions of sustained work and sleep loss. *Work Stress* 3:57-68.

Salamon, M., C. Euler, and O. Franzen. 1977. Perception of mechanical factors in breathing. In *Physical work and effort,* 101-14. *See* Borg 1977a.

Sargeant, A.J., and C.T. Davies. 1973. Perceived exertion during rhythmic exercise involving different muscle masses. *J. Human Ergol.* 2:3-11.

———. 1977. Perceived exertion of dynamic exercise in normal subjects and patients following leg injury. In *Physical work and effort,* 345-56. *See* Borg 1977a.

Schomer, H. 1986. Mental strategies and the perception of effort of marathon runners. *Int. J. Sport Psychol.* 17:41-59.

———. 1987. Mental strategy training programme for marathon runners. *Int. J. Sport Psychol.* 18:133-51.

Seip, R., D. Snead, E. Pierce, P. Stein, and A. Weltman. 1991. Perceptual responses and blood lactate concentration: Effect of training state. *Med. Sci. Sports Exerc.* 23:80-87.

Seliga, R., A. Bhattacharya, P. Succop, R. Wickstrom, D. Smith, and K. Willeke. 1991. Effect of work load and respirator wear on postural stability, heat rate, and perceived exertion. *Am. Indust. Hyg. Asso. J.* 52:417-22.

Shephard, R., H. Vandewalle, V. Gil, E. Bouhlel, and H. Monod. 1992. Respiratory, muscular, and overall perceptions of effort: The influence of hypoxia and muscle mass. *Med. Sci. Sports Exerc.* 24:556-67.

Sherrington, C.S. 1900. The muscular sense. In Schafer, E.A., ed., *Textbook of Physiology.* Edinburgh and London: Pentland.

Shiflett, S., and S.L. Cohen. 1982. The shifting salience of valence and instrumentality in the prediction of perceived effort, satisfaction and turnover. *Motivation Emotion* 6:65-77.

Sidney, K.H., and N.M. Lefcoe. 1977. The effect of ephedrine on the physiological and psychological responses to submaximal and maximal exercise in man. *Med. Sci. Sports* 9:95-99.

Sidney, K.H., and R.J. Shephard. 1977. Perception of exertion in the elderly, effects of aging, mode of exercise, and physical training. *Percept. Motor Skills* 44:999-1010.

Siegl, P., and K. Schultz. 1984. The Borg scale as an instrument for the detection of subjectively experienced stress in industrial medicine laboratory and field studies. *Zeitschr. gesamte Hygiene Grenzgebiete* 30:383-86.

Silverman, M., J. Barry, H. Hellerstein, J. Janos, and S. Kelsen. 1988. Variability of the perceived sense of effort in breathing during exercise in patients with chronic obstructive pulmonary disease. *Am. Rev. Respir. Dis.* 137:206-9.

Sjoberg, H. 1975. Relations between heart rate, reaction speed, and subjective effort at different work loads on a bicycle ergometer. *J. Human Stress* 1:21-27.

Sjoberg, H., M. Frankenhaeuser, and H. Bjurstedt. 1979. Interactions between heart rate, psychomotor performance and perceived effort during physical work as influenced by beta-adrenergic blockade. *Biol. Psychol.* 8:31-43.

Skinner, J.S., G. Borg, and E.R. Buskirk. 1969. Physiological and perceptual reactions to exertion of young men differing in activity and body size. In *Exercise and fitness,* ed. B.D. Franks, 53-66. Chicago: Athletic Institute.

Skinner, J.S., R. Hustler, V. Bergsteinova, and E.R. Buskirk. 1973a. Perception of effort during different types of exercise and under different environmental conditions. *Med. Sci. Sports* 5:110-15.

Skinner, J.S., R. Hustler, V. Bergsteinova, and E. R. Buskirk. 1973b. The validity and reliability of a rating scale of perceived exertion. *Med. Sci. Sports* 5:97-103.

Skrinar, G.S., S.P. Ingram, and K.B. Pandolf. 1983. Effect of endurance training on perceived exertion and stress hormones in women. *Percept. Motor Skills* 57:1239-50.

Smutok, M.A., G.S. Skrinar, and K.B. Pandolf. 1980. Exercise intensity: Subjective regulation by perceived exertion. *Arch. Phys. Med. Rehab.* 61:569-74.

Soule, R.G., and R.F. Goldman. 1973. Pacing of intermittent work during 31 hours. *Med. Sci. Sports* 5:128-31.

Soule, R., K. Pandolf, and R. Goldman. 1978. Energy expenditure of heavy load carriage. *Ergonomics* 21:373-81.

Sovijarvi, A.R., S. Rosset, J. Hyvarinen, A. Franssila, G. Graeffe, and M. Lehtimaki. 1979. Effect of air ionization on heart rate and perceived exertion during a bicycle exercise test. A double-blind cross-over study. *Eur. J. Appl. Physiol.* 41:285-91.

Spodaryk, K., U. Szmatlan, and L. Berger. 1990. The relationship of plasma ammonia and lactate concentrations to perceived exertion in trained and untrained women. *Eur. J. Appl. Physiol.* 61:309-12.

Squires, R., J. Rod, M. Pollock, and C. Foster. 1982. Effects of propranolol on perceived exertion soon after myocardial revascularization surgery. *Med. Sci. Sports Exerc.* 14:276-80.

Stamford, B.A. 1976. Validity and reliability of subjective ratings of perceived exertion during work. *Ergonomics* 19:53-60.

————. 1984. What's your exertostat? *Physician Sportsmed.* 12:203.

Stamford, B.A., and B.J. Noble. 1974. Metabolic cost and perception of effort during bicycle ergometer work performance. *Med. Sci. Sports* 6:226-31.

Stegemann, J., H.V. Ulmer, and K.W. Heinrich. 1968. Relationship between force and force perception as basis for the selection of energetically unfavorable pedalling frequencies in cycling. *Int. Z. Angew. Physiol.* 25:224-34.

Stephenson, L.A., M.A. Kolka, and J.E. Wilkerson. 1982. Perceived exertion and anaerobic threshold during the menstrual cycle. *Med. Sci. Sports Exerc.* 14:218-22.

Stevens, J.C., and W.S. Cain. 1970. Effort in isometric muscular contractions related to force level and duration. *Percept. Psychophysics* 8:240-44.

Stevens, J.C., and A. Krimsley. 1977. Build-up of fatigue in static work: Role of blood flow. In *Physical work and effort*, 145-56. *See* Borg 1977a.

Stevens, J.C., and J.D. Mack. 1959. Scales of apparent force. *J. Exper. Psychol.* 58:405-13.

Stevens, S.S. 1957. On the psychophysical law. *Psych. Rev.* 64:153-181.

Stevens, S.S. and E.H. Galanter. 1957. Ratio scales and category scales for a dozen perceptual continuaa. *J. Exper. Psychol.* 54:377-411.

Strindberg, L., and N.F. Petersson. 1972. Measurement of force perception in pushing trolleys. *Ergonomics* 15:545-54.

Sylva, M., R. Byrd, and M. Mangum. 1990. Effects of social influence and sex on rating of perceived exertion in exercising elite athletes. *Percept. Motor Skills* 70:591-94.

Tabata, I., and A. Kawakami. 1991. Effects of blood glucose concentration on ratings of perceived exertion during prolonged low-intensity physical exercise. *Japanese J. Physiol.* 41:203-15.

Tanaka, S. 1981. Perceived exertion during level and grade running on equivalent work intensities. In *Sporterziehung und Evaluation*, ed. H. Haag, 90-94. Schorndorf: Hofmann.

Teghtsoonian, R., M. Teghtsoonian, and J. Karlsson. 1977. The effects of fatigue on the perception of muscular effort. In *Physical work and effort*, 157-80. *See* Borg 1977a.

Tesch, P.A., and P. Kaiser. 1983. Effect of B-adrenergic blockade on O_2 uptake during submaximal and maximal exercise. *J. Appl. Physiol.* 54:901-5.

Thomas, S. 1980-81. Rating of perceived exertion—An alternative approach to monitoring training levels. In *Coaching science update*, 21-22.

Thomas, V., and T. Reilly. 1975. Circulatory, psychological and performance variables during 100 hours of paced continuous exercise under conditions of controlled energy intake and work output. *J. Human Move. Stud.* 1:149-55.

Toner, M.M., L.L. Drolet, and K.B. Pandolf. 1986. Perceptual and physiological responses during exercise in cool and cold water. *Percept. Motor Skills* 62:211-20.

Turkulin, K., B. Zamlic, and U. Pegan. 1977. Exercise performance and perceived exertion in patients after myocardial infarction. In *Physical work and effort*, 357-66. *See* Borg 1977a.

Ueda, T., and T. Kurokawa. 1991. Validity of heart rate and ratings of perceived exertion as indices of exercise intensity in a group of children while swimming. *Eur. J. Appl. Physiol.* 63:200-204.

Ueda, T., T. Kurokawa, K. Kikkawa, and T. Choi. 1993. Contribution of differentiated ratings of perceived exertion to overall exertion in women while swimming. *Eur. J. Appl. Physiol.* 66:196-201.

Ulin, S., T. Armstrong, S. Snook, and A. Franzblau. 1993a. Effect of tool shape and work location on perceived exertion for work on horizontal surfaces. *Am. Indust. Hyg. Asso. J.* 54:383-91.

Ulin, S., T. Armstrong, S. Snook, and W. Keyserling. 1993b. Perceived exertion and discomfort associated with driving screws at various work locations and at different work frequencies. *Ergonomics* 36:833-46.

Ulin, S., C. Ways, T. Armstrong, and S. Snook. 1990. Perceived exertion and discomfort versus work height with a pistol-shaped screwdriver. *Am. Indust. Hyg. Asso. J.* 51:588-94.

Ulmer, H. 1986. Perceived exertion as a part of a feedback system and its interaction with tactical behavior in endurance sports. In *The perception of exertion in physical work,* 317-26. *See* Borg and Ottoson 1986.

Ulmer, H.V., U. Janz, and H. Löllgen. 1977. Aspects of the validity of Borg's scale. Is it measuring stress or strain? In *Physical work and effort,* 181-96. See Borg 1977a.

Van Baak, M., F. Verstappen, and B. Oosterhuis. 1986. Twenty-four hour effects of oxprenolol Oros and atenolol on heart rate, blood pressure, exercise tolerance and perceived exertion. *Eur. J. Clin. Pharmacol.* 30:399-406.

Van Den Burg, M., and R. Ceci. 1986. A comparison of a psychophysical estimation and a production method in a laboratory and a field condition. In *The perception of exertion in physical work,* 35-46. *See* Borg and Ottoson 1986.

Van Herwaarden, C.L., R.A. Binkhorst, J.F. Fennis, and A. Van'T Larr. 1979. Effects of propranolol and metoprolol on haemodynamic and respiratory indices and on perceived exertion during exercise in hypertensive patients. *Br. Heart J.* 41:99-105.

Van Moorst, A., and P.S. Blitz. 1978. Physical fatigue and the perception of differences in load: A signal detection approach. *Proceedings of the 1978 International Symposium on Psychological Sport,* 58-68. Netanya, Israel.

Wang, Y., and W. Morgan. 1992. The effect of imagery perspectives on the psychophysiological responses to imagined exercise. *Behav. Brain Res.* 52:167-74.

Wangenheim, M., Borg, G., and Holzmann, P. 1987. A psychophysical study of work-related stress using observer ratings. *Upsal. J. Med. Sci.* 92:1-17.

Wangenheim, M., S. Carlsoo, B. Nordgren, et al. 1986. Perception of efforts in working postures. *Upsal. J. Med. Sci.* 91:53-66.

Ward, D., and O. Bar-Or. 1990. Use of the Borg scale in exercise prescription for overweight youth. *Can. J. Sport Sci.* 15:120-25.

Wardle, M. 1978. Psychophysical approach to estimating endurance in performing physically demanding work. *Human Factors* 20:745-47.

Wastl, P., H.V. Ulmer, and J. Deforth. 1982. Perceived exertion and strategy in 400 and 1500m running. *Leistungssport* 12:378-82.

Watt, B., and R. Grove. 1993. Perceived exertion. Antecedents and applications. *Sports Med.* 15:225-41.

Weiser, P.C., R.A. Kinsman, and D.A. Stamper. 1974. Task-specific symptomatology changes resulting from prolonged submaximal bicycle riding. *Med. Sci. Sports* 6:226-31.

Weiser, P.C., and D.A. Stamper. 1977. Psychophysiological interactions leading to increased effort, leg fatigue, and respiratory distress during prolonged, strenuous bicycle riding. In *Physical work and effort*, 401-16. *See* Borg 1977a.

West, D.M., C.G. Ellis, and E.M. Campbell. 1975. Ability of man to detect increases in his breathing. *J. Appl. Physiol.* 39:372-76.

Wiles, J., S. Bird, J. Hopkins, and M. Riley. 1992. Effect of caffeinated coffee on running speed, respiratory factors, blood lactate and perceived exertion during 1500-m treadmill running. *Br. J. Sports Med.* 26:116-20.

Wiles, J., R. Woodward, and S. Bird. 1991. Effect of pre-exercise protein ingestion upon VO_2, R and perceived exertion during treadmill running. *Br. J. Sports Med.* 25:26-30.

Wiley, R.L., and F.W. Zechman. 1966-67. Perception of added airflow resistance in humans. *Respir. Physiol.* 2:73-87.

Williams, D.H., and C. Williams. 1983. Cardiovascular and metabolic responses of trained and untrained middle-aged men to a graded treadmill walking test. *Br. J. Sports Med.* 17:110-16.

Williams, J., and R. Eston. 1986. Does personality influence the perception of effort? The results from a study of secondary schoolboys. *Phys. Ed. Rev.* 9:94-99.

Williams, M.A., and P.S. Fardy. 1979. Limitations in prescribing exercise from perceived exertion, onset of symptoms or fixed heart rates in cardiac patients. (Abstract). *Med. Sci. Sports* 11:111.

Williams, M.H., M. Lindhjem, and R. Schuster. 1978. The effect of blood infusion upon endurance capacity and ratings of perceived exertion. *Med. Sci. Sports* 10:113-18.

Wilmore, J.H., F.B. Roby, P.R. Stanforth, M.J. Buono, S.H. Constable, U. Tsao, and B.J. Lowdon. 1986. Ratings of perceived exertion, heart rate, and power output in predicting maximal oxygen uptake during submaximal cycle ergometry. *Physician Sportsmed.* 14:133-43.

Winborn, M., A. Meyers, and C. Mulling. 1988. The effects of gender and experience on perceived exertion. *J. Sport Exerc. Psychol.* 10:22-31.

Wong, D., P. Rechnitzer, D. Cunningham, and J. Howard. 1990. Effect of an exercise program on the perception of exertion in males at retirement. *Can. J. Sport Sci.* 15:249-53.

Wood, M.M., P.E. McCarthy, and J.E. Cotes. 1971. Perception of airway resistance in relation to breathlessness on exertion in chronic lung disease. *Scand. J. Respir. Dis.* 77 (Suppl.): 98-102.

Wrisberg, C., B. Franks, M. Birdwell, and D. High. 1988. Physiological and psychological responses to exercise with an induced attentional focus. *Percept. Motor Skills* 66:603-16.

Yamaji, K., Y. Yokota, and R. Shephard. 1992. A comparison of the perceived and the ECG measured heart rate during cycle ergometer, treadmill and stairmill exercise before and after perceived heart rate training. *J. Sports Med. Phys. Fitness* 32:271-81.

Yorio, J., R. Dishman, W. Forbus, K. Cureton, and R. Graham. 1992. Breathlessness predicts perceived exertion in young women with mild asthma. *Med. Sci. Sports Exerc.* 24:860-67.

Yoshitake, H. 1971. Relations between the symptoms and feeling of fatigue. *Ergonomics* 14:175-86.

Young, A.J., A. Cymerman, and K.B. Pandolf. 1982. Differentiated ratings of perceived exertion are influenced by high altitude exposures. *Med. Sci. Sports Exerc.* 14:223-28.

Zohar, D., and G. Spitz. 1981. Expected performance and perceived exertion in a prolonged physical task. *Percept. Motor Skills* 52:975-84.

2

CHAPTER

Psychophysics and the Effort Sense

Psychophysics is a term that may appear quite intimidating to one uninitiated in psychological measurement. It need not be. The term *psychophysics* has been used traditionally to designate the science associated with the study of human perception. More specifically, psychophysics is concerned with the relationship between physical stimuli and perceptual responses. In other words, psychophysics attempts to discover the laws that govern human perceptual response within a variety of sensory dimensions. The objectives of this chapter are threefold:

1. To acquaint the reader with a historical perspective relative to the science of psychophysics. The early work of classical psychophysicists like E. H. Weber (1795-1878) and G. T. Fechner (1801-1887) will be reviewed. In addition, the significant work of the father of modern psychophysics, S.S. Stevens, will be briefly critiqued.
2. To provide the reader with an elementary review of a variety of psychophysical methods that might be adapted for use in the study of perception of exertion during human movement. To date, with a few minor exceptions, the major measurement technique utilized by exercise scientists and clinicians has been the category scale commonly referred to as the Borg or RPE scale (Borg 1971). Other methods are available and perhaps preferential in certain experimental and clinical situations.
3. To illustrate how an elementary understanding of psychophysical methodology opens a greater variety of related literature to the new investigator. For example, there is a small but important body of literature concerned with the perception of heaviness generated by psychophysical methods not commonly utilized or published in the field of exercise and sport science.

A number of terms will be used throughout this chapter, as well as the entire book, which require explicit definitions so that we can communicate from a common semantic base.

Psychophysics—studies of the relationships between sensation and stimulus when both are measured as quantities (Marks 1974) or an exact theory of the relation of body and mind (Fechner 1860).

Sensation—a form of awareness assigned to the activation of a specific class of sense organs and the sensory mechanisms they feed into (Bartley 1970) a passive process.

Perception—the use of data provided by the sense organs to cope with conditions either outside or inside the body (Bartley 1970); an active process.

Can Subjective Reality Be Measured?

Questioning the measurability of subjective human response may appear incongruous for a book that promotes the study and application of human perception. We can assure you that the authors have found personal resolution to this question many years ago. However, there are some, scientists and laypeople alike, who challenge the validity and objectivity of such measurement. William James, famous 19th century American psychologist and philosopher, is said to have called psychophysics ''moonshiney,'' meaning that the measurement of subjective reality is whimsical. Such challenges need to be squarely faced, not ignored.

Western culture, dominated as it is with a mechanistic view of the physical world, is suspicious of any behavior that cannot be directly observed and measured. Indeed, perceptions cannot be directly verified by a scientific observer. This question has plagued psychophysics for more than 100 years. To a large degree, psychology depends on self-reports of human experience. Unlike the physical sciences, which can make direct recordings of the physical world, psychology largely depends on indirect measurements. Much of the collective energy of this discipline has been concerned with developing measurements that might overcome the complexities of recording psychic activity that has neurological origin and behavioral expression.

There can be little doubt that humans experience sensory stimulation arising from extrinsic and intrinsic sources, for example, environmental temperature and muscular discomfort, respectively. Sensations are interpreted—that is, perceptions are made—and we make important life decisions on the basis of these interpretations. Such a crucial human response like perception must be studied and applied to life needs. Our challenge as scientists and clinicians is to continually develop more sophisticated techniques to measure this complex human phenomenon. Since one of the goals of science is prediction, perhaps the ultimate source of validation for our work will be the accuracy and utility of our perceptual predictions. In other words, will our understanding of perceptual response provide us with correct and pragmatic human outcomes? In exercise science, perceptual measurements can be said to be valid if our ''numbers'' provide exercisers with data that help them to precisely and effectively adapt to various stimulus conditions.

Is There an Effort Sense?

The existence of the so-called "effort sense" is another complex question that we want to address at the outset. Sensory psychologists and physiologists quickly identify touch, taste, smell, hearing, and sight as the basic human senses. Specific sensory receptors have been identified, and physiological activity can be recorded from these receptors when they are impinged upon by pressure, food, odor, sound, or light. Exercise and sport scientists often refer to the *kinesthetic* or movement sense. Although not a basic sense in the classical tradition of psychophysics, nervous system structures have been identified that mediate kinesthesia. Effort or exertion is a complex sensory experience, which thus far has not been directly connected to a unique receptor or nervous system structure. Can we then call the experience of effort a sense?

P. A. Merton (1964), English physiologist, said "To admit its existence (effort sense) implies that we can acquire a knowledge of events outside the central nervous system without the use of sense-organs." In fact, using this logic, Sherrington (1900) rejected the notion of an effort sense. Merton's work, on the other hand, showed that subjects could tell how far they had moved a pointer even though their position sense had been removed. Such evidence points to the existence of an effort sense, even though its exact psychobiological explanation is still forthcoming.

The perception of effort that exercise and sport scientists and clinicians have come to associate with human movement is even more complex than the comparatively narrow field of study involving control of a small muscle group performing a simple task. For example, the effort experienced by a 10,000 meter runner during a race is a complicated process involving multiple physiological inputs modulated by several psychosocial variables. The identification of the physiological and psychological basis of the effort sense is an important scientific quest and must continue. The absence of absolute evidence to support an effort sense does not deny the fact that we do experience effort when we engage in physical activity. That experience must be studied so it can be understood and that understanding applied to human movement problems.

Classic Psychophysics: A Focus on Stimulus

Classical psychophysicists, like E.H. Weber and G.T. Fechner, were interested in measuring whether or not a subject could detect the presence of a sensory stimulus or a change in that stimulus. (Note that the response must be viewed in the context of a physical stimulus and not a perceptual response per se.) To make measurements, the classic psychophysicists needed a scale that described the sensory range. Since there was no physical yardstick to measure human perception, they developed scales with zero and final end points called thresholds.

The zero and terminal point at which a physical stimulus could be detected were termed the absolute thresholds. The zero point was referred to as the stimulus threshold and was distinguished from the terminal threshold, which is the highest point on the stimulus continuum that is detectable. In the case of sound frequencies, for example, an experimenter can determine both the lowest and highest frequency that is detectable by the human ear.

Another threshold of interest to the classical psychophysicists was referred to as the difference threshold (DL). The abbreviation DL comes from the German *differenz limen* used by G.T. Fechner. A synonym for DL is the term *just noticeable difference* (or jnd). As you might imagine, the DL is defined as the amount of change in the stimulus (i.e., in physical units) necessary to produce a jnd. The method used to determine a DL or jnd necessitates the use of a standard stimulus (SS) and a comparative stimulus (CS). The SS is presented and the subject is asked whether the CS is detectably different. Since difference threshold values are considered variable, their determination is not absolute. Thus, they are identified by a method of statistical approximation. By definition, in psychophysics, a DL or jnd is that CS value that is identified 50% of the time. Obviously, many CS values must be presented several times in order for this statistical approximation to be made. In the final analysis, the DL is associated with one physical stimulus only, that is, one identified 50% of the time.

As an example of the determination of the DL, let's use a bicycle ergometer experiment. Let's assume that the SS is 150 kpm/min (kilopond-meters per minute) and that the ergometer can be accurately incremented by 5 kpm/min. A presentation schedule is arranged so that various CS values, incremented in units of 5 kpm/min, are presented following the SS in both ascending and descending order. Each time a CS is presented the subject responds by saying yes or no, that is, yes, there is a noticeable difference in load or in associated exertion, or no, there is not. Following the completion of the presentation schedule, the percentage of yes and no responses are calculated for each CS. The CS value at which the majority of the subjects respond with a yes 50% of the time is designated as the DL. Although only limited work regarding exercise has been completed using these techniques, it appears that the DL for 300, 450, and 600 kpm/min of bicycle ergometer exercise approximates 36, 45, and 55 kpm/min, respectively (Noble, Smith, and Cafarelli 1975). This means that one would not expect subjects to change their perception of exercise load unless one incremented the ergometer intensity by at least these amounts. This type of experimental study needs to be undertaken across a wider range of ergometer exercise intensities and with other exercise modes as well.

Classic Psychophysical Methods

Three methods of measurement were used by the original psychophysicists to study human perception. The first method, used primarily to determine absolute thresholds, is called the *method of limits*. When the experimenter is interested in stimulus and terminal thresholds, there is no need to use a SS. Various CS values are presented in ascending and descending order with the object of determining the stimulus that is never perceived and the one always perceived.

Another classic method is called the *method of adjustment* (average error or equation). Using this technique the subject only makes judgments of equality. After the SS is presented the CS is manipulated by the subject until it is felt to be equal to the standard. The DL can be determined by the average error between the SS and the subject's selection of the apparently equal CS.

A third classic method is the *method of constant stimuli*. This method has been used in determining both absolute thresholds (stimulus and terminal) and difference thresholds. In this method, the experimenter repeatedly presents a number of stimuli in random order. The subject is asked only to judge whether or not the stimuli is perceived, i.e., yes or no, or is perceived to be different from the SS. This method was illustrated in the bicycle ergometer example given above.

Weber's Law

E.H. Weber was concerned with the apparent incongruity that exists between the physical world and how we psychologically experience that world. In fact, he found that the physical world and psychic interpretation of that world were not identical. However, Weber believed that human perceptions followed psychological laws, which, when discovered, would provide us with a means of predicting perceptual response. (Although Weber wrote extensively about these problems he did not explicitly formulate what we now call Weber's law. G.T. Fechner, a contemporary of Weber, interpolated the law from Weber's writings.) Weber postulated that the ratio of a given physical stimulus (S) to the amount that stimulus would have to change for a subject to detect a "just noticeable difference" (S) is a constant fraction (K). In other words, the ratio of the noticeable change in a stimulus to the stimulus itself is constant.

$$\text{Weber's Law: } \frac{\Delta S}{S} = K$$

How would this law apply to exercise on a bicycle ergometer? Let's take, for example, an exercise intensity of 150 kpm/min as a physical stimulus. Suppose that we discover that an increase in intensity of 25 kpm/min is required for a subject to detect a "just noticeable difference." We then compute K by dividing 25 by 150 (K = 0.17). Therefore, given a stimulus of 300 kpm/min we can predict the jnd to be 50 to maintain a constant K = 0.17. It's easy to see that Weber's law postulates a linear relationship between the stimulus and the change in sensory response.

Fechner's Law

Fechner's studies could not confirm the linear relationship predicted by Weber's law. He proposed that the ratio is not constant but increases with the logarithm of the stimulus. In other words, the jnd increases with increases in the stimulus, but not linearly. This means that as the stimulus increases, the jnd, denoted by Fechner as the response (R), increases logarithmically.

$$\text{Fechner's Law: } S = K \log R$$

Again, an exercise example might be helpful. If we find the jnd at a physical stimulus of 150 kpm/min to be 25 kpm/min, we would not expect a ratio of 0.17 when we increased the stimulus. For example, at a stimulus of 300 kpm/min we might find the jnd to be 75 kpm/min, which would result in a ratio of 0.25. Nevertheless, because the perceptual response (R) to the change in the stimulus rose logarithmically, the SR relationship is predictable.

The methods of Weber and Fechner were the so-called *indirect methods* of psychophysics. Neither utilized a direct measurement of the response. Instead, understanding of perceptual response was interpreted from the subject's *observation* of the change in the stimulus. It was believed that direct measurement of the perception was meaningless if not impossible. As mentioned earlier, arguments over the direct observability of subjective reality date back to the earliest days of psychophysical measurement.

Modern Psychophysics: A Focus on Response

Modern psychophysics dates back to the early 1930s and is coincident with the professional career of S.S. Stevens. Stevens was primarily interested in sensory processes. "Fundamental to the new psychophysics is the view that human subjects can make meaningful evaluations of the magnitudes of their sensory experiences, at least under certain conditions" (Marks 1974). In other words, subjects can make numerical judgments of their sensory experience. Modern psychophysics, then, studies the sensory response rather than the stimulus or change in the stimulus as was the case with classical psychophysics. The work of Stevens and other modern psychophysicists utilized the so-called direct methods. With these methods the measurement comes directly from the sensation rather than by extrapolations from measurements of the physical stimulus.

In modern psychophysical studies subjects are asked to *scale* sensation. *Scaling* refers to the use of numbers to differentiate among objects or events. Within the area of perceived exertion, we are interested in scaling, or assigning numbers to, the experience of exertion during physical movement. In order to scale correctly we need to know something about the nature of the numbers we use.

Types of Scales

We live in a world of scales. We rise in the morning to the clock, which is a scale. We look at the calendar, a scale of solar transition. We look out of the kitchen window at the thermometer, another scale. We open the morning paper to see how our favorite sports team is doing; the list of standings is a scale. These and other scales can be characterized by their ability to name, differentiate, and determine the magnitude of differences and to derive ratios.

The first and least discriminating scale is the *nominal scale*. This type of scale is limited to naming things. For example, the assignment of a student number is an example of the use of a nominal scale. The number is only a substitution for a name. It provides an important naming function but no other information. It tells us that student 007 is different from student 008 but nothing else.

An *ordinal scale* names an object or event but, in addition, tells us that it has more or less of a given quantity. The process of ranking is an example of ordinal scaling. Although such a scale differentiates according to quantity, it does not discriminate the magnitude of the difference. The results of a cross-country race can be expressed in terms of who finished first, second, third, and so on, but we don't know the time differences among the finishers with such a scale. The second place finisher may have been 2 sec or 2 min behind, but ranking does not inform us of this difference in magnitude of performance.

A still more sophisticated scale is the *interval scale*. The interval scale can name and differentiate quantity just like an ordinal scale, but, in addition, it tells us the magnitude of the differences. The Fahrenheit thermometer is an example of an interval scale. The numbers can differentiate different days by maximum temperature. We know that a day with a maximum temperature of 90° F is 5 degrees F hotter than a day of 85° F. Still, we cannot say that a day in which the maximum temperature is 80° F is twice as hot as a day of 40° F. The Fahrenheit thermometer does not have an absolute zero.

Scales that have an absolute zero are called *ratio scales* because we can use the numbers derived from these scales to make ratio statements. For instance, a ruler is a ratio scale. We can say that a measurement of 8" is twice as long as a measurement of 4". This type of scale gives us a maximum of information. It names, differentiates, tells differences, and provides ratios. Thus, the development of ratio scaling techniques in psychophysics opened a new era in the measurement of human perception.

Modern Psychophysical Methods

The modern era of psychophysical measurement has been marked by the development of a number of new methods to study perception. Some of these methods will be briefly described below. Moreover, examples of how these methods might be applied to human movement problems will be provided. Those interested in using these techniques will need to seek out a text that specializes in psychophysical measurement. It is not the intention of this book to provide detailed methodological explanations of the measurement procedures but only to acquaint the readers with techniques open to them. The examples, likewise, are not exhaustive but only attempt to provide a single, simple illustration.

Method of Equal Sense Distances (Bisection)

In the method of equal sense distances, two standards are presented in counterbalanced order. The subject's task is to bisect the distance between the two standards. For example, let the subject experience two exercise intensities on a bicycle ergometer, 300 and 900 kpm/min. Then, the subject must manipulate the ergometer resistance until it feels as if it is exactly between the two standards. A number of such manipulations would yield a plot of average bisection errors (x - 600), which are expressed as a function of stimulus level. Such a protocol might be effective for determining how well subjects can produce a requested exercise intensity. This technique may have application in exercise prescription studies.

Method of Equal-Appearing Intervals

In the method of equal-appearing intervals the experimenter presents all the stimuli at once. The subject must divide the stimuli into categories. Each stimulus is judged six times. The number of categories may or may not be preset. For example, present the subject with 14 hand weights (1.0, 1.5, 2.0, 3.5, 4.0, 4.5, 6.0, 6.5, 7.0, 8.5, 9.0, 9.5, 11.0, and 11.5 lbs) with the instruction to divide them into five categories according to heaviness. The group of 14 weights is presented six separate times. Numbers are generated by calculating the mean number of times each weight was placed in each category. For example, if the 2.0 lb weight was placed in category 1 (least heavy) four times and in category 2 twice, the experimenter would sum 1 + 1 + 1 + 1 + 2 + 2= 8 and divide by 6 (number of presentations). Thus, the 2.0 lb weight would be assigned the number 1.3. This type of experiment might be used to determine how well subjects discriminate heaviness. How many ounces does a baseball bat or tennis racquet have to vary before it is discriminated as heavier? One would think that such information may be of interest to equipment manufacturers.

Method of Fractionation

In the method of fractionation the subject is presented with a standard stimulus followed by a number of comparative stimuli. The subject's task is to identify the comparative stimulus that is a given fraction, say 50%, of the standard. For example, have the subject walk on a treadmill at 4.0 mph, the standard. Next, ask the subject to walk at several speeds (1.0, 1.5, 2.0, 2.5, and 3.0 mph) in random order with the task being to identify the comparative speed that is 50% of the standard. Such experiments will answer questions concerned with how well we can identify fractions of an experienced quantity. An adaptation of this method would require the subject to produce (perform) the required fraction. Coaches often request these productions of athletes. For example, a coach may ask a swimmer to produce laps at 85% or 90% of maximum speed (a standard). A question of scientific interest asks how accurately these productions can be made without time feedback.

Method of Magnitude Estimation

In the method of magnitude estimation the subject is presented with stimuli and asked to assign a numerical value to the perceived magnitude of each stimulus. The method need not utilize a standard (free magnitude estimation) or may employ a standard or anchor stimulus with a numerical value assigned by the experimenter. With the latter method, a standard stimulus is presented to the subject and assigned an arbitrary number, for example 10. As comparative stimuli are presented in random order, the subject allocates numbers on the basis of perceived intensity or magnitude. If the CS felt as if it were three times higher than the SS, he or she would report 30. When the results of such experiments are plotted, some responses are linear, some are positively accelerating, while others are negatively accelerating. If the same material is plotted using a log-log plot, the result for all sensory dimensions is a simple linear function (See Steven's power law). According to Stevens's power law, the exponent (n) of the power function derived from these log-log plots is the slope of the regression line and can be used as a rough description of the relationship. If the exponent is greater than 1.0, the perceptual intensity grows as a positively accelerating function of the stimulus. On the other hand, an exponent below 1.0 demonstrates a negatively accelerating function. For example, figure 2.1 shows the results of a magnitude estimation experiment using bicycle ergometer exercise. Subjects were requested to estimate the perceived intensity of both arm and leg exertion during leg exercise. The standard was set at 750 kpm/min and assigned the number 10. Exercise intensities were presented in random order. The upper panel (a) of figure 2.1 indicates that the perceptual response was slightly positively accelerating using a linear plot. On the other hand, the lower panel (b) shows a linear response with a log-log plot. The stimulus exponents (1.7 and 1.2) confirm the positive acceleration for both responses and defines the slope for each function (Noble et al. 1973).

Method of Rating

In the method of rating the subject is presented with stimuli to arrange into categories. This method is among the most common scaling procedures because it is easy to apply and explain. The Borg, or RPE, scale falls into this designation. Perceptions of exertion are separated into categories according to intensity, and a number is assigned to each. At the very least, this method can be considered an example of ordinal scaling, that is, perceptual intensities are ranked. At the most, perhaps a case can be made that Borg scale data responses are interval in nature, that is, there are equal intervals between intensities 7 and 8 and between 17 and 18. Certainly, it

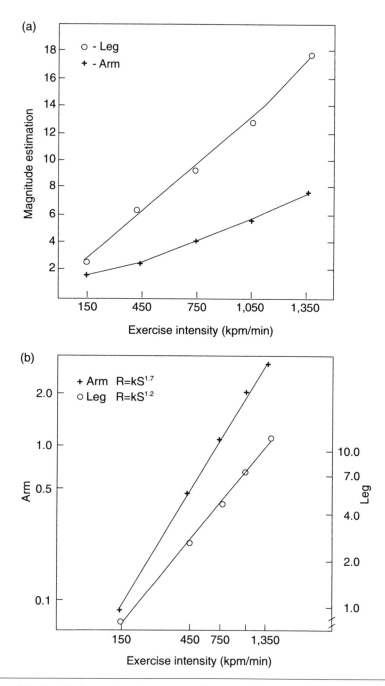

Figure 2.1   Positively accelerating perceptual response for arm and leg exercises using a (*a*) linear and (*b*) log-log plot.

cannot be said that the 15-graded Borg scale has ratio properties. This method of scaling will be discussed in more detail in the next chapter.

Method of Ranking

The method of ranking is like that of rating using ordinal data, except that it ranks categories of stimuli. The subject is presented with a series of stimuli that must be placed into categories based upon whether one stimulus is more or less intense than another. As with the method of rating, this method is popular because of its ease of application and interpretation.

Method of Paired Comparison

In the method of paired comparison the subject is presented with two stimuli at a time and is required to select the one that has the greater intensity.

Method of Cross-Modality Matching

In the method of cross-modality matching the intensity of one modality, say, handgrip force, is matched to the intensity of another modality, for example, perception of breathing resistance. An example is to request the subject to squeeze a hand dynamometer to a force that is equivalent to the intensity of the perception of breathlessness on the treadmill.

Stevens's Power Law

Although direct scaling methods began to appear in psychophysics by the late 19th century, it was not until the 1930s that these new methods became firmly established. These methods were mainly the so-called ratio methods, whereby subjects were asked to make direct, ratio judgments of sensation. For example, one might be asked to identify when a comparative stimulus doubled, halved, or reached a point three times greater than the standard stimulus. Stevens popularized the ratio method known as magnitude estimation, which proved to be useful in a variety of experimental protocols and sensory dimensions.

The earliest study using this type of scaling dealt with the perception of loudness of tones (Richardson and Ross 1930). The perception of loudness was found to grow as a power function of sound pressure. Subsequent work by Stevens (1936) as well as by others confirmed this finding. Therefore, Fechner's law was rejected. In fact, the sensation grows with the power of the stimulus, and each stimulus dimension was found to have a different power function. Since this relationship applied to more than two dozen different sensations, Stevens proposed this general power law:

$$\text{Steven's Power Law: } R = kS^n$$

where R is the magnitude of the sensation, k is a constant specifically associated
with the sensory dimension, S is the intensity of the physical stimulus, and *n* is
the exponent of the power function.

Figure 2.2 shows both the linear (a) and log-log (b) plots for seven sensory
dimensions. It can be noted that handgrip effort has an exponent *n* of 1.7.
Therefore, the sensory magnitude rises as a positively accelerating function of
the physical stimulus. It also can be noted that handgrip effort rises more acutely
than other sensory dimensions. The estimation of line length rises linearly (*n* =
1.0), while loudness is negatively accelerating (*n* = 0.67). All the sensory dimensions shown in figure 2.2 and several others comply with Stevens's power law.

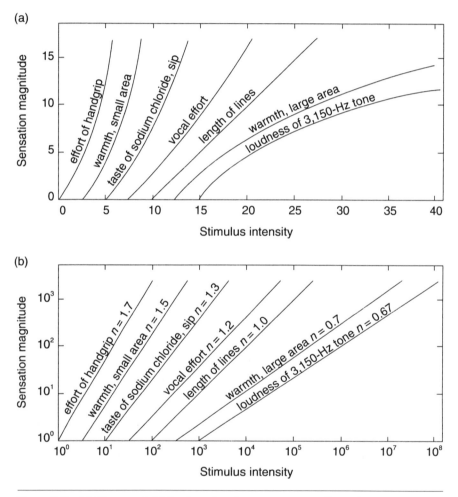

Figure 2.2   (*a*) Linear and (*b*) log-log plots for seven sensory dimensions.
Adapted from Stevens 1957.

Stevens (1957) further proposed that the power law could be extended to a general psychophysical law that states that "equal stimulus ratios produce equal sensation ratios."

The Incongruity of the Physical and Psychic Worlds

Why aren't we able to perceive the world exactly as it is presented to us physically? In other words, why do we perceive linearly presented physical stimuli in a positively or negatively accelerating fashion? If the human perceptual apparatus was a perfect system one would not expect such incongruity. In fact, it seems that perceptions are not exact imprints of the physical world.

However, if our methods for recording perceptions were more precise, response errors could be diminished. For instance, errors of *habituation* are common in psychophysical measurement. These errors occur when a subject "has made the same response a number of times in a row and continues to make that response even when it is no longer applicable" (Manning and Rosenstock 1968). The flip side of errors of habituation are the errors of *anticipation*. With this type of error the subject anticipates change when such change is not appropriate. The experimenter can minimize these two types of error by balancing the presentation of stimuli with ascending and descending trials. Another frequent error involves *time*. Time error occurs when the subject judges the second of two successively presented stimuli as either lesser (positive error) or greater (negative error) than the first. To guard against this error the experimenter must be careful to counterbalance the presentation of the standard and comparative stimuli. Counterbalancing is also important to protect against *space* error, which occurs when a subject is forced to make judgments nonpreferentially, for example, to pick up weights with a nondominant hand. Therefore, the experimenter plays an important role in reducing the degree of incongruity observed between the physical and psychic worlds. It is unlikely that the incongruity between perceptual and physical reality will ever be completely removed. It is possible that unconscious factors prevent congruity. Involvement of unconscious factors will be discussed in detail in a later chapter.

Differential Responses

Although the ratio methods are considered to be the gold standard of modern psychophysical methods, they are not entirely effective for determining perceptual differences between subjects. Since perceptual differences between subjects are a major focus of inquiry for exercise and sport scientists, magnitude estimation has not been the method of practical choice. Because of their ready application to differential human questions, rating methods, primarily the Borg scale, have been utilized almost exclusively. This is true even though rating methods such as the Borg scale do not have ratio properties. Because of its predominant use in exercise and sport science, the Borg scale will be the subject of the next chapter.

Summary

This chapter has been concerned with the psychophysical basis of the study of perception of effort. Psychophysics determines the relationship between physical stimuli and perceptual output. The laws that explain this relationship have changed several times in the past 100 years. In the 1800s, Weber postulated that the ratio of any physical stimulus (S) to the amount that stimulus would have to change for a subject to detect a just noticeable difference in its value (ΔS) is a constant. The linear relationship between the stimulus and the change in the stimulus indicated by Weber's law could not be confirmed by Fechner. He proposed that the ratio is not constant but increases with the logarithm of the stimulus. Later, the so-called modern psychophysicists, principally S.S. Stevens, found that Fechner's law did not hold across a number of sensory dimensions. Using direct methods, which provided numerical judgments of sensory responses, Stevens and others found that each sensation grows with a unique power of the stimulus. This power law has been shown to apply to more than two dozen different sensory dimensions.

The classical, indirect psychophysical techniques employed by Weber and Fechner consisted of three primary methods requiring the measurement of absolute thresholds and difference thresholds. The method of limits was used almost exclusively to measure absolute thresholds. In this method ascending and descending series of stimuli are presented to determine the stimulus never perceived and the one always perceived. With the method of adjustment the subject manipulates a comparative stimulus until it feels equal to a standard stimulus. Using the third method, constant stimuli, a given number of stimuli are repeatedly presented in random order, with subjects instructed to say whether or not the stimuli is perceived.

Modern psychophysicists have developed a number of new methods by which sensory dimensions can be measured. The most popular of these has been the ratio technique known as magnitude estimation. Utilizing this technique subjects are requested to assign a numerical value to the intensity of the perception. With this technique it is not only possible to establish equal intervals between numbers but, with the presence of an absolute zero, ratios can also be made.

References

Bartley, S.H. 1970. The homeostatic and comfort perceptual systems. *J. Psychol.* 75:157-162.

Borg, G. 1971. The perception of physical performance. In *Frontiers of fitness,* ed. R. J. Shephard, 280-94. Springfield, IL: Charles C Thomas.

Fechner, G.T. 1860. *Elemente der Psychophysik.* In D.H. Howes and E.G. Boring, eds., New York: Holt, Rinehart and Winston.

Manning, S.A., and E.H. Rosenstock. 1968. *Classical psychophysics and scaling.* New York: McGraw-Hill.

Marks, L.E. 1974. *Sensory processes: The new psychophysics.* New York: Academic Press.

Merton, P.A. 1964. Human position sense and sense of effort. *Symp. Soc. Exper. Biol.* 18:387-400.

Noble, B.J., G. Borg, E. Cafarelli,and K.F. Metz. 1973. Magnitude estimates of upper and lower body exertion during bicycle ergometry. In *18th International Congress of Applied Psychology.* Montreal, Canada.

Noble, B.J., S. Smith, and E. Cafarelli. 1975. Difference thresholds for bicycle ergometer exercise. Unpublished research.

Richardson, L.F., and J.S. Ross. 1930. Loudness and telephone current. *J. Genl. Psychol.* 3:288-306.

Sherrington, C.S. 1900. The muscular sense. In *Textbook of physiology,* ed. E.A. Schafer. Edinburgh and London: Pentland.

Stevens, S.S. 1936. A scale for the measurement of a psychological magnitude: Loudness. *Psychol. Rev.,* 43:405-16.

Stevens, S.S. 1957. On the psychophysical law. *Psychol. Rev.,* 64:153-81.

3

CHAPTER

The Borg Scale: Development, Administration, and Experimental Use

The preceding chapter presented ratio scaling methods—that is, scales that have an absolute zero and equal intervals to allow perceptions to be reported in ratios—as the gold standard of psychophysics. Despite this important measurement characteristic and the obvious advisability of employing ratio scaling when the goal is the description of general psychophysical functions, this method does not allow the possibility of making interindividual comparisons. Interindividual comparisons are the heart and soul of clinical evaluation and practice.

Gunnar Borg, trained in classic psychophysics, recognized from the beginning that the application of perceptual information to the evaluation of human performance rested not on classic or even modern psychophysical methods, but on scaling procedures that allow interindividual comparisons. To this end he even entered into a scientific debate with world famous psychophysicist S.S. Stevens (Borg 1982a).

Stevens had gone on record condemning the use of category scaling (Stevens 1971). However, Borg eloquently makes the point that magnitude estimation, for example, cannot be directly used in clinical settings when two subjects might rate a perceptual intensity as 50 and 75 but still feel the load to be ''slightly painful''; that is, the difference is in the use of numbers not in the perceptual intensity evaluated.

Thus, Borg developed a category scale in the early 1960s, now referred to as the Borg or rating of perceived exertion (RPE) scale, which continues to be used in the 1990s in both clinical and research settings.

The purposes of this chapter are twofold:

1. To trace the development of the Borg scale with emphasis on studies of its reliability and validity and on its correct administration.
2. To describe the utilization of the Borg scale within the sport and exercise science literature.

Development of the Borg Scale

The formation of a category scale is a complex process despite the apparent simplicity of the end product. This segment of the book traces Borg's deliberate attempts to develop a useful and effective scale from first generation to final form.

Assessment of Interindividual Differences

Borg's earliest publications reported results of investigations of *perceived pedal resistance* in which the ratio method called halving was utilized (Borg and Dahlstrom 1959, 1960). These studies supported earlier work by Stevens (1957), which showed that perception of muscular force followed a positively accelerating curve with an exponent of 1.7. Perhaps, the foundation for the development of Borg's category scale was established in his 1961 paper, "Interindividual Scaling and Perception of Muscular Force." Here Borg sets out his argument for the use of category scaling in the assessment of individual differences. He states that certain assumptions must be accepted for a scale to claim that it assesses individual differences:

- There is interindividual variation in the stimulus range; that is, maximal capacity varies among individuals.
- For every stimulus range there is a corresponding perceptive range.
- The intensity of an individual's perception is explicitly determined by its place in the perceptive range.
- The perceptive range may be set equal for all individuals.

This last point was considered the "main assumption." Certainly, the acceptance of this assumption is critical to the belief that a category scale can assess interindividual differences. Perhaps this point is best made by examining figure 3.1 (Borg 1961a). The figure shows hypothetical curves (O_1 and O_2) that might be observed in two separate subjects regarding the perception of weight. In this comparison the terminal threshold (S_t) is defined as the heaviest weight that can be lifted. Since subject O_2 is stronger, his or her S_t appears farther out on the stimulus continuum than the S_t for subject O_1. The terminal response (R_t), however, is set equal, because this is the point where each experiences *maximal* effort. Likewise, the stimulus threshold is set equal at $R = 0$ since one can theoretically imagine

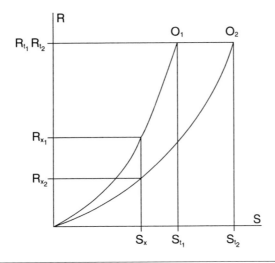

Figure 3.1   Interindividual comparison of perceptual response.
Reprinted from Borg 1961.

a weight too light for either subject to detect. As the stimulus increases, the response curves diverge according to the known psychophysical power law, and both terminate on a common R_t line. If the two subjects are compared at the same stimulus level (S_x), the resulting response should differ between individuals (R_{x_1} and R_{x_2}). The essential point remains that the perceptive range has been set equal. Thus, no matter what the physical capacities of the subjects that one wishes to compare, the range from the point at which the subjects cannot identify any response intensity to the point of maximal response intensity is equal. One might argue that the quantity of perceptual experience differs between individuals. But we must accept that, qualitatively, the perceptual ranges are equal; perceptual intensity can be set equal regardless of the experience base.

The First Category Scale

Stevens has written that category scales are partition scales that ''are created by requiring the subject to divide a segment of a continuum into parts'' (Stevens 1974). He further states that in its simplest form the category rating scale designates the categories with adjectives or by a finite set of numbers. Thus, it can be said that ''in category scaling, contiguous categories (usually numbers) are employed to mark off steps along whatever continuum is being scaled. Often, the subject is told that each step should correspond to a constant sensory interval.'' (Marks 1974).

Borg cites an unpublished 1961 manuscript, coauthored with Dahlstrom, entitled ''A Simple Rating Scale to Be Used in a Physical Work Test'' as the seminal

```
 0 –
 1 –
 2 –
 3 – Extremely light
 4 –
 5 – Very light
 6 –
 7 – Light
 8 –
 9 – Rather light
10 –
11 – Neither light nor laborious
12 –
13 – Rather laborious
14 –
15 – Laborious
16 –
17 – Very laborious
18 –
19 – Extremely laborious
20 –
```

Figure 3.2   21-graded rating scale.
Reprinted from Borg 1961.

appearance of his new scale. However, the first known use of the scale to appear in the public scientific press was later in 1961 (Borg 1961b). In this publication, the new 21-graded rating scale (fig. 3.2) was correlated with concomitantly measured pulse rate. The rating scale did not prove to be linearly related to either pulse rate or power output (S), making its validation suspect.

Heart Rate and Construction of the Scale

It is important at this point to digress for a moment to discuss two important points concerning the construction of the Borg scale. The first point concerns the use of pulse rate as a companion measure to perceived exertion. It is commonly accepted that pulse rate is a good general indicator of physical strain during exercise. Borg reasoned that a perceptual scale that produced results closely aligned with pulse rate would provide sound support for perceived exertion as a subjective indicator of physical strain. Likewise, a close linear association with pulse rate, as it increases with increasing power output, tends to substantiate the contention that Borg's scale is a category rating scale with interval properties (see earlier discussion). Although both types of scales use categories anchored with numbers, adjectives, or both, only the category scale can be considered to

```
 6 –
 7 – Very, very light
 8 –
 9 – Very light
10 –
11 – Fairly light
12 –
13 – Somewhat hard
14 –
15 – Hard
16 –
17 – Very hard
18 –
19 – Very, very hard
20 –
```

Figure 3.3   15-graded rating scale.
Reprinted from Borg 1971.

be an equal interval scale (Gamberale 1985). In fact, Borg constructed a 21-graded scale with the clear intent not only to closely align perceived exertion with pulse rate but, indeed, so that "the heart rate of a normal, healthy middle-aged man can be predicted if the RPE value is multiplied by 10; thus, RPE × 10 = HR" (Borg 1971).

Since the 21-graded scale was not linear with pulse rate, Borg designed a new 15-graded scale (fig. 3.3). He states, "In order to increase the linearity of the relationship between RPE values and work load and between RPE values and heart rates and at the same time to adjust the ratio of RPE values to heart rates, some modifications of the twenty-one-point scale were made" (Borg 1971). The scale is presented in quarto format which means it is "book size" of about 9 1/2 by 12 inches (Borg 1971). Many studies have subsequently confirmed the linear relationship between RPE and pulse rate using the 15-graded scale, even though the aforementioned prediction equation has not proven accurate.

Quantitative Semantics

How is a scale constructed so that perceptual ratings are linear with pulse rate and power output? This question brings us to the second point of concern regarding scale construction. The perceptual response is dependent on both the number of categories and the verbal definitions used to anchor each category (Gamberale 1985). Gamberale maintains that Borg was able to achieve linearity "by a careful choice of verbal categories" (Gamberale 1985). Undoubtedly, the reduction of categories from 21 to 15 also played a role. Let's take a closer look at the selection of verbal expressions.

Borg has made a little-known but major contribution to psychophysical measurement by the incorporation of the principles of quantitative semantics to scale development. Quantitative semantics is the science that deals with the meaning of words and the quantitative relationship between verbal expressions. Borg chose terms for the scale that were not only well defined but had a comparatively constant meaning between subjects (Borg 1962). He states, "If I want to construct a scale over the whole range of intensities, I can use the meaning of adjectives and adverbs and put them in the right place on a scale according to the meaning of the expressions" (Borg 1978).

Let's take an example from the continuum found in figure 3.4. In this case just five response categories are used. These categories span the continuum of physical sensation in a manner that might be used in a Likert scale. (For example, a 5-graded questionnaire scale that goes from *least acceptable*, "1", to *most acceptable*, "5".) "For ease in reporting and mathematical manipulation of the data, the categories are assigned a number according to semantic intensity from low to high (1 to 5)" (Maresh and Noble 1984). When Borg designed his category scales he selected "only well-defined terms with a comparatively good intersubjective, constant meaning" (Borg 1962). He further states,

> "When I adjust the efforts to a level that feels 'very light', 'rather strong' or 'very strong', I can do this with good precision knowing that there is a perfect rank order between these levels of intensity. Studies we have performed in quantitative semantics show that there are good possibilities to choose words that have about the same meaning among people according to the perceptual intensities 'behind' the words. This can be done according to the mean values of peoples' subjective ratings and the relative standard deviations (indicating the degree of preciseness of the words). If we, for instance, use words like 'very weak,' 'rather weak,' 'moderate' and 'somewhat strong' we know that these expressions do not only follow a rank order but also that the subjective interval between the expressions is fairly constant (Borg and Lindblad 1976)."

"The category scale that we in this way can construct is enough to satisfy the demands of an interval scale" (Borg 1978). This, of course, represents Borg's argument that his scale is a category scale; that is, the scale does not merely rank sensation categories but also satisfies the equal interval criterion.

No noticeable sensation	Light sensation	Moderate sensation	Strong sensation	Maximum sensation
1	2	3	4	5

Figure 3.4   Continuum of verbal expressions based on semantic intensity.
Reprinted from Maresh and Noble 1984.

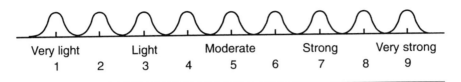

| Very light | | Light | | Moderate | | Strong | | Very strong |
| 1 | 2 | 3 | 4 | 5 | 6 | 7 | 8 | 9 |

Figure 3.5   Quantification of verbal expressions.

The way Borg worked with quantitative semantics is illustrated in figure 3.5. A number of words are selected and administered to a representative group of subjects who rate the intensity of each word's meaning. In so doing, each expression receives a mean score with a corresponding standard deviation. Thus, expressions can be selected that do not overlap others and represent equal quantitative intervals. In other words, the difference between "very light" and "light" and between "strong" and "very strong" represent equal semantic distances. Since the normal curves depicting the dispersion of intensity ratings for each expression do not overlap one another, it should not be possible for subjects to confuse the meaning of the expressions or, therefore, the intensity implied. The expressions, originally developed in Swedish, were cross-validated for possible cultural differences in English meaning during Borg's visit to the University of Pittsburgh in 1967 (Borg 1971). No differences were observed.

Thus, when Borg found that his 21-graded scale was curvilinear with heart rate and work load, he adjusted the numbers and nature of the expressions to achieve the desired linearity. The term "extremely light," 3 on the 21 scale, was changed to "very, very light," 7 on the 15 scale. "Rather light" and "neither light nor laborious," 9 and 11 on the old scale, both rather ambiguous terms, were altered to "fairly light" and "somewhat hard," 11 and 13 on the new scale. A major change, which probably contributed greatly to the move to increased linearity, was the change from the neutral term "neither light nor laborious" to the more assertive term "somewhat hard." This change also eliminated the bipolar nature of the scale.

The 21-Graded Scale

It is now appropriate to discuss the early experiments with the 21-graded scale in more detail. Figure 3.6 shows the results of Borg's earliest reported use of the 21-graded scale (Borg 1961b). He observed the growth of pulse rate and perceptual ratings as a function of power output (kpm/min). A sample of 12 medical students pedaled a bicycle ergometer for 6 min at each of five exercise stages: 100, 300, 600, 900, and 1,200 kpm/min. It can be seen that while pulse rate grows linearly with power output, perception showed a negative acceleration with power. The test-retest reliability computed in this experiment was .91. Although Borg stated that the agreement between the ratings and pulse rate in

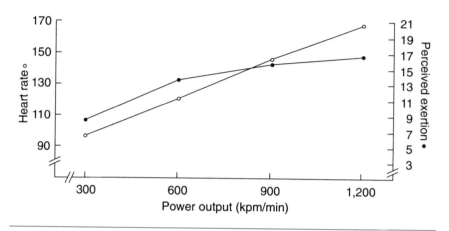

Figure 3.6   Heart rate–perceived exertion relationship on the 21-graded scale.

this experiment was "good," the ratings, in fact, did not grow linearly with
pulse rate or power output.

Similar data were collected on school children in 1959-60 but were not reported
until later (Borg and Dahlstrom 1962). This experiment was conducted in conjunction with P.O. Åstrand, who was testing the work capacity of school children
throughout Sweden. Again, the purpose was to examine the relationship between
the perceptual ratings and pulse rate using the 21-graded scale. In this study of
28 children, aged 14 and 15, the ratings were linearly related to both pulse rate
and power output. This result most likely encouraged Borg to use the scale in
the experiment with medical students previously described.

It is interesting to note that the 21-graded scale appears in Borg's publications
as late as 1970 (Borg and Linderholm 1970), despite the earlier recognition that
the perceptual ratings, in at least one sample, did not grow linearly with heart
rate and power output. In 1967, Borg and Linderholm reported the results of
their studies of the influence of age on perception of exertion (Borg and Linderholm 1967). In fact, the results indicated that perception was linear with heart
rate and power output in a group of 61 male lumber workers, as well as in several
other groups of males aged 18 to 20, 20 to 29, 30 to 39, 40 to 49, 50 to 59, 60
to 69, and 70 to 79 years. As others have shown, heart rate declined with age
at all power outputs. On the contrary, perceptual ratings either remained about
the same or increased with age. However, at given levels of perceived exertion,
heart rate declined with age. For example, 60-year-old men rated exercise as 17
on the Borg scale at a lower heart rate (e.g., 150) than 30-year-old men (e.g.,
180). When heart rate was plotted as a function of the ratings, a family of positive
linear responses were observed, with the younger groups selecting given ratings
at higher heart rates. This research indicated that perception of exertion was
responsive to the decline in maximal heart rate that occurs with increasing age.

Failure to be explicit about the incongruity of findings concerning the linearity of the 21-graded scale has led to some confusion among researchers and practitioners. Even now, some 25 years after the evolution to the new 15-graded scale, occasional use of the 21-graded scale is noted in scientific papers and clinical sites. Until such time as the 21-graded scale is shown to be as consistently linear as the 15-graded scale, a moratorium should be declared on its use and its corpus delicti reverently but appropriately buried. This is not to say that the 15-graded scale is the only measurement tool available. In fact, there are several scales and psychophysical techniques that might be used, depending on the purpose of the experiment or clinical application.

The 15-Graded Scale

The 15-graded scale is now referred to as the Borg scale or the RPE scale. As previously mentioned, it was developed to solve the problem of nonlinearity between perceptual ratings and both heart rate and power output observed with the 21-graded scale, even though this finding was not universally reported. Borg constructed the new scale in a very creative way. In addition to using sound principles of quantitative semantics, he decided that, if the scale was to be set linearly with heart rate, the scale numbers should be arranged to conform to the absolute heart rate quantities. He surmised that, since heart rate ranged from approximately 60 to 200 in a healthy group of young subjects, using digits aligned with these numbers might facilitate the prediction of heart rate from the RPE ratings (HR = RPE × 10). Although the prediction has long since been proven inadequate in a number of situations involving differing subjects, exercise modes, and environmental conditions, the scale numbers, 6 to 20, thought to be confusing by some, remain intact and quite functional. (Borg [1982b] has said that the prediction equation "was not intended to be taken too literally" because heart rate is effected by "age, type of exercise, environment, anxiety, and other factors.") Since heart rate can be considered an interval scale, from resting to maximum, and perceptual ratings are linear with heart rate, we might say that this relationship supports the contention that the Borg scale is a category scale because of its interval properties. In addition, as we mentioned earlier, the quantitative semantic basis of the category expressions also supports this contention.

The change to a 15-graded scale resulted in the linear relationship shown in figure 3.7 (Borg 1971). Correlations between heart rate and RPE, using the data from all exercise intensities of a graded exercise test, were .94 and .85 for tests on the bicycle ergometer and treadmill, respectively. Correlations at any one exercise intensity are usually found to be much lower. At any one intensity the variability of heart rates is usually greater than that of the perceptual ratings. Since there was no significant difference between the two correlations reported above, it was suggested that perceptual ratings may be independent of exercise mode. Later research, particularly with the use of the so-called differentiated

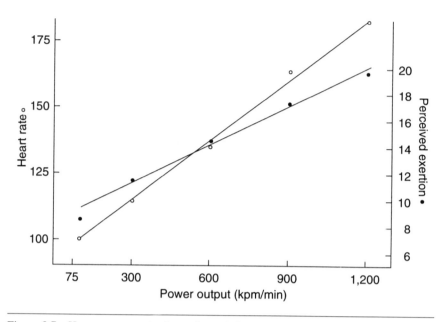

Figure 3.7   Heart rate–perceived exertion relationship using the 15-graded scale.
Reprinted from Borg 1971.

ratings, supports the opposite view, that is, that perceptions are dependent on
mode (Noble et al. 1986).

Category Scale or Rating Scale?

Whether the Borg scale is a category or rating scale is a somewhat esoteric
scientific question. It does address an important measurement issue that has been
confused from time to time. In fact, some of Borg's early work refers to his
scale as a rating scale (Borg 1961b), while only later is the term category scale
used (Borg 1973a). Gamberale (1985) has categorized the Borg scale as a rating
scale because, according to him, it does not meet the assumption of equal intervals
between categories (Gamberale 1985). Therefore, he would classify data received
from the Borg scale as ordinal rather than interval. As stated earlier, Borg said
in 1978 that the scale he constructed satisfied the demands of an interval scale
and, therefore, can be called a category scale (Borg 1978). The arguments that
favor classification as a category scale involve the development of the scale to
be linear with heart rate and the selection of category expressions based upon
quantitative semantics. Arguments that favor designation as a rating scale question
the preciseness of heart rate and adjective/adverb choice as a determinant of true
equal intervals on the scale. We believe that enough evidence exists to accept

the assumptions necessary to classify the Borg scale as a category scale. This topic could be the source of scholarly argument for some time, however.

Validity and Reliability

Establishment of validity and reliability is critical to the accepted scientific use of any measurement tool. It was particularly important in the case of measurement of effort perceptions. In the late 1960s, when the field of exercise and sport science was just gathering momentum, investigators were sensitive about measurements that might taint the quantitative image so important to its growth. Scientists, nurtured with a profound respect for the centimeter-gram-second system, still have a difficult time accepting the viability of a measurement derived from such a complex and unpredictable source as the human mind. To their credit, most exercise and sport scientists realize the complexity of human performance and the need for a multidisciplinary approach to performance problems. Still, the need for passing rigorous tests of validity and reliability faced those interested in the measurement of effort perceptions.

Thanks to the early efforts of James Skinner and his colleagues at Penn State, the first major effort to demonstrate the validity and reliability of the Borg scale was accomplished (Skinner et al. 1973). Validity was tested by having 16 male subjects ride a bicycle ergometer using two protocols. In one protocol they exercised through a series of power outputs presented progressively, from low to high intensity, in a manner we have come to accept as the standard procedure for a graded exercise test. The second protocol involved presenting the same power outputs in random order but with an intermittent administration. In the random order protocol the subjects exercised for 4 min at each exercise stage so that a steady-state response could be achieved. Then they rested for 8 min before the next power output was presented. This steady-state point is an extremely important detail. Just as we need to demonstrate steady state with heart rate or oxygen consumption at a given exercise intensity to ensure that we haven't measured a transient response, the same criterion is essential for perceptual responses. One can imagine a transience in perceptual intensity from the beginning of a stage until the achievement of metabolic steady state. In this investigation, the scale would be considered valid if the subject's perceptual ratings were not significantly different between the two protocols. That is to say, the scale would be valid in that subjects were not simply sensing the progressive change in power output and rating accordingly. Although power output may be involved, the subject must discriminate between the presentations presumably by rating changes in effort associated with changes in power output. There were no significant differences between the perceptual ratings recorded in the progressive and in the random protocols. Thus, the 15-graded scale was considered a valid assessment of perceptual response.

Reliability, on the other hand, was to be determined using a test-retest protocol. Reliability coefficients for the progressive and random tests were .80 and .78, respectively. This indicates that the variance accounted for in each case is 64% and 61%. With close to 40% of variance unexplained, one might challenge the reliability in this experiment. This criticism must certainly be accepted. Perspective can be achieved, however, by examining the reliability of heart rate under the same conditions. The coefficients were .87 and .91 for the progressive and the random protocols, respectively. In this case the accounted for variance is 76% and 83%. Even in the case of heart rate approximately 20% of the variance is unexplained. These results encouraged the continued use of the 15-graded scale.

In 1976, Bryant Stamford completed another assessment of the validity and reliability of the Borg scale. In this experiment, 14 female subjects completed bicycle ergometer tests arranged in progressive and oscillating (random) order similar to the procedure used by Skinner et al. (1973) just discussed. In addition, Stamford utilized 23 min of treadmill walking at a submaximal intensity, as well as tests involving stool stepping. Reliability coefficients, when ratings were requested at the end of a work test, were .90 for the progressive bicycle test, .71 for the oscillating test, .76 for stool stepping exercise, and .76 for the submaximal treadmill walking task. Although the coefficients were generally slightly lower than Skinner et al., the .90 for the progressive test is remarkable. Again, while not high, the reliability of the 15-graded scale is considered to be quite acceptable.

Validity was assessed in the Stamford study by examination of HR-RPE plots. Heart rate, an objective estimate of metabolic strain, was used as the criterion measure. While there was high interindividual variability in the HR-RPE coordinates at a given power output in the progressive test, the relationship was found to be linear. With regard to the oscillating and submaximal tasks a "close relationship between HR and RPE" was observed.

A more objective assessment of validity based on the HR-RPE relationship has been reported by Gamberale (1972). Using all the data of a progressive exercise test on the bicycle ergometer, a correlation of .94 was reported. Such a high relationship certainly supports the validity of the Borg scale.

Hogan and his collaborators (1980) at the Advanced Research Resources Organization examined the reliability and validity of perceived effort while performing various occupational tasks (Hogan, Ogden, Gebhardt, and Fleishman 1980). The Borg scale was not used but the results are relevant because they did use a 7-point category scale. The energy expenditure in 24 manual materials-handling tasks was directly measured, and perceived effort ratings were simultaneously requested from each subject. Intraclass correlations were computed to determine rater agreement, and the resulting reliability coefficient revealed a value of .83. The criterion measure for validity in this experiment was, of course, the actual measured energy expenditure of the task. The validity coefficient was computed to be .88. In a related study, Hogan and Fleishman (1979) reported a correlation of .83 between effort ratings and energy expenditure of 41 recreational activities (Hogan and Fleishman 1979). These studies lend support to the contention that the utilization of a category scale to measure perceived effort is both reliable and valid. The plasticity of reliability and validity from one condition or mode of exercise to another necessitates continuous experimental replication to be absolutely sure of the soundness of reported data and clinical diagnoses.

Borg's Category-Ratio Scale

It became clear to Borg, and others of us working in the field of perceived exertion, that the 15-graded scale may not always be appropriate for studies involving the sensation of certain physiological variables. Of particular concern were lactate accumulation and pulmonary ventilation. Unlike many other physiological variables studied in exercise physiology, these variables do not grow linearly with power output. Instead they increase in a positively accelerating fashion. (Some would argue that, in fact, lactate grows linearly after a relative plateau response, but certainly the response is not linear throughout the full range of power outputs.) Thus, if we are to understand the degree to which we perceive sensations associated with anaerobiosis, we must have a scale that grows like the physiological response.

Borg's first attempt to develop a category scale with ratio properties was prompted by more theoretical concerns (Borg 1973b). He wanted to develop a scale that satisfied the psychophysical requisites of ratio scaling but, at the same time, was capable of eliciting interindividual comparisons. At first a 20-graded scale (0-20) was developed (fig. 3.8). To do so, he combined quantitative semantics, the subjective intensity of expressions, with the known psychophysical properties of muscular effort (i.e., an exponent of 1.6). In his own words, the "knowledge of the physical intensities 'behind' the various verbal expressions has been used together with the knowledge of the general psychophysical function to identify the perceptual intensities for the expressions in question." Note that sensations of "light" effort can be scaled only in the first 25% of the categories, with the remaining 75% used for "somewhat hard" to "maximal exertion." With such a scale, perception of effort through about 50% of physiological effort is relegated to the smaller numbers, while the numbers rise more rapidly as soon as the sensations begin to be perceived as "somewhat hard." "Somewhat hard" on the 15-graded scale is 13, which is the midpoint (50th percentile) of the scale. Results of the early experiments with this method indicated "that the new category scale functioned fairly well as a ratio scale" but "that some slight changes of the scale are necessary to get it to come closer to an ordinary ratio scale" (Borg 1982a).

The next appearance of a category scale with ratio properties was in Borg's presentation at the International Congress of Applied Psychology at Leipzig in 1981. In his paper Borg (1982a) again took up the argument that standard ratio-scaling methods were incapable of producing interindividual comparisons so important to clinical evaluation (Borg 1982b). By this time, a revised scale, known as the CR-10 scale, had been developed that not only improved upon the inadequacies of the first attempt but met the criterion of being "a very simple scale" (fig. 3.9). To accomplish the simplicity the number of categories was

Perceived Exertion

```
 0 – Absolutely no feeling
       at all of exertion
 1 –
 2 – Very light
 3 –
 4 –
 5 –
 6 – Somewhat hard
 7 –
 8 –
 9 –
10 – Hard
11 –
12 –
13 –
14 – Very hard
15 –
16 –
17 –
18 – Very, very hard
19 –
20 – Maximal exertion
```

Figure 3.8   Borg's initial category-ratio scale.
Reprinted from Borg 1973.

```
 0   – Nothing at all
 0.5 – Extremely weak (just noticeable)
 1   – Very weak
 2   – Weak (light)
 3   – Moderate
 4   – Somewhat strong
 5   – Strong (heavy)
 6   –
 7   – Very strong
 8   –
 9   –
10   – Extremely strong (almost max)
 •   – Maximal
```

Figure 3.9   Borg's new category-ratio (CR-10) scale.
Reprinted from Borg 1982.

compressed to 12, including 0 for "nothing at all" and 0.5 for "extremely weak (just noticeable)." In addition to these changes the terms were changed from "light" and "hard" to "weak" and "strong." Pilot work indicated that there was still a ceiling effect, noted in the earlier scale; that is, subjects failed to use the top of the scale (10). Therefore, the term "maximal" was placed outside the scale, which the subject could use by freely assigning any number as in magnitude estimation. Empirical results showed that the new scale produced data that grew with an exponent of 1.6 and substantiated its ratio properties. Ratings from this scale were correlated with simultaneously recorded heart rate, resulting in a coefficient of .88. Borg concluded that "the simplicity of the scale should make it applicable in many different kinds of situations where estimates of subjective intensities are needed."

Noble et al. (1983) studied the relationship between category-ratio scale ratings and lactic acid accumulation (blood and muscle), as well as heart rate (Noble et al. 1983). It was hypothesized that, since lactate values rose in a positively accelerating fashion with power output, a scale devised to rise in a similar fashion should show parallel responses. Likewise, since heart rate grows linearly with power output, the responses should not be parallel. Perceptual ratings and blood lactate both increased with a similar quadratic (square) trend. Muscle lactate showed a cubic trend. One might expect a difference in response between blood and muscle lactate because of the need to maintain a gradient between the muscle and blood. Heart rate, as expected, showed a linear trend. The new category-ratio scale proved to be an efficient means of monitoring sensations associated with curveilinear physiological responses like lactate production. Presumably, such a result would also be found for pulmonary ventilation, although it has not yet been reported in the literature. The 15-graded scale might better be used when a direct relation with power output or physiological variables is desired.

Other Category Scales for Monitoring Perceived Effort

Psychophysical theory indicates that 7 to 10 categories within a scale is just as, if not more, satisfactory as many more categories. Likewise, it is believed that placement of maximal and minimal expressions is all that is necessary for a successful category scale. Therefore, in the early 1970s, the authors in consultation with psychologist Donald McBurney at the University of Pittsburgh, designed a 9-graded scale for use in measuring effort perceptions. This scale appears in figure 3.10. Note that the terminal expressions have been placed at 2 and 8 on the scale. This was done intentionally. So-called end effects are characteristic of category scales. That is to say, subjects tend to use the middle of the scale rather than the ends. When the absolute ends of the scale are not anchored with an expression, it makes it more likely that the terminal expressions will be used. An additional justification for the added numbers beyond the terminal expressions is that it is very possible that subjects can experience sensations greater than what they thought to be "maximal exertion" and less than they thought to be

```
1 –
2 – Not at all stressful
3 –
4 –
5 –
6 –
7 –
8 – Very, very stressful
9 –
```

Figure 3.10   9-graded scale.

```
1 – Very, very light
2 –
3 –
4 – Somewhat hard
5 –
6 –
7 – Very, very hard
```

Figure 3.11   7-graded scale.
Reprinted from Hogan and Fleishman 1979.

"no exertion at all'' (Maresh and Noble 1984). The additional number provides for flexibility within the scale. This scale proved to be both reliable and linear with heart rate and power output (Stamford and Noble 1974; Robertson et al. 1979).

Others have used similar scales for monitoring perceived effort. Hogan and Fleishman (1979) developed a 7-graded scale (fig. 3.11) for use in ergonomics research. "This scale is a direct conversion of the RPE scale, with the 7 anchors remaining identical but the numerical intervals reduced by half and beginning with '1' instead of '6.' '' This scale has proven to be a reliable measurement tool in occupational settings.

Borg (1973b) undertook the study of the comparative value of the various category scales developed by himself as well as by others. Correlation coefficients were computed between various scale ratings during two types of maximal tests. In one test, subjects rode the bicycle ergometer to exhaustion at a single power output (1,400 kpm/min). In the other, power output was varied every 6 min (300 kpm/min). Four scales were utilized: 21-graded scale, 15-graded scale, 9-graded scale (as discussed previously), and a line scale. In the case of the line scale (fig. 3.12), an 11-cm line marked on one end by "no exertion at all'' and, on the other, by "maximal exertion'' was marked by a pencil to indicate the degree to which the subject's exertion had progressed from "no exertion at all.'' In the single load maximal test, the correlations between the 21-graded scale and the

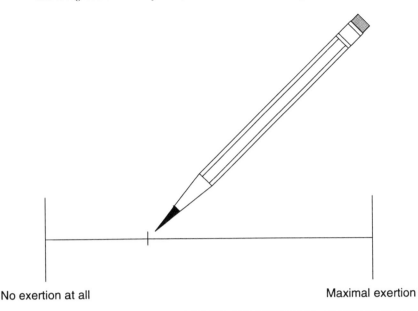

No exertion at all   Maximal exertion

Figure 3.12   Line scale with pencil mark reflecting how far the subject's exertion had progressed from "no exertion at all."

line scale and between the 21-graded scale and the 9-graded scale were .93 and .92, respectively. The same correlations were .83 and .92 during the graded exercise test. Each scale was also intercorrelated with heart rate. The 21-graded scale and 15-graded scale tended to be a little more highly correlated with heart rate. Borg's conclusion was that, since the correlations between rating scales were so high, the other scales were not contributing uniquely to the measurement of perceived exertion. In addition, since the correlations with heart rate were a little higher, Borg (1973b) proposed "that we use this scale [15-graded] in most cases." It might also be argued that these data support the use of the other scales in the study and application of perceived exertion.

Related Category Scales

It would be impossible to discuss all of the category scales that might be used in exercise and sport science. However, a few such scales have been used often enough as companion measurement tools to the Borg scale that they are worthy of mention. Figure 3.13 illustrates scales used with angina patients (angina scale), with chronic obstructive pulmonary disease patients (dyspnea scale) and for environmental studies (thermal and comfort scales) (American College of Sports Medicine 1986; Gagge, Stolwijk, and Hardy 1967). It is known that patients can distinguish between sensations arising from exercise and those that arise from

Angina scale

1+ Light, barely noticeable
2+ Moderate, bothersome
3+ Severe, very uncomfortable
4+ Most severe pain ever experienced in the past

Dyspnea scale

1 Mild—noticeable to patient—not to observer
2 Some difficulty—noticeable to observer
3 Moderate difficulty—but can continue
4 Severe difficulty—patient cannot continue

Thermal sensation

1 Cold
2 Cool
3 Slightly cool
4 Neutral
5 Slightly warm
6 Warm
7 Hot

Comfortable sensation

1 Comfortable
2 Slightly uncomfortable
3 Uncomfortable
4 Very comfortable

Figure 3.13   Related category scales.
Angina and dyspnea scales reprinted from American College of Sports Medicine 1986. Thermal and comfort scales reprinted from Gagge, Stolwijk, and Hardy 1967.

disease processes or the environment (Noble 1982; Pandolf et al. 1972). Therefore, it is a common practice in both clinical and experimental environments to present multiple scales for the assessment of a concert of sensations that might present themselves.

Which Scale to Use?

Perhaps the most asked question in recent years regarding the measurement of perceived exertion has been, Which scale do I use? The development of the new Borg scale (CR-10), in some ways has created more confusion than enlightenment. It is time that this question be directly addressed and the confusion dispelled. Borg himself (1982a) stated, ''the simplicity of the scale should make it applicable in many different kinds of situations where estimates of subjective intensities are needed.'' However, the fact remains that, during a graded exercise test, perceived exertion data using the category-ratio scale are positively accelerating. This nonlinearity does not invalidate the scale by any means, but it does make the data less useful in most practical settings. Indeed, the 15-graded scale has been received with such universality because of its linearity and, therefore, its ease of use. Some complain that the lack of equal distances between categories in the CR-10 scale and the use of the terms ''weak'' and ''strong'' are confusing to patients. On the other hand, the category-ratio scale can be very useful in certain experimental projects where ratio data is required or where the goal is to assess sensations related to pulmonary ventilation or lactate accumulation.

The study of human perception during exercise and sport has grown tremendously in the past 25 years. Much of this growth can be attributed to the experimental and practical attractiveness of Borg's 15-graded scale. However, just as exercise testing should not be limited to the Bruce protocol or the measurement of heart rate should not be restricted to the stethoscope, the measurement of perception should not be confined to the Borg scale. Future growth of this field will be a direct function of the creativity of investigators and practitioners as they seek to improve their ability to understand how humans perceive effort. This will entail the development of new measurement tools, the incorporation of little-used but already developed psychophysical methods, and the continued use and perfection of currently popular scales. An example of an innovative measurement of effort can be found in the work of Cafarelli and Bigland-Ritchie (1979). In this investigation a potentiometer linked to a digital display was used to measure effort sense.

Science has never grown without the refinement of its methods of measurement. We must be explicit and caution against throwing the baby out with the bathwater. The Borg scale has served us very well, as has the category-ratio scale for its purpose. These scales will be used effectively for many years to come. However, to progress we must always look to the development of new, more precise measurement instruments. The ultimate questions should always be: What is the goal of the measurement? How can I best measure perception? And, the corollary question: Can I develop a new technique, or is there a technique already developed, that can measure perception better?

Borg Scale Administration

The Borg scale has proven so handy and efficient that it is very easy to forget that established principles of administration must be followed. Of the several important points related to administration of the Borg scale, none is more important than the instructions provided to the patient, subject, or client.

Scale Instructions

We have observed some practitioner's instructions to consist only of ''This is a scale to tell us how you feel during exercise. When we ask you for a rating please pick a number." The fact that the scale is simple to understand makes it very "user friendly," but the example above may be better classified as user abuse. Following are six points that should be satisfied for adequate pretest or preexercise instruction (Maresh and Noble 1984).

1. **Define perceived exertion**. Perceived exertion can be defined as a method to determine the intensity of effort, stress, or discomfort that is felt during exercise. Ask the person to imagine walking from a slow pace to a very fast pace or from a low grade to a steep grade in gradual stages. Indicate that as the speed or grade is increased the body experiences a change in sensation that provides information that effort is increasing. Maresh and Noble believe that, as a general rule, those receiving instruction should be asked to attend to the physiological cues they experience from the physical effort expended. This is usually the relevant information one wishes to receive during both testing and training. That is to say, subjects should be instructed to monitor changes in physiological responses such as, for example, pulmonary ventilation.

2. **Anchor the perceptual range**. It is important to provide the subject or client with an understanding of the range of sensations that correspond to the scale you will be presenting to them. What is meant by 7 (very, very light)? What is meant by 19 (very, very strong)? Understanding the meaning of these near-extremes provides a context by which sensation intensities can be evaluated. One approach to anchoring the scale involves asking the client to try to remember the range of feelings previously experienced during similar exercise. For example, help them to recreate the easiest and most difficult exercise they have ever experienced. Based upon this re-creation, 7 and 19 on the scale can be anchored.

The scale can also be anchored by definition. Depending on your experimental or clinical goal, number 7 on the Borg scale can be anchored with a definition of rest (no exertion at all) or as the lowest exertion imaginable. In the former case, 7 is interpreted as the absence of effort, that is, a relative zero point. In the latter case, 7 would be more like a threshold of exertional perception. The point 19 on the scale is often anchored by explaining to the client that choice of this number should be reserved for feelings of maximal effort or the greatest effort imaginable. One may wish to describe 19 with an explanation of relative maximum, that is to say, maximum for the type of exercise the client is about to perform. One can imagine similar but distinctly different sensations associated with maximal effort while sprinting compared with performing technical maneuvers on the side of a mountain. One Wisconsin physician differentiates the instruction for 20 between farm and city patients prior to exercise testing. For the farmer he explains 20 as "the work that would be involved in chasing your prize dairy cow across the pasture and having to let it go because you just can't keep going." The city patient is instructed that 20 is "the work necessary to get to your house if it were on fire, but so much work that you just give up and say, 'Let it burn!'."

Anchors can be experienced rather than defined. The following protocol is designed to allow experimental subjects or clients to feel the two anchors of the scale during a cycling test. In fact, the anchor numbers are *assigned to* the sensations experienced while exercising at a very low level (7) and at a maximal level (19). (Prior to the actual test, explain that a rating of 6 should be assigned to any feelings of exertion that are less than those experienced while exercising at the extremely light intensity and a rating of 20 should be assigned to any feelings of exertion that are greater than those experienced during the extremely high exercise intensity.)

  a. Low anchor: "In order to acquaint you with the feelings of exertion that should be rated 7, we would like you to cycle at an extremely light intensity (0 kp, 50 rpm) for 3 min."
      i. Explain the anchoring test protocol. Begin the test. The scale should be in full view of the subject.
      ii. From 40 to 60 s of minutes 1 and 2 say: "Think about your feelings of exertion."
      iii. From 40 to 60 s of minute 3 say: "Think about your feelings of exertion and assign a rating of 7 to those sensations."
  b. High anchor: "In order to acquaint you with the feelings of exertion that should be rated 19, we would like you to cycle at an extremely high exercise intensity (set according to fitness level) until you reach exhaustion."
      i. Explain the anchoring test protocol. Begin the test. The scale should be in full view of the subject.
      ii. Beginning when the heart rate reaches 85% of age-related maximum, read the following instructions from 40 to 60 s of each minute until exhaustion: "When your feelings of exertion reach maximal intensity assign a rating of 19 to those sensations."

3. **Explain the nature and use of the scale.** Explain that when a response is requested, the patient should provide a number from the scale. They should imagine that each number from 6 through 20 represents a category of sensation ordered according to intensity. For example, the number 7 should be reported when the definition of category 6 is no longer met and the intensity has grown to the next possible level. The adjective-adverbial expressions are to be viewed as an aid to the selection of numbers. Words are known to show intensity as well as numbers. For example, the word *hard* represents an intensity that exceeds *light* and is less than *very hard*.

4. **Explain differentiated ratings.** Since the mid-1970s, differentiated ratings have become common in research, testing, and training. Differentiated ratings are specific to an anatomical area or sensation and distinguished from undifferentiated ratings, which are a gestalt of the overall sensation quality of the body (Pandolf 1982). Differentiated ratings have been used to segregate upper body sensations from lower body sensations during leg exercise. In this example, the goal is to have the subject provide sensation quantities from such consciously perceived qualities as ventilatory volume and respiratory rate as distinct from those cues arising from the working muscles themselves. It may be better to

name the source of the sensation more exactly such as cardiorespiratory or muscle discomfort, but a too finely graded specificity may select out a sensation that is of critical concern. For instance, muscle discomfort might exclude the sensation of joint discomfort. Some have used the terms *central* and *local* to differentiate between the qualities sought. Recently, research attempting to discover the physiological precursors for differentiated ratings has shown a preference for the terms *respiratory-metabolic* and *peripheral* signals. Word selection notwithstanding, instructions should include a clear explanation of what one is seeking if one asks an individual to differentiate their ratings.

5. **Correctness of perceptual responses**. In the mechanistic Western world we are inclined to accept those tangible qualities that can be documented by the centimeter-gram-second system as real, with qualities less quantifiable considered "unreal." Of course, we know that quantifiability does not dictate reality but only makes its documentation more accessible. Another tendency of our mechanistic world, especially reinforced by our educational system, is the need to be "right." When asked to provide a perception, people tend to want to be right. This assumes that there is a "right" and "wrong" perception. Since perceptions fall in the category of those things that are difficult to measure, perhaps even "unreal," the search for a right answer is a difficult one. In fact, as Borg (1970) has pointed out, "man reacts to the world as he perceives it and not as it 'really is'." We might say that, more often than not, as we carry on our daily routines we are governed by our perceptions and never question their validity. For example, we speed up and slow down based on how we feel without thinking about it or judging whether it is right or wrong. We just do it. However, when we are called upon to consciously monitor this process, we often become judgmental and question whether our perceptions are right or wrong. What scientists are interested in is the raw perception that occurs automatically in everyday life. In everyday life and in the scientific measurement of perceived exertion, there are no right or wrong answers; there are only answers. Borg (1978) has also stated that when stimulated by the challenge to the reliability of human perceptions he is more impressed by "the fantastic ability which man has to perceive things, how well man can discriminate changes in this complex system and that man can rely on his own sensations." Instructions should definitely include the admonition that there are no right or wrong answers.

6. **Answer participant's questions**. Answer any questions that the patient has concerning use of the Borg scale. The exact nature of instructions should be dictated by the purpose of the evaluation or measurement. Exercise program instructions may be somewhat different from those used prior to graded exercise testing. The instructions typically presented to patients prior to diagnostic testing may be different from those utilized in a specific research project. Instructions between research projects with different experimental goals may also be different. Regardless of the need to be specific, most of the preceding six points are usually appropriate to cover in some form. It is usually most efficient to prepare instructions in written or tape-recorded form so that clients and patients can read

or listen to them prior to making perceptual ratings. Following the reading, instructional reinforcements can be made and questions answered. Following is an example of experimental instructions reported by Robertson et al. (1979).

"All subjects underwent orientation sessions to establish the low and high rating scale standards. Prior to each exercise orientation, a tape-recorded definition of the perception of exertion and instructions for use of the Borg RPE scale were played. The instruction emphasized that the perceptual ratings should reflect sensations of exertion, stress, and/or discomfort. Rating standards were established for each exercise mode. The low standard was set equal to the feelings of exertion associated with pedalling and/or cranking the ergometer at 50 rev · min^{-1}, against a 0.08 watt resistance. The high standard equaled the sensations experienced during maximally exhaustive exercise on an ergometer. A rating of 7 was assigned to the low standard and a 19 to the high standard. Subjects were instructed to make their subjective assessments relative to their feelings of exertion associated with a rating of 7 and 19. A tape-recorded definition of perceived exertion and instructions for using the rating scale were played prior to each experimental trial. During testing, the perceptual ratings were measured from 15 to 45 s of each exercise minute. The rating scale was in full view of the subject during the entire test. As the respiratory valve prohibited a verbal rating response, a finger signal was employed. In this procedure a pointer was moved progressively from one scale category to the next, beginning with the lowest number. Subjects were instructed to extend the index finger of the right hand when the appropriate numerical rating was identified by the pointer. This technique made it possible to measure RPE during arm exercise where the hands were firmly gripped around the crank handles. Each rating was limited to a single numbered response. However, subjects were encouraged to use verbal expressions on the scale to aid in selecting the appropriate rating. Information as to the expected outcomes of the perceptual ratings was not provided."

Rating Practice

Other issues related to the administration of the Borg scale, as well as other psychophysical methods, are the question of the ability of subjects to use numbers and the problem of asking subjects to make perceptual judgments when this is not a customary activity. Such questions emphasize the advantage of rating practice sessions. This consideration is perhaps more appropriate for experimental projects and less appropriate for more practical uses of the scale. We have used rating practice in some experiments. One technique used was to ask subjects to judge line length. With this technique, the subject rates the length of test lines after viewing a standard line length. This method helps the investigator to know whether the concept of rating is understood and the extent to which accuracy is present. The goal is not to bias future tests by shaping an acceptable answering mode but to be sure that subjects have the ability to understand and execute instructions associated with perceptual experimentation. Experimenters should want subjects to rate perceptual intensity as naively as possible, but a certain minimal understanding of the scaling process is a reasonable expectation.

Experimental Use of the Borg Scale

Since its development, the 15-graded scale has been used in a variety of experimental situations. The purpose of this section is to provide the reader with a sampling of these experiments. It is not our intention to be exhaustive but to show the breadth of experimental use. These studies are largely descriptive in nature and are generally presented in chronological order beginning in 1971. Emphasis is not on the data generated but on how the scale was used to answer an experimental question.

Walking and Running Studies

The first of two studies dealing with the comparative response of perceived exertion during walking and running at the same velocity was presented at the International Congress of Applied Psychology in 1971 (Noble and Borg 1972). Earlier work by Boøje (1944) had shown that oxygen consumption during running at low velocities was greater than during walking. At about 5.0 mph the two curves intersected and from that point on the energy expenditure is greater for walking than for running. It was assumed that, because heart rate paralleled oxygen consumption during submaximal exercise, this variable would behave similarly. Likewise, since the Borg scale was designed to grow linearly with heart rate, it was hypothesized that perceived exertion would approximate the oxygen consumption response. The speed range in the first study was not sufficient to accept or reject the hypothesis. A replication study in 1973 (Noble et al. 1973) with appropriate speeds sampled supported the hypothesis. It is interesting to note that the results of this study challenged the role of heart rate in the setting of perceived exertion and supported a local factor, muscle and joint discomfort, in concert with central variables to explain perceived exertion.

Physical Training and Other Factors

Ekblom and Goldbarg, following the lead of Borg, published a classical study of perceived exertion in 1971. This study, conducted at the Gymnastics and Sports High School in Stockholm, observed the response of perceptual ratings to eight weeks of physical training, beta-adrenergic and parasympathetic blockade, arm versus leg exercise, cycling versus running, and swimming versus running. Basically, these investigators examined the relationship between heart rate (or oxygen consumption) and perceived exertion. They wanted to test the strength of these relationships when factors known to alter the heart rate (or oxygen consumption) response were introduced as experimental treatments. At given submaximal levels of oxygen consumption, RPE was not altered by blockade, and swimming perceptions were unchanged compared with running. When RPE was compared before and after training at given percentages of maximal oxygen consumption, no differences were noted. However, under conditions where muscle mass is a factor, for example, arm versus leg exercise and bicycling versus running, RPE is higher when a smaller muscle mass is involved.

Concentric Versus Eccentric Muscle Contractions

It is known that muscle fibers produce more tension when they are lengthened (eccentric contraction) than when they are shortened (concentric contraction). But when eccentric exercise is compared to concentric exercise at the same exercise intensity, each type of exercise produces the same total tension. Therefore, fewer muscle fibers are recruited during eccentric exercise. In addition, even though tension may be equal when these two types of contraction are compared at the same exercise intensity, eccentric contraction results in lower oxygen consumption. This knowledge led Henriksson, Knuttgen, and Bonde-Peterson (1972) to hypothesize that perceived exertion would be less during eccentric contractions performed at the same exercise intensity as concentric contractions. This hypothesis was confirmed. Also, when perception was compared at equal oxygen consumption levels, eccentric contractions produced greater ratings of perceived exertion.

Muscle Mass

Sargeant and Davies (1973) conducted a series of experiments that extended the work of Ekblom and Goldbarg (1971). Exercise comparisons were made in which muscle mass was manipulated as an independent variable. One-arm exercise was compared with two-arm exercise, and one-leg exercise with two-leg exercise. As might be expected, perceived exertion varied with limb volume; that is, at the same absolute exercise intensity, RPE was greater with the lower muscle mass. However, when exercise was compared at the same relative percentage of aerobic power, no differences were observed.

Temperature

The group at the Human Energy Research Laboratory at the University of Pittsburgh, after Borg's visit in 1967, conducted a number of studies to test the hypothesis that perceived exertion was principally a response to heart rate. In one of those studies temperature was manipulated to evaluate the heart rate/ perceived exertion hypothesis (Pandolf et al. 1972). It is known that temperature increases heart rate above that induced by exercise 1 beat for each increment of 1° C. Exercise treatments were compared in which exercise intensity was equal but heart rate was artificially augmented by increased temperature. It was assumed that if perceived exertion followed heart rate, the RPE would be greater in the heat treatments. However, RPE did not reflect the change in heat-induced heart rate but followed increases in exercise intensity.

Chronic Obstructive Lung Disease

The Borg scale has been proven effective not only during exercise therapy for various patient groups, but also in clinical research. One example compared patients suffering from chronic obstructive lung disease (COPD) with a control group (Löllgen, Ulmer, and von Nieding 1977). Both groups performed bicycle ergometer exercise using four power outputs and four pedal rates. Correlations to determine the relationship among RPE, power output, and heart rate were found to be lower in COPD patients than in controls. At the same power output, RPE decreased with an increase in pedal rate in control subjects. Patients decreased their RPE from 40 to 60 to 80 rpm but increased at 100 rpm.

Altitude

The U.S. Army Institute of Environmental Medicine maintains an Altitude Division to study human adaptation to hypobaric environments. In keeping with their mission, in 1979 several investigators reported on studies of perception of effort at high altitude (Horstman, Weiskopf, and Robinson 1979). Twenty young males (mean age = 19.8 yr) were tested at sea level to determine responses to 60%, 80%, and 95% of $\dot{V}O_2$max and exercise to exhaustion at 85% $\dot{V}O_2$ max. Subsequently, the subjects were transported to 4,300 m (Pike's Peak, Colorado) where all tests were repeated within 48 hr of initial hypobaric exposure. Perceived exertion was significantly lower at high altitude for exercise performed at 60% and 80% $\dot{V}O_2$max and at a time point equal to 25% of the endurance test at 85% $\dot{V}O_2$ max. No other perceptual comparisons were significantly different. It should be noted that, since $\dot{V}O_2$ max was reduced at 4,300 m by 19%, the absolute power output for exercise at various percentages of $\dot{V}O_2$max at altitude was decreased.

Psychology

It goes without saying that understanding perceptual response to exercise and sport is not only a physiological matter. During the first 10 years of the study of perceived exertion in the United States, experiments that concentrated on psychological issues were conspicuous by their sparsity. A study published in 1980 by Rejeski and Ribisl is typical of a growing number of articles in recent years stressing mediation of perceived exertion by psychological factors. The experimental protocol involved two trials in which subjects ran on a treadmill at 85% of $\dot{V}O_2$ max. During the first trial, exercise duration was 20 min. In the following trial, exercise was terminated at 20 min, even though subjects were told that they would run for 30 min. Perceived exertion was significantly lower in the "30-min" trial from minute 2 through minute 15. This was the case even though no differences were observed in heart rate, respiratory rate, or pulmonary minute volume. Expectation of exercise duration apparently can modulate perceptual response.

Menstruation

Whether the menstrual cycle influences performance or certain physiological and psychological variables related to performance has been a concern of scientists for many years. The issue of whether cyclic changes associated with menstruation might affect one's subjective evaluation of effort has been experimentally tested. In one study a group ($N = 12$) of college-age females (19-23 yr) were tested premenstruation (within 48 h of onset), at day 1 of menstruation (within 24 h following onset), and midcycle (within 48 h of cycle midpoint; Higgs and Robertson 1981). Testing consisted of treadmill running at 90% and 100% of $\dot{V}O_2$max at each cycle point. RPE was not altered at 90% but was found to be significantly higher for the precycle and day 1 phases at the 100% level.

Sleep Deprivation

Most of us have experienced the sensation of reduced performance following sleep loss. But, is performance really reduced? Likewise, is sleep loss accompanied by a reduction in physiological function and perception? Martin and Gaddis (1981) studied the effect of 30 h sleep loss on responses to bicycle ergometer exercise. In addition to the sleep loss protocol, subjects exercised following a normal sleep condition to control for training, learning, habituation, and accumulated fatigue. Oxygen consumption, carbon dioxide production, pulmonary ventilation, heart rate, and blood pressure were unchanged by sleep loss. However, the sleep loss perturbation resulted in a significant increase in perceived exertion.

Gender

Inevitably scientists ask the question of whether gender is a factor in human function. The study of perceived exertion is no different. Males and females have been compared while walking and running submaximally and maximally on a treadmill (Noble, Maresh, and Ritchey 1981). When perceived exertion was compared at absolute levels of oxygen consumption (L/min), females experienced more intense exercise sensations. However, when the data was expressed in relative terms (%$\dot{V}O_2$ max), no differences were found. Differences in $\dot{V}O_2$max between genders probably explain the differences observed at absolute levels.

Circadian Rhythms

In the late 1970s and early 1980s considerable interest was shown in variations that may accompany solar or lunar cycles. Confirmation of such variations has important implications for testing and training. In one attempt to unravel this complex question, repeat treadmill exercise was administered so that data points were established every two hours from 12:00 (noon) until 10:00 A.M. (Faria and Drummond 1982). No significant difference in aerobic power was observed over the 24-h period. Perceived exertion was higher at heart rates of 130, 150, and 170 during the 2:00 P.M. and 4:00 P.M. testing sessions compared with those held at 8:00 P.M., 10:00 P.M., and 12:00 midnight.

Occupational Tasks

Exercise science would not be complete unless it incorporated tasks that one encounters in occupational settings. The assessment of the severity of materials handling tasks is a tedious and expensive matter. The use of a simple procedure like the rating of physical effort as a predictor of severity was undertaken by one group of investigators (Asfour et al. 1983). Perceived exertion proved to be linear with heart rate and oxygen consumption during the handling of materials. Correlations between RPE and oxygen consumption of about .70 led this group to promote perceived exertion as a predictor of physiological severity in occupational settings.

Aging

Not only do we find that an increasing percentage of our population is found in older age categories, but a growing number of older men and women are exercising on a daily basis. Methods to monitor and control exercise intensity in order to maintain safety is of interest to both practitioners and scientists. A sample of 105 women and 97 men was tested using a 600-m walk and a 2-min walk in place (Miller et al. 1985). Heart rate and perceived exertion were measured. Although HR-RPE correlations were significant, they were quite low without high predictive value. Using the authors words, "the low correlation values obtained may illustrate the difficulty encountered when exercise intensity does not consist of progressively increasing workloads."

Growth

To be maximally useful, the concept of perceived exertion should be an effective assessment tool for school-age children. To confirm perceived exertion relationships found in adult populations, 30 adolescent boys were tested on a bicycle ergometer at three submaximal power outputs (Eston and Williams 1986). Correlations between perceived exertion and power output and between perceived exertion and heart rate were .78 and .74, respectively. Since these values approximate those found with adults, the concept of assessing perceived exertion was recommended for adolescent boys.

Postscript

It must be noted again that the foregoing discussion of the literature was not intended to be exhaustive. It is intended to be only illustrative of the various settings and samples in which perceived exertion has been a dependent variable. We have not editorialized these contributions nor have the results been the primary focus.

Summary

Ratio scaling methods are considered to be the gold standard for describing the growth of perceptual response as a function of physical stimulation. However, ratio scaling has little clinical value, because it does not produce data that provides a basis for making interindividual comparisons. Borg recognized this deficiency and developed the theoretical framework for the assessment of interindividual differences. The theory involves the acceptance of four assumptions: There is interindividual variation in the stimulus range; every stimulus range has a corresponding perceptive range; intensity of perception is determined by its place in the perceptive range; and the perceptive range can be set equal for all individuals. This work led to the development of a category scale for the determination of interindividual differences in perceived exertion during exercise.

Initially, the category scale consisted of 21 grades (0-20). The scale was constructed with the explicit intent to provide perceptual data that was linear with heart rate and power output. Experience with the scale indicated that in some situations perception did not grow linearly with heart rate. Therefore, a 15-graded scale (6-20) was developed to correct this lack of linearity. Even though the initial intent was to predict heart rate from the scale ratings by multiplying the RPE by 10, a number of studies have shown that this prediction is inaccurate. However, the heart rate–perceived exertion linearity remains and serves as a major argument for classifying the scale as a category scale that provides equal interval perceptual data. The use of quantitative semantics for the

choice and placement of category expressions also supports the classification of
Borg's scale as a category scale with interval properties.

The 15-graded Borg scale has been studied to determine its validity and
reliability. Validity criteria have consisted of comparing perceptual responses in
protocols in which power output was presented progressively and at random,
correlating perceived exertion with heart rate, and correlating perceived exertion
with energy expenditure. In all cases the scale proved to be a valid assessment
of perceived exertion. Reliability was assessed using test-retest paradigms. Reliability coefficients ranged from .71 to .91. Thus, the 15-graded scale can be
considered a reliable measure of perceived exertion as well.

Several other category scales have been developed to measure perceived
exertion. One is a 9-graded scale anchored only at the extremes. This scale was
highly correlated (.92) with the 21-graded scale during a graded exercise test.
Another scale, 7-graded, has been used successfully in occupational contexts and
shows a solid relationship with energy expenditure (.70). A line scale, in which
intensity of perception is indicated by pencil marks made perpendicular to a
horizontal line anchored on each end with "no exertion at all" and "maximal
exertion," respectively, has also been shown to be effective in the measurement
of perceived exertion.

In recent years, Borg developed a category scale with ratio properties that has
the advantages of ratio scales but also can be used for assessing interindividual
differences. The scale was developed to be simple, with 12 grades and a general
maximal category within which the subject is free to make magnitude estimations.
Expressions have been appropriately arranged so that data is positively accelerating, approximating the exponent (1.6) commonly found with muscular effort. This
scale is also appropriate for assessing sensations that may arise from physiological
variables that do not grow linearly with power output, such as lactic acid accumulation and pulmonary ventilation.

Many practitioners and exercise scientists have asked which of the two scales,
15-graded or category-ratio, is most appropriate for clinical and experimental
work. In a theoretical sense the correct answer is neither. Many scales and
measurement methods are available and should be selected on the basis of the
clinical or experimental objective. The 15-graded scale has been used widely
and with considerable success in practical settings. Although Borg supports the
category-ratio scale as simple and effective in a variety of settings and situations,
it does not seem to be as easily understood as the 15-graded scale. It is our
recommendation that in most clinical testing and training contexts the 15-graded
scale is the scale of choice. The category-ratio scale can be used effectively for
specialized purposes, such as the assessment of respiratory distress. The general
rule for scale selection, however, must always be to use the scale that matches
the clinical or experimental need.

Preparation of subjects and clients through the presentation of comprehensive
instructions is critical to the correct use of category scales. Instructions should
include: an explanation of the concept of perceived exertion, illustrations of the
anchor expressions used to describe the perceptive range, an explanation of

how the numbers and expressions are to be used, comment on how ratings are differentiated if such ratings are to be requested, encouragement of subjects and clients to rate naively without making judgments or evaluating correctness, and a request that questions should be asked if the instructions are the least bit confusing.

The final section of this chapter has been devoted to providing examples of the spectrum of experimental uses for Borg's 15-graded category scale. No attempt was made to be exhaustive or to review literature per se but to provide a view of the breadth and nature of the use of the RPE scale. The following experimental uses were noted: walking and running, physical training, concentric and eccentric exercise, effect of muscle mass, temperature, chronic obstructive pulmonary disease, altitude, psychological factors, menstruation, sleep deprivation, gender, circadian rhythms, occupational tasks, aging, and growth.

References

American College of Sports Medicine. 1986. *Guidelines for graded exercise testing and exercise prescription.* Philadelphia: Lea and Febiger.

Asfour, S.S., M.M. Ayoub, A. Mital, and N.J. Bethea. 1983. Perceived exertion of physical effort for various manual handling tasks. *Am. Indust. Hyg. Asso. J.* 44:223-28.

Bøje, O. 1944. Energy production, pulmonary ventilation, and length of steps in well-trained runners working on a treadmill. *Acta Physiol. Scand.* 7:362.

Borg, G. 1961a. Interindividual scaling and perception of muscular force. *Kungliga Fysiografiska Sallskapets i Lund Forhandlingar* 31:117-25.

———. 1961b. Perceived exertion in relation to physical work load and pulse-rate. *Kungliga Fysiografiska Sallskapets i Lund Forhandlingar* 31:105-15.

———. 1962. Physical performance and perceived exertion. Lund, Sweden: Gleerup.

———. 1970. Perceived exertion as an indicator of somatic stress. *Scand. J. Rehab. Med.* 2:92-98.

———. 1971. The perception of physical performance. In R.J. Shephard (Ed.), *Frontiers of fitness,* 280-94. Springfield, IL: Charles C Thomas.

———. 1973a. *A note on a category scale with "ratio properties" for estimating perceived exertion.* Reports from the Institute of Applied Psychology, no. 36. Stockholm: Univ. of Stockholm.

———. 1973b. Perceived exertion: A note on "history" and methods. *Med. Sci. Sports* 5:90-93.

———. 1978. Psychological assessments of physical effort. In *Proceedings of the 1978 International Symposium on Psychological Assessment in Sport,* 49-57. Netanya, Israel: Wingate Institute for Physical Education and Sport.

———. 1982a. A category scale with ratio properties for intermodal and interindividual comparisons. In *Psychophysical judgment and the process of perception,* ed. H. Geissler and P. Petzold, 25-34. Berlin: VEB Deutscher Verlag der Wissenschaften.

————. 1982b. Psychophysical bases of perceived exertion. *Med. Sci. Sports Exerc.* 14:377-81.

Borg, G., and H. Dahlstrom. 1959. Psykofysisk undersokning avarbete pacykeler-gometer. *Nord. Med.* 62:1383.

————. 1960. The perception of muscular work. *Umea Vetensk. Bibiotekskr.* 5:1-26.

————. 1962. A pilot study of perceived exertion and physical working capacity. *Acta Soc. Med. Upsal.* 67:21-27.

Borg, G., and I. Lindblad. 1976. *The determination of subjective intensities in verbal descriptions of symptoms.* Reports from the Institute of Applied Psychology, no. 75. Stockholm: Univ. of Stockholm.

Borg, G., and H. Linderholm. 1967. Perceived exertion and pulse rate during graded exercise in various age groups. *Acta Med. Scand.* 472 (Suppl.): 194-206.

————. 1970. Exercise performance and perceived exertion in patients with coronary insufficiency, arterial hypertension and vasoregulatory asthenia. *Acta Med. Scand.* 187:17-26.

Cafarelli, E., and B. Bigland-Ritchie. 1979. Sensation of static force in muscles of different length. *Exper. Neurol.* 65:511-525.

Ekblom, B., and A.N. Goldbarg. 1971. The influence of physical training and other factors on the subjective rating of perceived exertion. *Acta Physiol. Scand.* 83:399-406.

Eston, R.G., and J.G. Williams. 1986. Exercise intensity and perceived exertion in adolescent boys. *Br. J. Sports Med.* 20:27-30.

Faria, I.E., and B.J. Drummond. 1982. Circadian changes in resting heart rate and body temperature, maximal oxygen consumption and perceived exertion. *Ergonomics* 25:381-86.

Gagge, A.P., J.A.J. Stolwijk, and J.D. Hardy. 1967. Comfort and thermal sensations and associated physiological responses at various ambient temperatures. *Environ. Res.* 1:1-20.

Gamberale, F. 1972. Perceived exertion, heart rate, oxygen uptake and blood lactate in different work operations. *Ergonomics* 15:545-54.

————. 1985. The perception of exertion. *Ergonomics* 26:299-308.

Henriksson, J., H.G. Knuttgen, and F. Bonde-Peterson. 1972. Perceived exertion during exercise with concentric and eccentric muscle contractions. *Ergonomics* 15:537-44.

Higgs, S.L., and L.A. Robertson. 1981. Cyclic variations in perceived exertion and physical work capacity in females. *Can. J. Appl. Sport Sci.* 6:191-96.

Hogan, J.C., and E.A. Fleishman. 1979. An index of the physical effort required in human task performance. *J. Appl. Psychol.* 64:197-204.

Hogan, J.C., G.D. Ogden, D.L. Gebhardt, and E.A. Fleishman. 1980. Reliability and validity of methods for evaluating perceived physical effort. *J. Appl. Psychol.* 65:672-79.

Horstman, D.H., R. Weiskopf, and S. Robinson. 1979. The nature of the perception of effort at sea level and high altitude. *Med. Sci. Sports* 11:150-54.

Löllgen, H., H.V. Ulmer, and G. von Nieding. 1977. Heart rate and perceptual response to exercise with different pedalling speed in normal subjects and patients. *Eur. J. Appl. Physiol.* 37:297-304.

Maresh, C., and B.J. Noble. 1984. Utilization of perceived exertion ratings during exercise testing and training. In *Cardiac rehabilitation: Exercise testing and prescription,* ed. L.K. Hall, 155-73. Great Neck, N.Y.:Spectrum.

Marks, L.E. 1974. *Sensory processes: The new psychophysics.* New York: Academic Press.

Martin, B.J., and G.M. Gaddis. 1981. Exercise after sleep deprivation. *Med. Sci. Sports Exerc.* 13:220-23.

Miller, G.D., R.D. Bell, M.L. Collins, and T.B. Hoshizaki. 1985. The relationship between perceived exertion and heart rate of post 50 year-old volunteers in two different walking activities. *J. Human Move. Stud.* 11:187-95.

Noble, B.J. 1982. Clinical applications of perceived exertion. *Med. Sci. Sports Exerc.* 14:406-11.

Noble, B.J., and G. Borg. 1972. Perceived exertion during walking and running. In *Proceedings of the 17th International Congress of Applied Psychology,* ed. R. Piret, 387-92. Brussels.

Noble, B.J., G. Borg, I. Jacobs, R. Ceci, and P. Kaiser. 1983. A category-ratio perceived exertion scale: Relationship to blood and muscle lactate and heart rate. *Med. Sci. Sports Exerc.* 15:523-28.

Noble, B.J., W.J. Kraemer, J.G. Allen, J.S. Plank, and L.A. Woodard. 1986. The integration of physiological cues in effort perception: stimulus strength vs. relative contribution. In *The perception of exertion in physical work,* eds. G. Borg, and D. Ottoson, 83-96. Dobbs Ferry, NY: Sheridan House.

Noble, B.J., C.M. Maresh, and M. Ritchey. 1981. Comparison of exercise sensations between females and males. In *Women and sports: An historical, biological, physiological and sports medicine approach,* ed. J. Borms, M. Hebbelinck, and A. Venerando, 175-79. Basel: Karger.

Pandolf, K.B. 1982. Differentiated ratings of perceived exertion during physical exercise. *Med. Sci. Sports Exerc.,* 14:397-405.

Pandolf, K.B., E. Cafarelli, B.J. Noble, and K.F. Metz. 1972. Perceptual responses during prolonged work. *Percept. Motor Skills* 35:975-85.

Rejeski, W.J., and P.M. Ribisl. 1980. Expected task duration and perceived effort: An attributional analysis. *J. Sport Psychol.* 2:227-36.

Robertson, R.J., R.L. Gillespie, J. McCarthy, and K.D. Rose. 1979. Differentiated perceptions of exertion: Part 1. Mode of integration of regional signals. *Percept. Motor Skills* 49:683-89.

Sargeant, A.J., and C.T. Davies. 1973. Perceived exertion during rhythmic exercise involving different muscle masses. *J. Human Ergol.* 2:3-11.

Skinner, J.S., R. Hustler, V. Bergsteinova, and E.R. Buskirk. 1973. The validity and reliability of a rating scale of perceived exertion. *Med. Sci. Sports* 5:97-103.

Stamford, B.A. 1976. Validity and reliability of subjective ratings of perceived exertion during work. *Ergonomics* 19:53-60.

Stamford, B.A., and B.J. Noble. 1974. Metabolic cost and perception of effort during bicycle ergometer work performance. *Med. Sci. Sports* 6:226-31.

Stevens, S.S. 1957. On the psychophysical law. *Psychol. Rev.* 64:153-81.

———. 1971. Issues in psychophysical measurement. *Psychol. Rev.* 78:426-50.

———. 1974. Perceptual magnitude and its measurement. In *Handbook of perception: Psychophysical judgment and measurement,* eds. C. Carterette and M.P. Friedman, 361-89. New York: Academic Press.

4

CHAPTER

Physiological Models of Exertional Symptoms and Perceptions: Historical and Conceptual Development

The assumption that sensations associated with physical exercise have physiological origins is central to the clinical and pedagogical application of scaled perceptions of exertion. Perceptual responses are an expression of the sensory link between external stimuli arising from physical work and internal responses reflecting physiological functions (Noble 1977). During exercise, perceptual and physiological responses appear as interlocking domains. Information regarding the quality and quantity of exercise performance is provided through the functional interdependence of these domains (Noble 1977). In turn, regulatory decisions based on sensory feedback allow the adjustment of exercise intensity to achieve a prescribed metabolic demand. By recognizing the mediating role of physiological processes in shaping the effort sense, scaled perceptions of exertion can be used as a subjective adjunct to standard clinical and laboratory measurements in

1. assessing exercise tolerance,
2. prescribing exercise intensity,
3. determining the effect of a therapeutic exercise intervention, and
4. guiding the time course of a graded exercise test.

It is the purpose of this chapter to explore theoretical and empirical models that link perceptual and physiological processes during exercise performance. Consideration will be given to the evolution of conceptual models that link discrete underlying physiological events with exertional symptoms and perceptions and to differentiation of perceptual signals of exertion.

Exertional Symptomatology

The effort sense is a complex psychophysiological process that integrates a large number of exertional symptoms, each having one or more physiological mediators. Borg and Lindblad (1976) noted that the linguistic expression of these exertional symptoms forms a *perceptual reality*, allowing for a more global measurement of both physiological and psychological determinants of exercise performance. As an example, exertional symptoms can be used to subjectively determine exercise tolerance during clinical evaluations, to assess the effects of exercise training and rehabilitative therapy, and to provide a basis for comparison of perceptual responses between different work tasks, environmental conditions, and clinical states (Borg, Karlsson, and Lindblad 1976).

One of the earliest attempts to systematically categorize subjective symptoms of exercise-induced fatigue was undertaken by Weiser and Stamper (1977). Their experiments examined self-reported sensory experience during prolonged cycle ergometer exercise. It was assumed that a general correspondence existed between self-reported changes in exertional symptomatology and physiological processes that induce fatigue. The results of these investigations form the foundation for our understanding of the link between perceptual signals of exertion and underlying physiological events. Theoretical models that describe this linkage have their origins in the study of exertional symptomatology.

Subjective Symptoms of Fatigue

Among the most pronounced symptoms of exertional intolerance is the sensation of fatigue (Weiser, Kinsman, and Stamper 1973). Subjective correlates of fatigue are complex, reflecting the integration of many discrete sensations having different physiological origins (Weiser, Kinsman, and Stamper 1973). When measuring symptoms during exercise, a multidimensional statistical procedure such as key cluster analysis is necessary. Weiser, Kinsman, and Stamper (1973) used this statistical procedure to identify key symptom clusters based on self-reported responses to a scaled adjective check list, the Physical Activity Questionnaire (PAQ). The PAQ contains 63 adjectives scaled in a 5-point Likert system. The adjectives reflect various states of mood, somatic discomfort, and arousal. They are classified according to three broad clusters: fatigue, task aversion, and motivation. The adjectives that constitute the fatigue cluster are directly associated with physiological limitations to exercise performance (Weiser, Kinsman, and Stamper 1973; Bartley 1964). Each adjective was rated separately prior to and at the end of cycle ergometer endurance tests performed at an intensity equivalent to either 56% (Weiser, Kinsman, and Stamper 1973) or 65% of peak oxygen uptake ($\dot{V}O_2$ peak) (Weiser and Stamper 1977). For both intensities, cycle ergometer exercise was terminated by the subjects at the point of subjectively intolerable fatigue. Key cluster analysis identified three relatively unique subsets of fatigue, namely, leg fatigue, general fatigue, and cardio-pulmonary fatigue (fig. 4.1; Weiser, Kinsman, and Stamper 1973, 83). A fourth set of symptoms labeled task aversion was also identified but was not directly associated with physical fatigue. The leg fatigue subcluster was presumed to be task specific for cycle ergometer exercise. However, all subclusters demonstrated a modest degree of interdependence. That is, task aversion was somewhat related to both general fatigue ($r = .57$) and leg fatigue ($r = .26$), while the relation between leg fatigue and general fatigue ($r = .82$) was much stronger, accounting for 66% of the common variance between the two symptom subsets.

Horstman et al. (1979) provided independent validation for Weiser's classification of exertional symptoms during dynamic exercise. When measured at selected time points during submaximal (80% $\dot{V}O_2$ peak) cycle ergometer exercise, subjective symptoms of fatigue and exertional intolerance in the legs (i.e., aches, cramps, pain, fatigue, muscular and articular heaviness) and cardiorespiratory system (i.e., sensations of dyspnea) were shown to be strong predictors of submaximal endurance performance. It was concluded that subjective symptoms arising from muscles, joints, and the cardiorespiratory system operate in consort with physiological processes to set the upper limits of endurance performance. Table 4.1

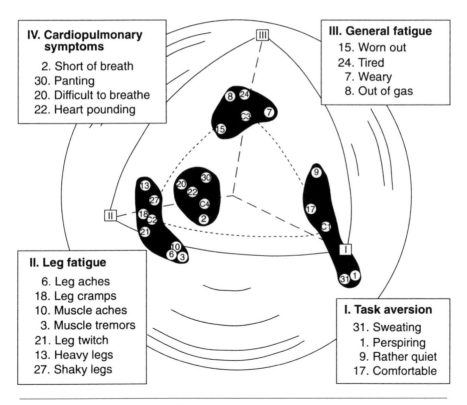

Figure 4.1   Spherical analysis (SPAN) diagram of four clusters at end-of-ride.
Adapted from Weiser, Kinsman, and Stamper 1973.

Table 4.1   Categories of Exertional Symptoms During Dynamic Exercise

Symptom categories		
Effort/fatigue	Pain/discomfort	Cardiopulmonary exertion
Leg fatigue[a]	Leg pain/aches[a, b, c]	Chest pain[a]
Nonspecific fatigue[b, c, d, f]	Joint pain/aches[a, b]	Dyspnea[a, b]
Heaviness[b]	Headaches[a]	Heart pains[a]
Leg effort[c]	Cramps[b]	Panting[a]
	Muscle pain[b]	Breathing difficulties[a, h, i]
	Pain[c, g]	Cardiorespiratory effort[e]

[a]Borg, Karlsson, and Lindblad 1976. [b]Horstman et al. 1979. [c]Morgan 1973. [d]Hueting and Sarphati 1966; Hueting and Poulus 1970. [e]Noble et al. 1983. [f]Nieman et al. 1987. [g]Droste et al. 1991. [h]Maresh et al. 1993. [i]Yorio et al. 1992.

lists various symptoms that are associated with exertional intolerance during dynamic exercise.[1] These symptoms can be grouped into three broad categories: effort/fatigue, pain/discomfort, and cardiopulmonary exertion. The categories are consistent with the symptom clusters identified by Weiser and colleagues. When viewed collectively, these symptoms provide construct validity for a multidimensional array of self-reported subjective responses during exercise that are generalizable across a wide range of population subsets. The generalizability of these symptoms permits their use in defining the subjective components that constitute the perceptual experience during physical exertion.

Physiological Models of Sensory Processing During Exercise

Kinsman and Weiser were among the first to develop a model describing the sensory link between subjective symptoms and physiological events during exercise. This model (fig. 4.2) uses a pyramidal format to classify levels of sensory processing that extend from the underlying physiological substrata to a global report of exertional sensations for the overall body. A unique conceptual feature of the Kinsman-Weiser model is that it positions exertional symptom clusters within a vertical sensory pathway. Subjective sensations of fatigue are then linked directly with their underlying physiological mediators. The model contains five

[1]The symptom clusters described by Weiser and discussed previously are not included.

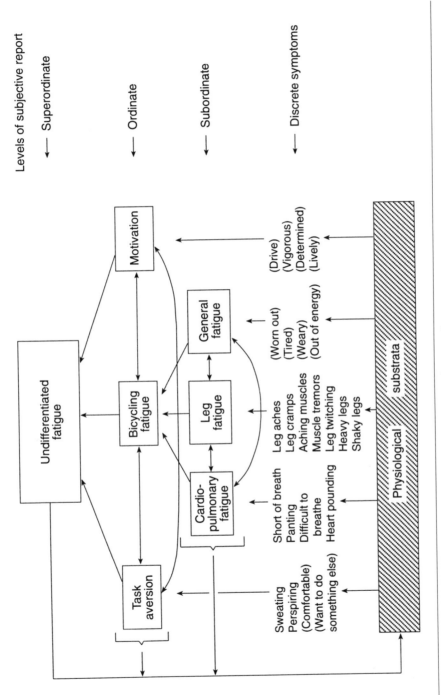

Figure 4.2 Pyramidal schema for subjective symptomatology during exercise.
Reprinted from Weiser and Stamper 1977.

levels of psychobiological responsiveness. To appreciate the neuromotor and behavioral flow of sensory experience during exercise, the pyramidal schema should be examined from base to peak.

The base of the pyramid contains the underlying *physiological substrata*. This basic level comprises various physiological processes that serve as mediators for subjective symptoms of fatigue and exertional intolerance during cycle exercise. The next level in ascending order contains *discrete symptoms* that have their origins in the underlying physiological substrata. These symptoms define a broad range of sensory experiences during cycle exercise, such as perceived shortness of breath, muscle aches, and weariness. At the *subordinate* level, discrete symptoms are grouped into subclusters that define mode-specific (i.e., cardiopulmonary, leg, and general) fatigue during cycle exercise. The various mode-specific subclusters combine at the *ordinate* level of sensory processing to form a primary symptom cluster labeled bicycling fatigue. Primary symptom clusters associated with task aversion and motivation are also formed at the ordinate level. The *superordinate* level is located at the peak of the pyramid and is the terminus for vertical flow of sensory information. At this level the three primary symptom clusters are integrated into a global report of undifferentiated fatigue for the body overall. Subjective reports at the superordinate level involve the vertical integration of a variety of discrete symptoms each having a different intensity weighting (Robertson et al. 1979a). It is believed that this perceptual integration process is controlled by the central nervous system. However, the specific neuromotor mechanism that regulates this integration process is not totally understood.

Validation of the Kinsman-Weiser Physiological Model

The theoretical basis of the Kinsman-Weiser model assumed that sensations of fatigue were as important as physiological determinants of fatigue in setting the limits of exercise performance (Kinsman and Weiser 1976). In this context, limiting factors for exercise performance are not exclusively physiological or biochemical. Rather, the decision to continue or discontinue exercise is based on subjective symptoms that have their origins in underlying physiological events. These physiological events involve both the contractile functions of peripheral skeletal muscle and cardiorespiratory responses. During an exercise challenge, functional changes in the neuromuscular and cardiorespiratory systems increase symptom severity, thereby subjectively setting the limits of endurance performance. This assumption was validated by scaling exertional symptoms during prolonged cycle ergometer exercise at a power output equivalent to 65% $\dot{V}O_2$ peak (Weiser and Stamper 1977). Ergometer performance was volitionally terminated by the subject at the point exercise could no longer be subjectively tolerated.

Electromyography (EMG) of the vastus lateralis was used as a marker of motor unit recruitment, while respiratory rate was used to indicate a change in ventilatory drive. Increases in these physiological measures were considered indicative of muscular and cardiorespiratory stress. Leg fatigue symptom severity increased as EMG amplitude decreased ($r = -.731$ to $-.955$), and cardiorespiratory distress symptoms increased as respiratory rate increased ($r = .519$ to $.938$). Multiple regression analysis indicated that the intensity of exertional symptoms (leg fatigue, motivation, perceived effort, general fatigue, and cardiopulmonary distress) reported after 6 min of exercise accounted for 76% of the variance in cycle ergometer endurance performance, that is, total ride time. These findings provided initial validation of a model that linked discrete sensations of exertion with specific underlying physiological events during dynamic exercise (Kinsman, Weiser, and Stamper 1973).

Differentiated Model of Perceptual Signals

Precision in scaling exertional signals during exercise can be enhanced by differentiating perceptual reports according to their specific physiological mediators (Pandolf, Bruse, and Goldman 1975; Pandolf 1982; Robertson et al. 1979a, 1979b). Differentiated exertional signals provide a more concise definition of the physiological and/or symptomatic processes that shape the perceptual context during exercise. In turn, the clinical and experimental application of the perceptual response takes on a more precise focus.

Pandolf (1982) and Pandolf, Bruse, and Goldman (1975) have proposed a modification of the Kinsman-Weiser theoretical model of sensory reporting that includes the concept of differentiated exertional signals. The modification involves a reclassification of the exertional symptoms that constitute the subordinate level of sensory reporting. In addition to a general exertion symptom cluster, two differentiated clusters are identified: local muscular exertion and cardiopulmonary exertion. Each of these clusters is directly related to the physical exertion cluster at the ordinate level. Based on this classification, discrete exertional symptoms can be differentiated according to physiological mediators that are specific to either the active muscles and joints or to the cardiopulmonary and aerobic metabolic systems. This classification of differentiated symptoms is an extension of Ekblom and Goldbarg's (1971) hypothesis that the effort sense is shaped by *local* perceptual signals reflecting feelings of muscular and articular discomfort and by *central* signals of cardiopulmonary exertion, that is, perceived tachycardia, tachypnea, and dyspnea. In a similar manner Borg's (1962) initial description of the effort sense proposed that the complex of sensations encountered during dynamic exercise is related to the muscle and circulatory systems. More recently, the term *peripheral* has replaced local when referring to physiological mediators that have their origins in the muscles and joints of involved limbs. The term *respiratory-metabolic* has replaced central perceptual responsiveness.

In an applied context, differentiated exertional sensations are anatomically regionalized to those body compartments that are involved in the exercise performance. The link between differentiated perceptual signals and underlying physiological mediators is then specific to a particular body region. The anatomical regionalization of differentiated perceptions of exertion is particularly useful when developing exercise prescriptions for varied recreational, occupational, and home environments. As the mode of physical activity varies between such environments, so do the involved muscle groups. Therefore, to provide an effective and clinically appropriate cardiovascular stimulus, an exercise prescription must be mode specific. Quite often, differentiated perceptual signals that are anatomically regionalized to involved musculature are used as an adjunct to target physiological responses in regulating mode-specific exercise prescriptions.

Models That Include a Perceptual-Cognitive Reference Filter

Certain types of exertional symptoms are not specifically related to physiological processes. These nonspecific symptoms constitute the clusters labeled task aversion and motivation in the Kinsman-Weiser model. Located at the ordinate level of sensory processing, these clusters reflect psychological factors. The various components of these psychological symptom clusters interact to form a *perceptual style* (Robertson et al. 1977). In doing so, they systematically influence exertional sensations at all levels of subjective reporting. It is apparent that these symptom clusters contribute to perceptual responsiveness at a point more fundamental than the ordinate level, necessitating revision of the original Kinsman-Weiser model. This revised construct is presented here as a third-generation model that reorders the sequence of sensory processing during exercise (fig. 4.3). The symptom clusters labeled task aversion and motivation have been combined into a single conceptual classification called the *perceptual-cognitive reference filter.*[2] This filter contains a catalog of *sensory context* reflecting a broad range of psychological and cognitive processes. These processes are not directly related to the underlying physiological substrata. Nevertheless, they systematically account for individual differences in perceptual responses during physical exercise.

From an operational standpoint, the perceptual-cognitive reference filter is positioned at the subordinate level of sensory processing. Such positioning illustrates the role of the filter in modulating sensory signals as they travel from their physiological or neuromotor origins to conscious expression of both differentiated and undifferentiated exertional perceptions.

Comparatively little is known about the components of the perceptual-cognitive reference filter or how these components function to influence the effort sense. It is likely that the filter is developmental, expanding in scope and maturing in both precision and efficiency as the individual's movement-related experiences become more varied. A partial list of the cognitive controls that constitute the reference filter

---

[2]Various labels such as the percepto-stat (Morgan and Pollock 1977), perceptual information system (Borg and Lindblad 1976), symptom experience catalog (Borg and Lindblad 1976), absolute perceptual frame of reference (Borg and Lindblad 1976), and the perceptual reference filter (Noble 1977) have also been used to describe the psychological symptom clusters that constitute the subordinate level of sensory processing.

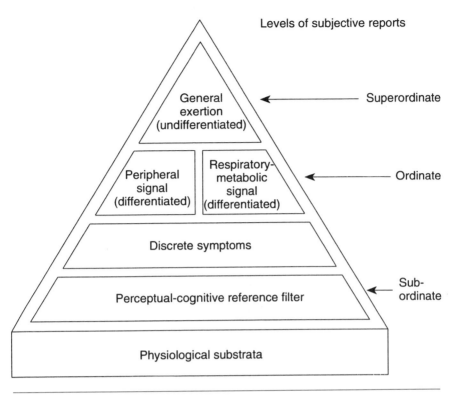

Figure 4.3   Revised model of sensory reporting with the perceptual-cognitive reference filter appearing at the subordinate level.

is presented in table 4.2. These cognitive controls operate independently or in consort to form a bank of stored data through which perceptual signals are filtered (Noble 1977). Operationally, the filter provides an absolute set of references against which the intensity of the perceptual signal is compared and subsequently modulated (Borg and Lindblad 1976). The net effect is to systematically influence perceptual style, accounting for interindividual differences in the intensity of scaled sensory responses during exercise. As such, identification of the individual components of the filter and subsequent quantification of the way in which they shape sensory experience is a prerequisite to accurate clinical interpretation of exertional perceptions. The role of the perceptual-cognitive reference filter in shaping sensory responsiveness during exercise is explored more fully in chapter 8, which deals with the influence of psychological factors in the setting of perceived exertion.

Summary

This chapter explored the evolutionary development of physiological models that explain the perceptual experience during dynamic exercise. The first-generation

Table 4.2   Possible Components of the Perceptual-Cognitive Reference Filter

Component[a]	Reference
Stimulus intensity modulation	Robertson et al. 1979a, 1979b
Lifelong athletic or exercise experience	Noble et al. 1986
Pain tolerance	Robertson et al. 1977; Ryan and Kovacic 1966

Clinical status
  Psychosomatic illness
  Fear/anxiety
	Borg and Lindblad 1976

Psychopathology	Morgan 1973
Attentional focus	Robertson et al. 1978; Hueting and Poulus 1970; Hueting and Sarphati 1966
Exercise motivation	Weiser, Kinsman, and Stamper 1973
Task value	Weiser, Kinsman, and Stamper 1973
Cultural patterns	Noble 1977
Personality characteristics, e.g., extroversion/introversion	Morgan 1973
Mental references	Borg and Lindblad 1976
Premeasurement perceptions and cues	Borg and Lindblad 1976
Dissociative/associative cognitive strategy	Morgan and Pollock 1977
Sensory experience	Morgan and Pollock 1977
Mood states, e.g., depression, neuroticism, anxiety	Morgan 1973
Task aversion	Weiser, Kinsman, and Stamper 1973
Comfort zone	Morgan 1973

[a]Each component of the perceptual-cognitive reference filter can systematically increase or decrease the intensity of the exertional signal.

models considered only exertional symptoms such as task aversion and generalized fatigue. The second- and third-generation models conceptualized the role of physiological mediators in shaping perceptual signal strength. These later models recognized that the expression of the exertional signal reflects interindividual differences in perceptual style and that the actual rating can occur on either the differentiated or undifferentiated level. When examined collectively these models provide the theoretical and empirical foundation for a global conceptualization of the perceptual experience during dynamic exercise. This global model is presented in chapter 12.

References

Bartley, S.H. 1964. *Fatigue: Mechanism and management.* Springfield, IL: Charles C Thomas.

Borg, G. 1962. Physical performance and perceived exertion. In *Studia psychologia et paedagogica,* vol. 11, 1-35. Lund, Sweden: Gleerup.

Borg, G., J.G. Karlsson, and I. Lindblad. 1976. *Quantitative variation of subjective symptoms during ergometer work.* Reports from the Institute of Applied Psychology, no. 72. Stockholm: Univ. of Stockholm.

Borg, G., and I. Lindblad. 1976. *The determination of subjective intensities in verbal descriptions of symptoms.* Reports from the Institute of Applied Psychology, no. 75. Stockholm: Univ. of Stockholm.

Droste, C., M.W. Greenlee, M. Schreck, and H. Roskamm. 1991. Experimental pain thresholds and plasma beta-endorphins levels during exercise. *Med. Sci. Sports Exerc.* 23:334-41.

Ekblom, B., and A.N. Goldbarg. 1971. The influence of physical training and other factors on the subjective rating of perceived exertion. *Acta Physiol. Scand.* 83:399-406.

Horstman, D.H., W.P. Morgan, A. Cymerman, and J. Stokes. 1979. Perception of effort during constant work to self-imposed exhaustion. *Percept. Motor Skills* 48:1111-26.

Hueting, J.E., and A.J. Poulus. 1970. Amphetamine, performance, effort and fatigue. In *Proceedings of Netherlands Society for Physiology and Pharmacology,* 11th Federation Meeting of Medical-Biological Societies.

Hueting, J.E., and H.R. Sarphati. 1966. Measuring fatigue. *J. Appl. Psychol.* 50:535-38.

Kinsman, R.A., and P.C. Weiser. 1976. Subjective symptomatology during work and fatigue. In *Psychological aspects of fatigue*, ed. E. Simonson and P.L. Weises, 336-405. Springfield, IL: Charles C Thomas.

Kinsman, R.A., P.C. Weiser, and D.A. Stamper. 1973. Multidimensional analysis of subjective symptomatology during prolonged strenuous exercise. *Ergonomics* 16:211-26.

Maresh, C.M., M.R. Deschenes, R.L. Seip, L.E. Armstrong, K.L. Robertson, and B.J. Noble. 1993. Perceived exertion during hypobaric hypoxia in low- and moderate altitude natives. *Med. Sci. Sports Exerc.* 25:945-51.

Morgan, W.P. 1973. Psychological factors influencing perceived exertion. *Med. Sci. Sports* 5:97-103.

Morgan, W.P., and M.L. Pollock. 1977. Psychologic characterization of the elite distance runner. *Ann. N.Y. Acad. Sci.* 301:382-403.

Nieman, D.C., K.A. Carlson, M.E. Brandstater, R.T. Naegele, and J.W. Blankenship. 1987. Running endurance in 27-h-fasted humans. *J. Appl. Physiol.* 63:2502-9.

Noble, B.J. 1977. Physiological basis of perceived exertion: A tentative explanatory model. Unpublished report.

Noble, B.J., G. Borg, I. Jacobs, R. Ceci, and P. Kaiser. 1983. A category-ratio perceived exertion scale: Relationship to blood and muscle lactates and heart rate. *Med. Sci. Sports Exerc.* 15:523-29.

Noble, B.J., W.J. Kraemer, J.G. Allen, J.S. Plank, and L.A. Woodard. 1986. The integration of physiological cues in effort perception: Stimulus strength vs.

relative contribution. In *Perception of exertion in physical work,* ed. G. Borg and D. Ottoson, 83-96. London: Macmillan.

Pandolf, K.B. 1982. Differentiated ratings of perceived exertion during physical exercise. *Med. Sci. Sports Exerc.* 14:397-405.

Pandolf, K.B., R.L. Burse, and R.F. Goldman. 1975. Differentiated ratings of perceived exertion during physical conditioning of older individuals using leg-weight loading. *Percept. Motor Skills* 40:563-74.

Robertson, R.J., R.L. Gillespie, E. Hiatt, and K. Rose. 1977. Perceived exertion and stimulus intensity modulation. *Percept. Motor Skills* 45:211-18.

Robertson, R.J., R.L. Gillespie, J. McCarthy, and K. Rose. 1978. Perceived exertion and the field-independence-dependence dimension. *Percept. Motor Skills* 46:495-500.

————. 1979a. Differentiated perceptions of exertion: Part I. Mode of integration of regional signals. *Percept. Motor Skills* 49:683-89.

————. 1979b. Differentiated perceptions of exertion: Part II. Relationship to local and central physiological responses. *Percept. Motor Skills* 49:691-97.

Ryan, E.D., and C.R. Kovacic. 1966. Pain tolerance and athletic participation. *Percept. Motor Skills* 22:383-90.

Weiser, P.C., R.A. Kinsman, and D.A. Stamper. 1973. Task specific symptomatology changes resulting from prolonged submaximal bicycle riding. *Med. Sci. Sports* 5:79-85.

Weiser, P.C., and D.A. Stamper. 1977. Psychophysiological interactions leading to increased effort, leg fatigue, and respiratory distress during prolonged, strenuous bicycle riding. In *Physical work and effort,* ed. G. Borg, 401-16. New York: Pergamon Press.

Yorio, J.M., R.K. Dishman, W.R. Forbus, K.J. Cureton, and R.E. Graham. 1992. Breathlessness predicts perceived exertion in young women with mild asthma. *Med. Sci. Sports Exerc.* 24:860-67.

II
P A R T

Physiological and Psychological Mediators

The application of perceived exertion in clinical and competitive settings requires knowledge of the underlying physiological and psychological processes being subjectively monitored and evaluated. Physiological responses to an exercise stimulus mediate the intensity of perceptual signals of exertion by acting individually or collectively to alter tension-producing properties of skeletal muscle. In turn, changes in peripheral and respiratory muscle tension are monitored through a final common neurophysiological pathway that transmits exertional signals from the motor to sensory cortex. It is this neurophysiological signal that is consciously interpreted by the sensory cortex as effort sensation. This sensory continuum contains a feedback loop wherein scaled perceptual reports are interactively linked with physiological and neurological events in order to determine the appropriateness of an exertional response under varying performance and clinical conditions.

An important feature of this psychophysiological model concerns the classification of physiological events that mediate perceptual signals. The classification system includes *respiratory-metabolic, peripheral* and *nonspecific* physiological mediators. *Respiratory-metabolic* mediators comprise a cluster of physiological responses that influence ventilatory drive during exercise.[1] *Peripheral* physiological mediators are

---

[1]The term *respiratory-metabolic* is used in place of the previously applied term *central* when describing physiological mediators for the effort sense. This change in terminology is suggested for two reasons. First, the term respiratory-metabolic is connotatively consistent with those physiological events that influence breathing. Secondly, the term *central* normally refers to the central nervous system and thus its use is confusing when applied to respiratory-metabolic processes.

localized to the limbs and trunk. A third class, termed *nonspecific* mediators, is composed of generalized or systemic physiological events that are not directly linked to either peripheral or respiratory-metabolic signals. Nevertheless, these nonspecific mediators do contribute to effort sensations during exercise.

The juxtaposition of peripheral and respiratory-metabolic exertional signals can be examined as a time-series event. Under most circumstances, peripheral signals are transmitted from the beginning of exercise and continue to influence exertional sensations throughout the performance. Respiratory-metabolic factors act as an amplifier or gain modifier that potentiates the peripheral signal. The potentiating input from respiratory-metabolic factors begins approximately 30-100 s after the start of exercise, the time period corresponding to that required for cardiorespiratory adaptation. At present, it is not known if and to what extent nonspecific physiological factors influence the relative strength and time of onset of the other types of signal mediators.

In addition to physiological mediators it is recognized that selected psychological factors also systematically influence the effort sense. These factors are generally classified as either *situational* or *dispositional*, accounting for varying degrees of interindividual differences in perceived exertion during dynamic exercise.

Part II contains five chapters. Chapter 5, "Respiratory-Metabolic Mediators of Exertional Perceptions," considers the role of ventilatory drive, oxygen uptake and heart rate in mediating the intensity of the perceptual signal. A model is proposed to explain how some or all of these mediators act in an integrated manner to shape the effort sense. A threshold that marks the relative metabolic rate at which the respiratory-metabolic mediators begin to systematically shape the intensity of exertional perceptions is also considered.

Chapter 6, "Peripheral and Nonspecific Physiological Mediators," examines the effect of alterations in blood pH, lactic acid concentration and glucose on the intensity of the exertional signal during short and long duration exercise. Consideration is also given to the peripheral mediating role of regional blood flow and muscle fiber type. Nonspecific perceptual mediators such as catecholamines, β-endorphins and both skin and body core temperature are also discussed.

Chapter 7 examines the final common pathway for exertional perceptions. Feedforward and feedback neurophysiological pathways for the exertional signal are explained. Consideration is also given to the possible interaction between these two pathways in transmitting and shaping the perceived intensity of exertion.

Chapter 8 considers the influence of psychological factors on the setting of perceived exertion. Specific attention is given to the role of both situational and dispositional psychological factors in determining individual differences in "perceptual style" during physical exercise. The integrative role of a perceptual-cognitive reference filter is also examined.

Chapter 9 explores the role of the unconscious in effort perceptions. This chapter initially considers the physiological basis of the unconscious and then briefly reviews the classical psychological theories of Freud and Jung. The role of the unconscious in setting the intensity of the exertional experience during physical exercise is then examined from the standpoint of both the rater and observer.

5

CHAPTER

Respiratory-Metabolic Mediators of Exertional Perceptions

The physiological processes that are thought to function as mediators for the respiratory-metabolic signal of exertion include ventilatory drive ($\dot{V}_E$), oxygen consumption ($\dot{V}O_2$), carbon dioxide excretion ($\dot{V}CO_2$), heart rate (HR), and blood pressure (Robertson 1982; Jones 1984; Mihevic, Gliner, and Horvath 1981; Pandolf 1983; Pandolf et al. 1984). The comparative importance of each of these physiological processes in mediating the respiratory-metabolic signal of exertion is described in the following sections. Mechanisms underlying the final common neurophysiological pathway for this perceptual signal are considered in chapter 7.

Ventilatory Drive

The sensory link between $\dot{V}_E$ and respiratory effort has been established in a number of investigations that employed simple and multiple regression analyses. While these correlational investigations do not indicate causality, they do provide evidence for a functional relation between ventilatory responses to exercise and respiratory effort. For example, Yorio et al. (1992) found breathlessness to be a strong independent predictor of RPE in young women with mild asthma when exercising between 75% and 85% of their peak oxygen uptake. Correlation coefficients ranging from $r = .61$ to $r = .94$ have been found between RPE and both $\dot{V}_E$ and respiratory rate (RR) (Borg 1976; Edwards et al. 1972; Kamon, Pandolf, and Cafarelli 1974; Noble et al. 1973; Pandolf et al. 1972; Sargeant and Davies 1973; Skinner, Borg, and Buskirk 1969; Smutok, Skrinar, and Pandolf 1980; Sargeant and Davies 1977; Toner, Drolet, and Pandolf 1986). In addition, $\dot{V}_E$ and RR were consistently among the first variables to enter a stepwise multiple regression analysis to predict RPE during treadmill and cycle ergometer exercise in neutral and hot environments (table 5.1; Noble et al. 1973; Sargeant and Davies 1973).

Table 5.1 Results of the Multiple Regression Analyses at 5, 15, and 30 Min in the Neutral and Heated Conditions

Time point	Step	Independent variable	R	$R^2 \times 100$
Neutral				
	1.	$\dot{V}_E$	.559	31.2
	2.	$\dot{V}_E$, $\dot{V}O_2$	.679	48.1
	3.	$\dot{V}_E$, $\dot{V}O_2$, RQ	.732	53.5
5 min	4.	$\dot{V}_E$, $\dot{V}O_2$, RQ, RR	.767	58.8
	5.	$\dot{V}_E$, $\dot{V}O_2$, RQ, RR, HR	.805	64.5
	6.	$\dot{V}_E$, $\dot{V}O_2$, RQ, RR, HR, $\dot{V}CO_2$	.807	65.1
	7.	$\dot{V}_E$, $\dot{V}O_2$, RQ, RR, HR, $\dot{V}CO_2$, T_r	.808	65.3
	8.	$\dot{V}_E$, $\dot{V}O_2$, RQ, RR, HR, $\dot{V}CO_2$, T_r, T_s	.813	66.0
	1.	$\dot{V}_E$	.745	55.5
	2.	$\dot{V}_E$, $\dot{V}CO_2$	.831	69.0
	3.	$\dot{V}_E$, $\dot{V}CO_2$, HR	.852	72.6
15 min	4.	$\dot{V}_E$, $\dot{V}CO_2$, HR, T_s	.886	78.5
	5.	$\dot{V}_E$, $\dot{V}CO_2$, HR, T_s, RQ	.890	79.3
	6.	$\dot{V}_E$, $\dot{V}CO_2$, HR, T_s, RQ, $\dot{V}O_2$	.893	79.7
	7.	$\dot{V}_E$, $\dot{V}CO_2$, HR, T_s, RQ, $\dot{V}O_2$, T_r	.895	80.1
	8.	$\dot{V}_E$, $\dot{V}CO_2$, HR, T_s, RQ, $\dot{V}O_2$, T_r, RR	.896	80.2
	1.	RR	.651	41.1
	2.	RR, $\dot{V}_E$	.650	42.2
	3.	RR, $\dot{V}_E$, T_r	.668	45.6
30 min	4.	RR, $\dot{V}_E$, T_r, $\dot{V}O_2$	.677	45.8
	5.	RR, $\dot{V}_E$, T_r, $\dot{V}O_2$, HR	.701	49.2
	6.	RR, $\dot{V}_E$, T_r, $\dot{V}O_2$, HR, RQ	.717	51.5
	7.	RR, $\dot{V}_E$, T_r, $\dot{V}O_2$, HR, RQ, T_s	.727	52.8
	8.	RR, $\dot{V}_E$, T_r, $\dot{V}O_2$, HR, RQ, T_s, $\dot{V}CO_2$	.729	53.1

(continued)

The strongest evidence in support of ventilatory drive as a physiological mediator for respiratory-metabolic signals of exertion is found when pulmonary ventilation is experimentally manipulated to determine if RPE demonstrates a corresponding change. Hypnosis (Morgan et al. 1976), induced erythrocythemia (Robertson et al. 1982), hypoxia (Robertson et al. 1986), hyperoxia (Pederson and Welch 1977), and variations in cycle pedaling frequency (Robertson et al. 1979b) and testing mode (Franklin et al. 1983) have all been used to experimentally perturb ventilatory responses for this purpose. Let us examine the findings of several of these experiments.

Robertson et al. (1982) used autologous red blood cell (RBC) infusion to experimentally perturb $\dot{V}_E$ during cycle ergometer exercise. The erythrocythemia

Table 5.1   *(continued)*

Time point	Step	Independent variable	R	$R^2 \times 100$
Heated				
	1.	$\dot{V}_E$	.563	31.7
	2.	$\dot{V}_E$, T_s	.658	43.2
	3.	$\dot{V}_E$, T_s, HR	.752	56.6
5 min	4.	$\dot{V}_E$, T_s, HR, T_r	.811	65.9
	5.	$\dot{V}_E$, T_s, HR, T_r, $\dot{V}CO_2$	.848	71.9
	6.	$\dot{V}_E$, T_s, HR, T_r, $\dot{V}CO_2$, RR	.904	81.7
	7.	$\dot{V}_E$, T_s, HR, T_r, $\dot{V}CO_2$, RR, $\dot{V}O_2$	.905	81.9
	8.	$\dot{V}_E$, T_s, HR, T_r, $\dot{V}CO_2$, RR, $\dot{V}O_2$, RQ	.917	84.1
	1.	$\dot{V}_E$	.675	45.5
	2.	$\dot{V}_E$, RR	.745	55.5
	3.	$\dot{V}_E$, RR, T_r	.800	64.0
15 min	4.	$\dot{V}_E$, RR, T_r, $\dot{V}O_2$	.833	69.4
	5.	$\dot{V}_E$, RR, T_r, $\dot{V}O_2$, T_s	.875	76.6
	6.	$\dot{V}_E$, RR, T_r, $\dot{V}O_2$, T_s, HR	.917	84.0
	7.	$\dot{V}_E$, RR, T_r, $\dot{V}O_2$, T_s, HR, RQ	.918	84.2
	8.	$\dot{V}_E$, RR, T_r, $\dot{V}O_2$, T_s, HR, RQ, $\dot{V}CO_2$	.918	84.2
	1.	RR	.483	23.3
	2.	RR, T_s	.549	30.2
	3.	RR, T_s, HR	.629	39.5
30 min	4.	RR, T_s, HR, T_r	.695	48.3
	5.	RR, T_s, HR, T_r, $\dot{V}CO_2$	.700	49.0
	6.	RR, T_s, HR, T_r, $\dot{V}CO_2$, $\dot{V}_E$	.762	58.0
	7.	RR, T_s, HR, T_r, $\dot{V}CO_2$, $\dot{V}_E$, RQ	.836	69.9
	8.	RR, T_s, HR, T_r, $\dot{V}CO_2$, $\dot{V}_E$, RQ, $\dot{V}O_2$	.875	76.6

Reprinted from Noble et al. 1973.

that occurs with RBC reinfusion increases arterial oxygen content and consequently reduces $\dot{V}_E$ for a constant submaximal power output or total body $\dot{V}O_2$. The purpose of the experiment was to determine if RPE-Chest (RPE-C) changed in parallel with the post-reinfusion attenuation of $\dot{V}_E$. Pulmonary ventilation decreased from pre- to post-reinfusion at a power output equivalent to 45% $\dot{V}O_2$max, while RPE-C was unaffected by artificial expansion of the RBC mass (fig. 5.1). A different pattern of sensory responsiveness emerged at a power output equivalent to 70% $\dot{V}O_2$max. Both $\dot{V}_E$ and RPE-C were lower during the post-reinfusion than during the pre-reinfusion tests, suggesting a causal link between the two processes.

Pulmonary ventilation has also been shown to mediate perceptual signals when respiratory response to exercise is perturbed by altering ambient oxygen pressure

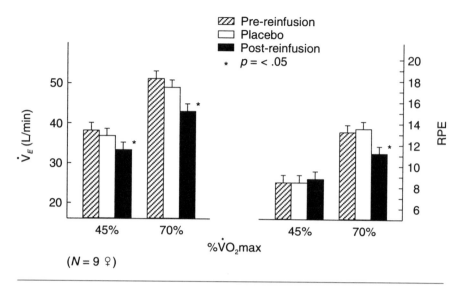

Figure 5.1   Effect of induced erythrocythemia on the relationship between rated perceived exertion (RPE) and ventilation ($\dot{V}_E$).
Reprinted from Robertson 1982.

(Robertson et al. 1982; Pederson and Welch 1977; Maresh et al. 1993). During submaximal exercise, pulmonary ventilation decreases while breathing a hyperoxic gas mixture and increases while breathing a hypoxic gas mixture. Assuming $\dot{V}_E$ is a perceptual signal mediator, RPE should exhibit corresponding changes. By example, Young, Cymerman, and Pandolf (1982) examined perceptual and ventilatory responsiveness during exercise at an altitude of 4,300 m. Ventilatory drive and the perceived intensity of cardiorespiratory exertion were elevated at high altitude as compared with sea level conditions when responses were measured at the same relative metabolic rate. The reciprocal of this perceptual response was seen during exercise under hyperoxic conditions. At a given $\%\dot{V}O_2$max, both $\dot{V}_E$ and RPE were significantly lower when breathing a hyperoxic (50% O_2 in N_2) as compared with an approximate normoxic (25% O_2 in N_2) gas mixture (Pederson and Welch 1977).

Experimental evidence derived under a variety of performance and environmental conditions strongly supports the role of $\dot{V}_E$ in mediating respiratory-metabolic signals of perceived exertion. However, it appears that ventilation functions as an important signal mediator at higher but not lower relative metabolic rates. The possibility that the respiratory-metabolic signal of exertion is dependent on metabolic rate is discussed in more detail later in this chapter.

Respiratory Rate and Tidal Volume

The role of respiratory rate (RR) and tidal volume (TV) in mediating perceptual signals has been examined using a variety of experimental perturbations. Robertson

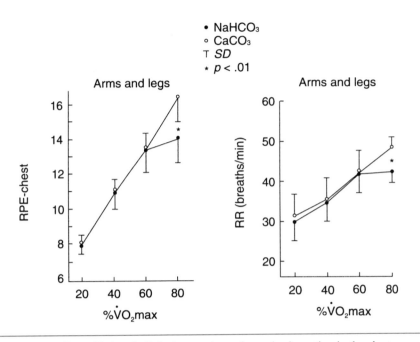

Figure 5.2   Effect of induced alkalosis on ratings of perceived exertion in the chest (RPE-Chest) and respiratory rate (RR) during arm and leg exercise. At a given %V̇O₂max, means that are connected by an * are significantly ($p < .01$) different.
Reprinted from Robertson and Metz 1986.

et al. (1979a, 1979b) found that RR and RPE-C were higher at slower compared with faster pedaling rates, while TV was the same for all pedaling conditions. In an analogous finding, both RR and RPE decreased during submaximal exercise (80% $\dot{V}O_2$peak) when alkalosis was induced by NaHCO₃ ingestion (Robertson and Metz 1986; fig 5.2). Tidal volume was not affected by the experimental perturbation. It would appear that adjustments in RR during dynamic exercise are one of the primary physiological mediators for respiratory-metabolic signals of exertion (Robertson et al. 1986).

Evidence supporting the role of TV as a perceptual signal mediator is comparatively limited. Bakers and Tenney (1970) were among the first to show that changes in lung volume could be accurately perceived. However, these experiments were conducted with the subject in a resting state. Goslin and Rorke (1986) noted that when external loads were transported using a backpack, both TV and RPE were higher at faster (1.69 m/s) than at slower (1.35 m/s) speeds. Respiratory rate did not differ between speeds. In the presence of such limited information, it is not entirely clear what role TV plays in mediating the respiratory-metabolic signal of exertion (Robertson 1982). More extensive experimentation using controlled laboratory perturbation of TV is needed to answer this question.

Respiratory Gases

The demand for breathing is regulated in large part by metabolic requirements for tissue oxidation ($\dot{V}O_2$) and carbon dioxide excretion (VCO_2). These two determinants of pulmonary gas exchange serve as physiological mediators for the respiratory-metabolic signal of exertion.

Oxygen Uptake ($\dot{V}O_2$)

Perceptual signals associated with $\dot{V}O_2$ are mediated by the ventilatory drive required to support aerobic metabolism. As ventilatory drive intensifies in response to a greater aerobic energy requirement, the consequent increase in developed inspiratory muscle tension is consciously perceived as a signal of respiratory-metabolic exertion. Correlation coefficients for the relation between $\dot{V}O_2$ and RPE range from $r = .76$ to $r = .97$ for both intermittent and continuous arm and leg exercise (Edwards et al. 1972; Sargeant and Davies 1973; Smutok, Skrinar, and Pandolf 1980; Sargeant and Davies 1977; Toner, Drolet, and Pandolf 1986; Goslin and Rorke 1986).

A number of investigations noted a lack of correspondence between $\dot{V}O_2$ and RPE when the aerobic metabolic requirement of an exercise task was experimentally manipulated (Cafarelli 1977; Pandolf 1983; DeMello et al. 1987; Löllgen, Graham, and Sjogaard 1980; Pandolf and Noble 1973). Recognizing this inconsistency, it is likely that the role of aerobic metabolism in mediating exertional sensations can be more clearly defined by the relative (i.e., %$\dot{V}O_2$max) rather than the absolute $\dot{V}O_2$ (Sargeant and Davies 1973; Robertson 1982; Berry et al. 1989; Pandolf et al. 1984). As an example, the dependence of RPE on the relative aerobic requirement is seen when perceptual comparisons are made between normoxic and normobaric hypoxic environments. At a constant submaximal $\dot{V}O_2$, RPE is lower during normoxia than hypoxia (fig. 5.3; Robertson et al. 1982). Upon initial consideration, it appears that $\dot{V}O_2$ and RPE are independent. However, $\dot{V}O_2$max is attenuated during acute hypoxia exposure. Therefore, the absolute $\dot{V}O_2$ that is used as a reference point represents a lower relative aerobic metabolic rate under the normoxic than under simulated altitude conditions. The perceptual responses appear to have been mediated by the relative level of $\dot{V}O_2$. This assumption is confirmed when RPE is reported as a function of %$\dot{V}O_2$max. Using a constant %$\dot{V}O_2$max as a reference, RPE is the same between normoxic and hypoxic conditions (fig. 5.3). These data indicate that the relative rather than the absolute $\dot{V}O_2$ may play the more important role in mediating the strength of the respiratory-metabolic signal of exertion during dynamic exercise. In support of this conclusion, overall body RPE (RPE-O) can be predicted with a reasonable degree of accuracy using the relative oxygen uptake according to the following equation: RPE-O = $5.59 + 15\%$ $\dot{V}O_2$max; $r = .94$ (Davies and Sargeant 1979).

Evidence supporting the relative oxygen uptake as a perceptual signal mediator is not totally consistent. The investigations listed in table 5.2 examined the relation

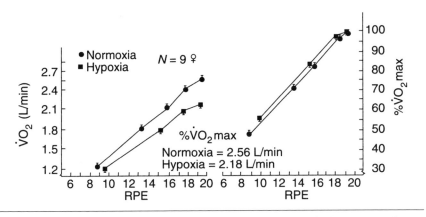

Figure 5.3   Effect of acute normobaric hypoxia on the relationship between rated perceived exertion (RPE) and the absolute ($\dot{V}O_2$) and relative (%$\dot{V}O_2$max) oxygen uptake. Reprinted from Robertson 1982.

between %$\dot{V}O_2$max and RPE using a broad range of experimental procedures to perturb the aerobic metabolic requirement. For each of the citations listed in the top panel, scaled perceptual responses differed between the various experimental perturbations when comparisons were made at an absolute $\dot{V}O_2$ or power output (PO). Such differences were not apparent when a constant %$\dot{V}O_2$max or %POmax was used as a reference for perceptual comparisons. These experimental findings indicate that the intensity of respiratory-metabolic exertional signals during dynamic exercise is mediated by the %$\dot{V}O_2$max. Those investigations listed in the bottom panel of table 5.2 did not find RPE to be dependent on %$\dot{V}O_2$max, rejecting the relative metabolic rate as a perceptual signal mediator. Notable among this latter group are investigations that compared perceptual responses under selected conditions of heat and cold stress (Toner, Drolet, and Pandolf 1986; Pivarnik and Senay 1986). Apparently, the relation between RPE and %$\dot{V}O_2$max is distorted when heat flux is altered by changes in environmental temperature. Under these conditions, the emergence of comparatively strong nonspecific signal mediators related to skin temperature and thermal comfort may filter out a portion of the respiratory-metabolic signal. The dependence of RPE on the relative metabolic rate is consequently dampened.

The relation between RPE and %$\dot{V}O_2$max is also distorted when perceptual responses are compared at the blood lactate inflection point (Purvis and Cureton 1981; DeMello et al. 1987). Rated perceptions of exertion are reasonably constant at the lactate inflection point even though the %$\dot{V}O_2$max at which blood lactate begins to accumulate varies widely between individuals who differ in functional aerobic power and state of training. This observation prompted the suggestion that the onset of blood lactate accumulation might be a more appropriate reference than %$\dot{V}O_2$max when comparing perceptual responses between individuals who

Table 5.2   Relative Level of Oxygen Consumption as a Mediator of Perceived Exertion: Research Summary

Investigation (author)	Exercise type	Perturbation factor[a]
Supporting evidence		
Bar-Or and Reed (1986)	Cycle/treadmill	Fitness/body fat
Bar-Or and Reed (1986)	Ergometer/arms & legs	Neuromuscular disease
Berry et al. (1989)	Treadmill walk/run	Exercise mode, aerobic fitness
Davies and Sargeant (1979)	Treadmill	Atropine/practolol
Docktor and Sharkey (1971)	Treadmill walk	Exercise training
Ekblom and Goldbarg (1971)	Cycle/treadmill	Exercise mode & training
Haskvitz et al. (1992)	Cycle	Aerobic training
Hetzler et al. (1991)	Cycle/treadmill	Exercise mode
Horstman et al. (1979)	Treadmill walk/run	Exercise mode
Noble, Maresh, and Ritchey (1981)	Treadmill walk/run	Gender differences
Pandolf (1986)	Cycle/arms & legs	Exercise mode
Pivarnik, Grafner, and Elkins (1988)	Cycle	Exercise mode, ambient temperature
Pollock, Jackson, and Foster (1986)	Cycle/arms & legs	Exercise mode
Robertson et al. (1982)	Cycle	RBC reinfusion
Sargeant and Davies (1973)	Cycle (1 & 2 limbs)	Exercise mode & limb volume
Sargeant and Davies (1977)	Cycle	Limb volume
Seip et al. (1991)	Cycle	Training status
Sidney and Shephard (1977)	Cycle/treadmill	Age, exercise mode, training
Sidney and Shephard (1977)	Cycle/treadmill Walk	Gender differences
Skinner et al. (1973)	Cycle	Body fat
Sovijarvi et al. (1979)	Cycle/Negative air ionization	
Young, Cymerman, and Pandolf (1982)	Cycle	High altitude
Nonsupporting evidence		
DeMello et al. (1987)	Treadmill	Functional exercise capacity, lactate inflection point
Hill et al. (1987)	Treadmill/cycle	Interval/continuous training
Mihevic et al. (1981)	Cycle	Aerobic fitness
Myles and Saunders (1979)	Treadmill	Light & heavy external loads
Pivarnik and Senay (1986)	Cycle	Exercise training, heat stress
Purvis and Cureton (1981)	Cycle	Gender/lactate inflection point

[a]Procedure used to experimentally manipulate $\%\dot{V}O_2max$.

differ in aerobic fitness (DeMello et al. 1987; Haskvitz et al. 1992; Seip et al. 1991; Hetzler et al. 1991).

In general, experimental evidence indicates that for most exercise conditions, the relative metabolic rate functions as a mediator for respiratory-metabolic signals of exertion. The functional link between $\%\dot{V}O_2max$ and RPE has important implications for perceptually regulated exercise prescriptions as well as laboratory assessment of exercise performance. That is, establishing a relation between $\%\dot{V}O_2max$ and RPE is a prerequisite for perceptually prescribed exercise intensity using estimation-production procedures (see chapter 11). The relative oxygen uptake is also an important physiological reference when RPE is used to predict or evaluate exercise tolerance. Finally, the relative oxygen uptake is a useful metabolic marker with which to compare RPE when different types of exercise modes or limb volumes are involved (Sargeant and Davies 1973).

Carbon Dioxide Excretion (VCO_2)

Ventilatory excretion of CO_2 during exercise serves as a signal mediator for respiratory-metabolic perceptions of exertion. Cafarelli and Noble (1976) were among the first to study the functional link between VCO_2 and perceptual responsiveness during exercise. A hypercapnic breathing mixture was used to perturb $\dot{V}_E$ at exercise intensities equivalent to 54% and 71% $\dot{V}O_2max$. At 54% $\dot{V}O_2max$, $\dot{V}_E$ was higher when subjects breathed an air mixture enriched with 3.5% CO_2 (fig 5.4). RPE did not differ between normocapnic and hypercapnic conditions. However, at 71% $\dot{V}O_2max$, both $\dot{V}_E$ and RPE were higher during the hypercapnic condition. These data suggest that during higher intensity exercise, a greater ventilatory drive secondary to the increased demand for CO_2 excretion mediates respiratory-metabolic signals of exertion.

More recently, Robertson et al. (1986) used $NaHCO_3$ ingestion to examine the mediating effect of ventilatory buffering on respiratory-metabolic signals of exertion. The alkalotic shift in blood pH that attends $NaHCO_3$ ingestion attenuates the drive for respiratory excretion of CO_2 during high-intensity exercise. A corresponding reduction is noted in the intensity of respiratory-metabolic sensations of exertion. In the Robertson et al. (1986) experiment, ventilation, RR, and RPE-C did not differ between acid-base conditions at lower exercise intensities where respiratory buffering of metabolic acidosis is limited. However, both respiratory function and RPE-C were attenuated under induced alkalosis at 80% $\dot{V}O_2max$. At higher exercise intensities, ventilatory excretion of CO_2 to buffer metabolic acidosis would appear to serve as a physiological mediator for respiratory-metabolic signals of exertion.

Heart Rate

Evidence supporting heart rate (HR) as a physiological mediator for respiratory-metabolic signals of exertion is not consistent and in some cases may be misleading (Robertson 1982). While intrathoracic pressure changes during myocardial contractions may be consciously monitored at rest, it is unlikely that HR is

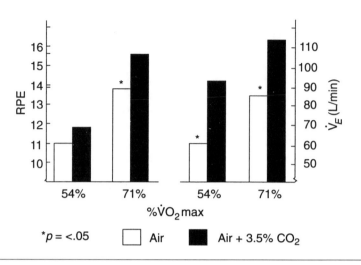

Figure 5.4   Effect of hypercapnia on rated perceived exertion (RPE) and pulmonary ventilation ($\dot{V}_E$) during running.
Reprinted from Robertson 1982.

perceived during exercise. However, from a historical perspective, a large amount of research pertaining to the physiological basis of exertional perceptions has explored HR as a signal mediator. For this reason, the relation between HR and respiratory-metabolic signals of exertion is considered here.

The format for the Borg RPE scale (Borg 1962) provided the first suggestion that HR might serve as a perceptual signal mediator. Because the RPE scale has categories ranging from 6 to 20, a given perceptual rating can be multiplied by a factor of 10 to approximate the exercise HR. The validity of the RPE × 10 ratio is acceptable for younger and middle-aged men during exercise at comparatively high power outputs (Mihevic, Gliner, and Horvath 1981) but is questionable for children and adolescents (Bar-Or 1977).

The majority of the evidence linking HR with perceptual signals of exertion is derived from correlational data. Borg's (1962) initial efforts to validate the RPE scale yielded a correlation of $r = .85$ between HR and RPE responses to progressively increasing power outputs. Correlation coefficients ranging from $r = .42$ to $r = .94$ have been found between HR and RPE while lifting weights (Gamberale 1972), pushing a wheelbarrow (Gamberale 1972), riding a cycle ergometer (Borg 1973; Edwards et al. 1972; Gamberale 1972; Löllgen, Ulmer, and von Nieding 1977; Eston and Williams 1986), transporting external weights (Skinner et al. 1973, Goslin and Rorke 1986), treadmill walking (Skinner et al. 1973), performing one- and two-limb exercise (Gamberale 1972; Sargeant and Davies 1973), and immersed in cold water (Toner, Drolet, and Pandolf 1986). The relation between HR and RPE is approximately the same in younger and older age groups (Eston and Williams 1986).

The foregoing correlational evidence suggests that HR may function as a perceptual signal mediator. However, correlational data cannot be used to infer causality. A substantial amount of experimental evidence shows a general lack of correspondence between HR and RPE when one or the other variable has been experimentally manipulated during dynamic exercise. As an example, Pandolf (1977) demonstrated that during submaximal exercise, HR increased as a function of increasing environmental temperature, while RPE was unchanged by heat stress (fig. 5.5). The literature reviews of Robertson (1982) and Pandolf (1983) should be consulted for a more specific description of those investigations that demonstrate a lack of correspondence between HR and RPE during exercise. When the experimental evidence is examined collectively, it can be concluded that HR does not appear to function as a physiological mediator for respiratory-metabolic signals of exertion.

Blood Pressure

It is possible that mechanisms involving CNS regulation of vascular smooth muscle mediate perceptual signals of exertion through a neurological pathway

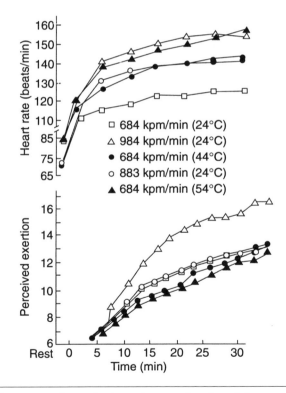

Figure 5.5   Heart rate and perceived exertion as a function of time at various physical work loads and environmental temperatures.
Reprinted from Pandolf 1977.

not yet defined (Pandolf 1983). In this regard, a relation between scaled perceptual responses and systemic blood pressure has been found by some investigators (Juhani, Pekka, and Timo 1986; Pandolf 1986) and not by others (Squires et al. 1982, Perkins et al. 1991).

Threshold for the Respiratory-Metabolic Signal

Ventilatory drive does not appear to be a potent perceptual signal mediator at lower exercise intensities (Edwards et al. 1972; Robertson et al. 1982). However, at a critical metabolic rate between 45% and 75% $\dot{V}O_2$max, sensory signals associated with ventilatory drive begin to intensify and are readily perceived. Not coincidentally, the blood lactate inflection point also occurs within this range of exercise intensities. As isocapnic buffering of metabolic acidosis is initiated at the lactate inflection point (Wasserman 1978) the comparatively sudden onset of signals reflecting respiratory-metabolic exertion may in part be linked to an exponential increase in CO_2 excretion (Jones 1984). In support of this hypothesis, a strong correlation has been noted between RPE and $\dot{V}_E/\dot{V}O_2$, the latter variable being directly related to respiratory excretion of CO_2 (Pandolf 1986). Corroborating evidence in support of a threshold for the onset of respiratory-metabolic sensations of exertion is provided by Cafarelli and Noble (1976) and Robertson et al. (1986), who observed that ventilatory drive functioned as a perceptual signal mediator at high but not low metabolic rates. Similarly, $\dot{V}_E$, $\dot{V}O_2$, and HR do not become statistically significant predictors of RPE-C until exercise intensity exceeds 75% $\dot{V}O_2$max (Noble et al. 1986).

In contrast, Killian and Jones (1984) question a threshold for the sudden increase in respiratory-metabolic perceptual signal. They report that normal subjects and pulmonary patients are consistently able to scale perceptions of respiratory effort while at rest under resistive loading conditions and during low-level exercise. Therefore, the concept of a finite metabolic threshold for the onset of the respiratory-metabolic signal of exertion remains unclear.

Integrative Model

Ventilatory drive and the requirements for oxygen uptake and carbon dioxide excretion appear to be the most important physiological mediators for respiratory-metabolic signals of exertion. The trilevel model presented in figure 5.6 describes the effect of respiratory-metabolic signal mediators when juxtaposed with peripheral mediators (Robertson 1982). In level I, the metabolic rate is less than 50% $\dot{V}O_2$max, and the symptomatic responses reflect an awareness of movement. The strength of the respiratory-metabolic signal at this level is minimal. As the metabolic rate approaches the lactate inflection point (i.e., 50-70% $\dot{V}O_2$max), exercise is perceived to be effortful but tolerable. The transition from level I to II corresponds to a change in ventilatory response from exercise hyperpnea to isocapnic buffering (Wasserman 1978). At this level, the respiratory-metabolic signal begins to intensify. When level III is attained, the metabolic rate is in excess of 70% $\dot{V}O_2$max. The activity may be considered painful or unpleasant and at the highest exercise intensities may be terminated because of these intolerable subjective symptoms. The transition from level II to III is accompanied by a change in ventilatory response from isocapnic buffering to a respiratory compensation of metabolic acidosis (Wasserman 1978). At level III, respiratory-metabolic signals of exertion are very strong and contribute significantly to the overall body perception of exertion (Robertson et al. 1979b).

When exercise is performed in normoxic environments and in the absence of lung disease, the strength of the respiratory-metabolic signal of exertion is usually lower than that of the peripheral muscle signal at all submaximal intensities. In contrast, respiratory-metabolic signal strength is equal to or greater than the peripheral signal during exercise in hypoxic environments (Young, Cymerman, and Pandolf 1982) or when forced breathing patterns are necessitated by an activity such as swimming (Noble et al. 1986). During exercise, patients with lung disease also report sensations of respiratory effort that are comparatively more intense than peripheral exertional signals, often terminating the performance because of unbearable breathlessness or dyspnea (Killian 1985).

The perceived magnitude of respiratory effort increases as a positively accelerating power function of added resistive loads, with the relation having an exponent of 1.6 (Gamberale et al. 1978). The order of magnitude of this exponent is similar to that reported for total body muscular effort (Borg 1962; Borg 1982), suggesting commonality in the underlying neurophysiological pathways for both types of sensations. This possibility is explored in chapter 7, which examines the final common pathway for perceptual signals of exertion.

Level	Symptoms	Metabolic intensity %$\dot{V}O_2$max	Relative contribution		
			Respiratory-metabolic		Peripheral
			$\dot{V}_E$	%$\dot{V}O_2$max	
I	Movement awareness	< 50	Limited	Proportional	Dominant
II	Discomfort tolerance	50-70	Moderate	Proportional	Dominant
III	Noxious pain avoidance	> 70	Significant	Proportional	Dominant

Figure 5.6   Model of the potentiating relationship between respiratory-metabolic and peripheral signals of exertion at low (level I), moderate (level II), and high (level III) metabolic rates.
Reprinted from Robertson 1982.

Summary

This chapter considered three possible physiological mediators for the respiratory-metabolic signal of perceived exertion. Both experimental and clinical evidence strongly supports ventilatory function as a physiological mediator for the respiratory-metabolic signal. It appears that the perceptual mediating influence of ventilatory drive is not especially pronounced until moderate exercise intensities associated with the lactate inflation point are achieved. Oxygen uptake exerts a mediating effect on perceptual signal strength when expressed in relative (i.e., %$\dot{V}O_2$max) but not absolute (i.e., L/min) terms. When experimentally perturbed, RPE and exercise heart rate do not change proportionally, which calls into question the role of cardiac frequency in mediating the intensity of the respiratory-metabolic perceptual signal.

References

Bakers, J.H., and S.M. Tenney. 1970. The perception of some sensations associated with breathing. *Respir. Physiol.* 10:85-92.

Bar-Or, O. 1977. Age related changes in exercise perception. In *Physical work and effort,* ed. G. Borg, 255-266, New York: Pergamon Press.

Bar-Or, O., and S.L. Reed. 1986. Ratings of perceived exertion in adolescents with neuromuscular disease. In *The perception of exertion in physical work,* ed. G. Borg and D. Ottoson, 137-48. London: Macmillan.

Berry, M.J., A. Weyrich, R. Roberds, and K. Krause. 1989. Ratings of perceived exertion in individuals with varying fitness levels during walking or running. *Eur. J. Appl. Physiol. Occup. Physiol.* 58 (5):494-99.

Borg, G. 1962. Physical performance and perceived exertion. In *Studia psychologia et paedagogica,* vol. 11, 1-35. Lund, Sweden: Gleerup.

————. 1973. *A note on a category scale with "ratio properties" for estimating perceived exertion.* Reports from the Institute of Applied Psychology, no. 366. Stockholm: Univ. of Stockholm.

————. 1976. *Perception of panting during ergometer work.* Reports from the Institute of Applied Psychology, no. 73. Stockholm: Univ. of Stockholm.

————. 1982. Psychophysical bases of perceived exertion. *Med. Sci. Sports Exerc.* 14:377-81.

Cafarelli, E. 1977. Peripheral and central inputs to the effort sense during cycling exercise. *Eur. J. Appl. Physiol.* 37:181-89.

Cafarelli, E., and B.J. Noble. 1976. The effect of inspired carbon dioxide on subjective estimates of exertion during exercise. *Ergonomics* 19:581-89.

Davies, C.T., and A.J. Sargeant. 1979. The effects of atropine and practolol on the perception of exertion during treadmill exercise. *Ergonomics* 22:1141-46.

DeMello, J.J., K.J. Cureton, R.E. Boineau, and M.M. Singh. 1987. Ratings of perceived exertion at the lactate threshold in trained and untrained men and women. *Med. Sci. Sports Exerc.* 19:354-62.

Docktor, R., and B. Sharkey. 1971. Note on some physiological and subjective reactions to exercise and training. *Percept. Motor Skills* 32:233-34.

Edwards, R.H.T., A. Melcher, C.M. Hesser, O. Wigebtz, and L.G. Ekelund. 1972. Physiological correlates of perceived exertion in continuous and intermittent exercise with the same average power output. *Eur. J. Clin. Invest.* 2:108-14.

Ekblom, B., and A.N. Goldbarg. 1971. The influence of physical training and other factors on the subjective rating of perceived exertion. *Acta Physiol. Scand.* 83:399-406.

Eston, R.G., and J.G. Williams. 1986. Exercise intensity and perceived exertion in adolescent boys. *Br. J. Sports Med.* 20:27-30.

Franklin, B.A., L. Vander, D. Wrisley, and M. Rubenfire. 1983. Aerobic requirements of arm ergometry: Implications for exercise testing and training. *Physician Sportsmed.* 11:81-90.

Gamberale, F. 1972. Perception of exertion, heart rate, oxygen uptake and blood lactate in different work operations. *Ergonomics* 15:545-54.

Gamberale, F., I. Holmér, A.S. Kindblom, and A. Nordström. 1978. Magnitude perception of added inspiratory resistance during steady-state exercise. *Ergonomics* 21:531-38.

Goslin, B.R., and S.C. Rorke. 1986. The perception of exertion during load carriage. *Ergonomics* 29:677-86.

Haskvitz, E.M., R.L. Seip, J.Y. Weltman, A.D. Rogol, and A. Weltman. 1992. The effect of training intensity on ratings of perceived exertion. *Int. J. Sports Med.* 13:377-83.

Hetzler, R.K., R.L. Seip, S.H. Boutcher, E. Pierce, D. Snead, and A. Weltman. 1991. Effect of exercise modality on ratings of perceived exertion at various lactate concentrations. *Med. Sci. Sports Exerc.* 23:88-92.

Hill, D.W., K.J. Cureton, S.C. Grisham, and M.A. Collins. 1987. Effect of training on the rating of perceived exertion at the ventilatory threshold. *Eur. J. Appl. Physiol.* 56:206-11.

Horstman, D.H., W.P. Morgan, A. Cymerman, and J. Stokes. 1979. Perception of effort during constant work to self-imposed exhaustion. *Percept. Motor Skills* 48:1111-26.

Jones, N.L. 1984. Dyspnea in exercise. *Med. Sci. Sports Exerc.* 16:14-19.

Juhani, I., S. Pekka, and A. Timo. 1986. Strain while skiing and hauling a sledge or carrying a backpack. *Eur. J. Appl. Physiol.* 55:597-603.

Kamon, E., K. Pandolf, and E. Cafarelli. 1974. The relationship between perceptual information and physiological responses to exercise in the heat. *J. Human Ergol.* 3:45-54.

Killian, K.J. 1985. The objective measurement of breathlessness. *Chest* 88 (Suppl.): 84S-90S.

Killian, K.J., and N.L. Jones. 1984. The use of exercise testing and other methods in the investigation of dyspnea. *Clin. Chest Med.* 5:99-108.

Löllgen, H., T. Graham, and G. Sjogaard. 1980. Muscle metabolites, force, and perceived exertion bicycling at varying pedal rates. *Med. Sci. Sports Exerc.* 12:345-51.

Löllgen, H., H.V. Ulmer, and G. von Nieding. 1977. Heart rate and perceptual responses to exercise with different pedalling speed in normal subjects and patients. *Eur. J. Appl. Physiol.* 37:297-304.

Maresh, C.M., M.R. Deschenes, R.L. Seip, L.E. Armstrong, K.L. Robertson, and B.J. Noble. 1993. Perceived exertion during hypobaric hypoxia in low- and moderate-altitude natives. *Med. Sci. Sports Exerc.* 25:945-51.

Mihevic, P.M. 1983. Cardiovascular fitness and the psychophysics of perceived exertion. *Res. Q. Exerc. Sport* 54:239-46.

Mihevic, P.M., J.A. Gliner, and S.M. Horvath. 1981. Perception of effort and respiratory sensitivity during exposure to ozone. *Ergonomics* 24:365-74.

Morgan, W.P., K. Hirta, G.A. Weitz, and B. Balke. 1976. Hypnotic perturbation of perceived exertion: Ventilatory consequences. *Am. J. Clin. Hypn.* 18:182-90.

Myles, W.S., and P.L. Saunders. 1979. The physiological cost of carrying light and heavy loads. *Eur. J. Appl. Physiol.* 42:125-31.

Noble, B.J., W.J. Kraemer, J.G. Allen, J.S. Plank, and L.A. Woodard. 1986. The integration of physiological cues in effort perception: Stimulus strength vs. relative contribution. In *The perception of exertion in physical work,* ed. G. Borg and D. Ottoson, 83-96. London: Macmillan.

Noble, B.J., C.M. Maresh, and M. Ritchey. 1981. Comparison of exercise sensations between females and males. In *Women and sports: An historical, biological, physiological and sports medicine approach,* ed. J. Borms, M. Hebbelinck, and A. Venerando, 175-79. Basel: Karger.

Noble, B.J., K.F. Metz, K.B. Pandolf, and E. Cafarelli. 1973. Perceptual responses to exercise: A multiple regression study. *Med. Sci. Sports* 5:104-9.

Pandolf, K.B. 1977. Psychological and physiological factors influencing perceived exertion. In *Physical work and effort,* ed. G. Borg, 371-84. New York: Pergamon Press.

———. 1983. Advances in the study and application of perceived exertion. *Exerc. Sport Sci. Rev.* 11:118-58.

———. 1986. Local and central factor contributions in the perception of effort during physical exercise. In *The perception of exertion in physical work,* ed. G. Borg and D. Ottoson, 97-110. London: Macmillan.

Pandolf, K.B., D.S. Billings, L.L. Drolet, N.A. Pimental, and M.N. Sawka. 1984. Differentiated ratings of perceived exertion and various physiological responses during prolonged upper and lower body exercise. *Eur. J. Appl. Physiol.* 53:5-11.

Pandolf, K.B., E. Cafarelli, B.J. Noble, and K.F. Metz. 1972. Perceptual responses during prolonged work. *Percept. Motor Skills* 35:975-85.

Pandolf, K.B., and B.J. Noble. 1973. The effect of pedalling speed and resistance changes on perceived exertion for equivalent power outputs on the bicycle ergometer. *Med. Sci. Sports* 5:132-36.

Pederson, P.K., and H.G. Welch. 1977. Oxygen breathing, selected physiological variables and perception of effort during submaximal exercise. In *Physical work and effort*, ed. G. Borg, 385-400. New York: Pergamon Press.

Perkins, R.K., J.E. Sexton, R.D. Solberg-Kassel, and L.H. Epstein. 1991. Estimates of type A behavior do not predict perceived exertion during graded exercise. *Med. Sci. Sports Exerc.* 23:11:1283-88.

Pivarnik, J.M., T.R. Grafner, and E.S. Elkins. 1988. Metabolic, thermoregulatory, and psychophysiological responses during arm and leg exercise. *Med. Sci. Sports Exerc.* 20:1-5.

Pivarnik, J.M., and L.C. Senay. 1986. Effect of endurance training and heat acclimation on perceived exertion during exercise. *J. Cardiopul. Rehab.* 6:499-504.

Pollock, M.L., A.S. Jackson, and C. Foster. 1986. The use of the perception scale for exercise prescription. In *The perception of exertion in physical work*, ed. G. Borg and D. Ottoson, 161-78. London: Macmillan.

Purvis, J.W., and K.J. Cureton. 1981. Ratings of perceived exertion at the anaerobic threshold. *Ergonomics* 24:295-300.

Robertson, R.J. 1982. Central signals of perceived exertion during dynamic exercise. *Med. Sci. Sports Exerc.* 14:390-96.

Robertson, R.J., J.E. Falkel, A.L. Drash, A.M. Swank, K.F. Metz, S.A. Spungen, and J.R. LeBoeuf. 1986. Effect of blood pH on peripheral and central signals of perceived exertion. *Med. Sci. Sports Exerc.* 18:114-22.

Robertson, R.J., R. Gilcher, K. Metz, T. Allison, H. Bahnson, G. Skrinar, A. Abbott, R. Becker, and J. Falkel. 1982. Effect of induced erythrocythemia on hypoxia tolerance during physical exercise. *J. Appl. Physiol. Respir. Environ. Exerc. Physiol.* 53:490-95.

Robertson, R.J., R.L. Gillespie, J. McCarthy, and K.D. Rose. 1979a. Differentiated perceptions of exertion: Part I. Mode of integration of regional signals. *Percept. Motor Skills* 49:683-89.

———. 1979b. Differentiated perceptions of exertion: Part II. Relationship to local and central physiological responses. *Percept. Motor Skills* 49:691-97.

Robertson, R.J., and K.F. Metz. 1986. Ventilatory precursors for central signals of perceived exertion. In *The perception of exertion in physical work*, ed. G. Borg and D. Ottoson, 111-21. London: Macmillan.

Sargeant, A.J., and C.T. Davies. 1973. Perceived exertion during rhythmic exercise involving different muscle masses. *J. Human Ergol.* 2:3-11.

———. 1977. Perceived exertion of dynamic exercise in normal subjects and patients following leg injury. In *Physical work and effort*, ed. G. Borg, 345-56. New York: Pergamon Press.

Seip, R.L., D. Snead, E.F. Pierce, P. Stein, and A. Weltman. 1991. Perceptual responses and blood lactate concentration: Effect of training state. *Med. Sci. Sports Exerc.* 23:80-87.

Sidney, K.H., and R.J. Shepard. 1977. Perception of exertion in the elderly, effects of aging, mode of exercise, and physical training. *Percept. Motor Skills* 44:999-1010.

Skinner, J.S., G. Borg, and E.R. Buskirk. 1969. Physiological and perceptual reactions to exertion of young men differing in activity and body size. In *Exercise and fitness,* ed. B.D. Franks, 53-66. Chicago: Athletic Institute.

Skinner, J.S., R. Hustler, V. Bersteinova, and E.R. Buskirk. 1973. Perception of effort during different types of exercise and under different environmental conditions. *Med. Sci. Sports* 5:110-55.

Smutok, M.A., G.S. Skrinar, and K.B. Pandolf. 1980. Exercise intensity: Subjective regulation by perceived exertion. *Arch. Phys. Med. Rehab.* 61:569-74.

Sovijarvi, A.R., S. Rosset, J. Hyvarinen, A. Franssila, G. Graeffe, M. Lehtimcki. 1979. Effect of air ionization on heart rate and perceived exertion during a bicycle exercise test. A double-blind cross-over study. *Eur. J. Appl. Physiol.* 41:285-91.

Squires, R.W., J.L. Rod, M.L. Pollock, and C. Foster. 1982. Effects of propranolol on perceived exertion after myocardial revascularization surgery. *Med. Sci. Sports Exerc.* 14:276-80.

Toner, M.M., L.L. Drolet, and K.B. Pandolf. 1986. Perceptual and physiological responses during exercise in cool and cold water. *Percept. Motor Skills* 62:211-20.

Wasserman, K. 1978. Breathing during exercise. *New Engl. J. Med.* 298:780-85.

Yorio, J.M., R.K. Dishman, W.R. Forbus, K.J. Cureton, and R.E. Graham. 1992. Breathlessness predicts perceived exertion in young women with mild asthma. *Med. Sci. Sports Exerc.* 24:860-67.

Young, A.J., A. Cymerman, and K.B. Pandolf. 1982. Differentiated ratings of perceived exertion are influenced by high altitude exposures. *Med. Sci. Sports Exerc.* 14:223-28.

6

CHAPTER

Peripheral and Nonspecific Physiological Mediators

Peripheral signals of exertion during dynamic exercise are mediated by physiological events in active muscles and joints. Recent evidence indicates that a class of physiological mediators called *nonspecific* also has an important effect on perceptual responsiveness during exercise. Because several peripheral and nonspecific factors exert their sensory influence through interrelated physiological events, both classes of mediators are discussed in this chapter.

Peripheral Mediators

Peripheral physiological mediators are primarily regionalized to exercising muscles in the limbs, trunk, and upper torso (including the shoulder and neck). Physiological processes that are thought to mediate the intensity of peripheral exertional perceptions are (1) metabolic acidosis (pH and lactic acid), (2) fast- and slow-twitch contractile properties of skeletal muscle fiber, (3) muscle blood flow, and (4) blood-borne energy substrates (i.e., glucose, free fatty acids, glycerol).

Metabolic Acidosis

The intensity of peripheral exertional perceptions has been linked to acidotic shifts in blood pH and to the appearance of lactic acid in blood and muscle. The following sections consider evidence that both supports and refutes these factors as physiological mediators for peripheral perceptual signals.

Blood pH

During high-intensity dynamic exercise, shifts in blood pH are thought to mediate peripheral perceptions of exertion in active limbs (Kostka and Cafarelli 1982; Robertson et al. 1986). An examination of some of the research upon which this observation is based may be helpful. Robertson et al. (1986) used $NaHCO_3$ ingestion to alter blood pH responses during arm and leg exercise at relative metabolic rates ranging from 20% to 80% $\dot{V}O_2max$. Differentiated ratings of exertion were determined for the active and inactive limbs during both arm and leg exercise. By varying limb involvement between different exercise modes, it was possible to directly link blood pH shifts with differentiated peripheral perceptions arising from active muscle mass. Blood pH was higher following ingestion of $NaHCO_3$ than $CaCO_3$ (i.e., a placebo) for all exercise modes (fig. 6.1; Robertson et al. 1986). During arm exercise at 80% $\dot{V}O_2max$, the differentiated rating of exertion for the arms (RPE-A) was lower under the alkalotic than under the placebo condition. RPE-A was not affected by blood acid-base shifts during leg exercise. The reciprocal was seen for the leg rating; that is, RPE-L was lower under alkalosis during leg exercise but did not differ from the placebo condition during arm exercise. These findings indicate that shifts in blood pH during high-intensity exercise (i.e., 80% $\dot{V}O_2max$) mediate peripheral exertional sensations in active muscle. The higher the blood pH (i.e., lower [H^+] concentration), the less intense are the peripheral perceptions of exertion arising from involved body

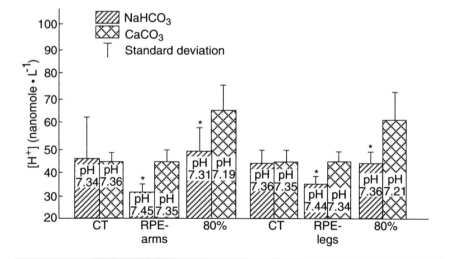

Figure 6.1   Effect of induced alkalosis on venous blood [H^+] and pH at control (CT), preexercise (Pre), and 80% $\dot{V}O_2max$. At each sampling period, an * indicates that means are significantly different ($p < .01$) between acid-base conditions.
Reprinted from Robertson et al. 1986.

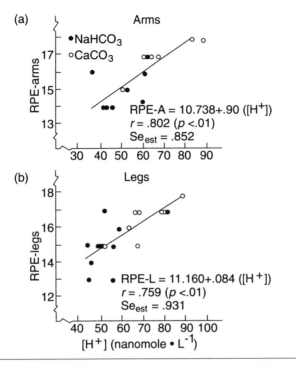

Figure 6.2 Regression analysis of the relationship between blood [H⁺] and differentiated ratings of perceived exertion (RPE) during separate (*a*) arm and (*b*) leg exercise at 80% $\dot{V}O_2$max.
Reprinted from Robertson et al. 1986.

regions (fig. 6.2). It is interesting that differentiated ratings of exertion for both the arms and legs were not affected by changes in blood pH when the relative exercise intensity was below 80% $\dot{V}O_2$max, suggesting a threshold effect.

The reciprocal of the above findings has been reported by Kostka and Cafarelli (1982); that is, when acidotic shifts in blood pH were induced by NH_4Cl ingestion, exertional perceptions were intensified. When viewed in juxtaposition, the investigations of Robertson et al. (1986) and Kostka and Cafarelli (1982) provide convincing support for blood pH as a physiological mediator of peripheral perceptions of exertion. The mediating effect of blood pH on peripheral signals occurs at higher but not lower exercise intensities. That is, neither alkalotic (Robertson et al. 1986) nor acidotic (Kostka and Cafarelli 1982) shifts in blood pH influence peripheral perceptual responses during exercise that is performed at relatively low metabolic rates. Metabolic acidosis is usually minimal below the lactate inflection point (50-70% $\dot{V}O_2$max). As a result, blood acid-base status does not begin to mediate the intensity of peripheral exertional signals until a metabolic marker, such as the lactate inflection point, is reached (Robertson et al. 1986).

Once the lactate inflection point is attained, a shift in blood pH of approximately 0.10 units is most likely needed to mediate the intensity of exertional perceptions. Kostka and Cafarelli (1982) did not find an attenuation in effort sensation when blood pH increased by only 0.04 units following $NaHCO_3$ ingestion. In contrast, Robertson et al. (1986) observed an attenuation in perceptual intensity when blood pH increased by 0.10 units under induced alkalosis. Apparently, shifts in blood pH that are substantially less than 0.10 units are not sufficient to mediate peripheral exertional signals.

Further confirmation of blood pH as a mediator of perceptual intensity is presented in figure 6.3 (Robertson et al. 1992). Both RPE and blood pH were measured during a 12-min supine recovery period following four different treadmill test protocols. The postexercise abatement of metabolic acidosis was comparatively more rapid following the least aggressive (1 MET increment per stage) than following the most aggressive (4 MET increment per stage) protocol. The abatement of exertional perceptions was also faster for the least aggressive than the most aggressive protocol. These findings suggest that a causal link between the intensity of exertional perceptions and blood pH exists during recovery from exercise as well as during exercise.

A few investigations question the role of blood pH as a physiological mediator for peripheral exertional perceptions. Robertson et al. (1979b) found that during cycling at a constant power output, differentiated ratings of perceived exertion for the legs (RPE-L) were higher at slower pedaling rates than at faster ones, while blood pH was unaffected by pedaling rate. Similarly, Poulus, Docter, and Westra (1974) observed that sensations of fatigue intensified as a function of elapsed exercise time despite "normalization" of blood pH via continuous infusion of $NaHCO_3$. In both experiments, peripheral perceptual ratings and blood pH were independent responses during exercise. It is not entirely clear why the results of these experiments and those of Robertson et al. (1986) and Kostka and Cafarelli (1982) are inconsistent.

The physiological mechanism underlying blood pH as a mediator for peripheral perceptions of exertion involves a disruption in contractile and energy-producing properties of skeletal muscle (Kostka and Cafarelli 1982; Poulus, Docter, and Westra 1974; Robertson et al. 1986). This mechanism assumes that blood pH shifts are indicative of corresponding shifts in muscle pH and that blood and tissue acid-base alterations occur within a comparatively similar time frame (Jones et al. 1977; Sutton, Jones, and Toews 1981). The relative acidosis that accompanies high-intensity exercise inhibits the activity of intermediate glycolytic enzymes such as phosphofructokinase and lactate dehydrogenase. Glycolytic production of ATP for myofibril contraction is interrupted, causing fatigue of metabolically active muscle (Jones et al. 1977; Sutton, Jones, and Toews 1981). As muscles fatigue, motor unit recruitment and firing frequency increase (Cafarelli 1977; Kostka and Cafarelli 1982; Löllgen, Graham, and Sjogaard 1980). These increases in motor unit activation are monitored by the sensory cortex (McCloskey et al. 1983). The greater the magnitude of motor unit activation, the more intense are the exertional signals arising from peripheral skeletal muscle.

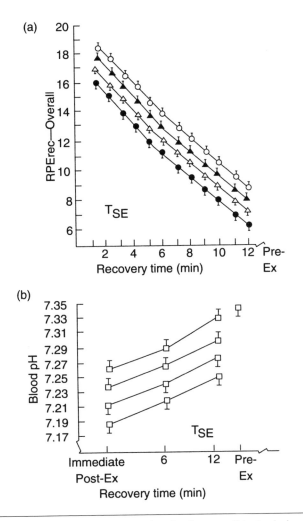

Figure 6.3   (*a*) Ratings of perceived exertion for the overall body during recovery (RPErec-Overall) from maximal treadmill exercise and (*b*) blood pH following maximal treadmill exercise using four different protocols. Values are means ± *SE* for treadmill protocols A (●), B (○), C (▲), and D (△). The preexercise value is an average of the four protocols.
Reprinted from Robertson et. al. 1992.

Blood Lactic Acid

Blood lactic acid concentration [Hla] is thought to mediate the intensity of peripheral perceptions of exertion in active limbs during high-intensity exercise (Allen and Pandolf 1977; Noble et al. 1983; Young, Cymerman, and Pandolf

1982). However, unlike blood pH, the specific role of [Hla] in mediating perceptions of exertion is not clearly understood (Robertson et al. 1988). Substantial correlational evidence suggests a link between blood [Hla] and rated perceptions of exertion for the body overall and for differentiated responses in the arms and legs (Pandolf 1983). In contrast, experimental paradigms that manipulated [Hla] to determine if exertional perceptions exhibited corresponding changes have not consistently demonstrated a causal relation between variables (Pandolf 1983). A more extensive examination of this inconsistent evidence is helpful in determining the extent to which blood [Hla] influences the intensity of exertional perceptions.

Correlational and Experimental Evidence.   Considerable correlational evidence suggests that blood [Hla] is related to the intensity of both undifferentiated and differentiated perceptions of exertion. Correlation coefficients for the relation between [Hla] and RPE range from .42 to .84 for exercise on a treadmill, stationary cycle, and arm ergometer (Skrinar, Ingram, and Pandolf 1983; Edwards et al. 1972; Allen and Pandolf 1977; Morgan and Pollock 1977; DeMello et al. 1987; Robertson et al. 1979a, 1979b; Borg, Ljunggren, and Ceci 1985; Ljunggren, Ceci, and Karlsson 1987). The relation between blood [Hla] and perceived exertion during both continuous and intermittent exercise can be expressed as [Hla] = 0.64 RPE − 4.6; r = .83 (Edwards et al. 1972). In general, RPE increases as a negatively accelerating function of blood [Hla] in trained and untrained men and women during both cycle and treadmill exercise (Pederson and Welch 1977; DeMello et al. 1987; Borg, Hassmen, and Lagerstrom 1987; Skrinar, Ingram, and Pandolf 1983). As an example, figure 6.4 shows that RPE increases as a

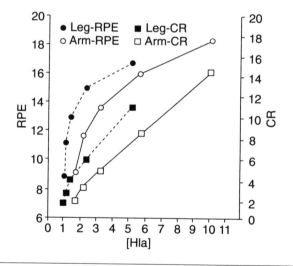

Figure 6.4   Relationships between ratings of perceived exertion, rated on the RPE scale and the CR scale, and blood lactate ([Hla]; mmol/L) for leg and arm exercises. Reprinted from Borg, Hassmen, and Lagerstrom 1987.

negative function of venous blood [Hla] during arm and leg exercise using both the Borg 10-graded category-ratio scale and the Borg 15-graded category scale (Borg, Hassmen, and Lagerstrom 1987). In addition, blood [Hla] is consistently among the first variables to enter multiple regression equations to predict RPE during dynamic exercise (Johansson 1986; Pandolf 1986; Borg, Ljunggren, and Ceci 1985).

The comparatively strong correlation between [Hla] and RPE that is seen under a variety of exercise conditions suggests that the appearance of lactate in blood mediates the intensity of peripheral exertional perceptions. However, the identification of a physiological mediator for perceived exertion requires that a specific cause-and-effect relation be established between variables. Such a causal relation cannot be inferred solely from correlational evidence. The findings of experimental investigations that manipulate [Hla] to determine if corresponding changes occur in perceived exertion must also be examined. A considerable amount of this experimental evidence both refutes and supports blood [Hla] as a physiological mediator for the intensity of exertional perceptions.

Refuting Evidence. A substantial number of psychophysiological experiments have shown that perturbation of blood [Hla] does not yield corresponding changes in the intensity of scaled exertional perceptions (Skrinar, Ingram, and Pandolf 1983; Löllgen, Graham, and Sjogaard 1980; Stamford and Noble 1974; Robertson et al. 1979b; Allen and Pandolf 1977; Pederson and Welch 1977; Bergh et al. 1986; Moffatt and Stamford 1978; Allen et al. 1985; Sargeant and Davies 1973; Young, Cymerman, and Pandolf 1982; Essig, Costill, and Van Handel 1980; the literature review of Pandolf 1983 should be consulted for a more comprehensive list of these experiments). Such experiments question the role of blood [Hla] in mediating the intensity of peripheral exertional perceptions. This conclusion is underscored in a particularly extensive experiment reported by Löllgen, Graham, and Sjogaard (1980). Measurements were obtained for both RPE and anaerobic metabolism using a paradigm wherein power output on a cycle ergometer was kept constant while pedaling frequency varied (i.e., 40, 60, 80, and 100 rpm). A parabolic relation was found between RPE and pedal frequency ($r = .79$; fig. 6.5). In contrast, changes in blood [Hla] as well as muscle ATP, creatine phosphate, phosphagen, and nicotinamide adenine dinucleotide were independent of pedal frequency. These data indicate that neither blood [Hla] nor changes in muscle metabolites mediate exertional perceptions during moderate- to high-intensity (70-100% $\dot{V}O_2max$) exercise.

Supporting Evidence. Several different lines of experimental evidence support blood [Hla] as a physiological mediator for rated perceptions of exertion (Edwards et al. 1972; Gamberale 1972; Young, Cymerman, and Pandolf 1982; Horstman et al. 1979; Noble et al. 1983; Borg, Ljunggren, and Ceci 1985; Borg, Hassmen, and Lagerstrom 1987; Ekblom and Goldbarg 1971; DeMello et al. 1987; the review by Pandolf 1983 should be consulted for a more extensive list of these investigations). As an example, Noble et al. (1983) reported that blood [Hla] and

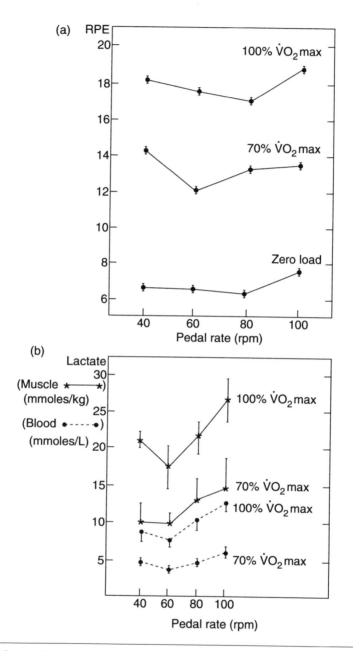

Figure 6.5 (a) Rating of perceived exertion (RPE) during unloaded pedaling, and sub-maximal (70% V̇O₂max) and maximal (100% V̇O₂max) exercise intensity at varying pedal rates and (b) muscle (*) and blood (dots) lactate during submaximal and maximal exercise (means ± SE).

Reprinted from Löllgen, Graham, and Sjogaard 1980.

rated perceptions of exertion for the legs (RPE-L) increased as a positively accelerating function of power output during progressive cycle ergometer exercise (fig. 6.6). The exponents of the functions for blood [Hla] (2.2) and RPE-L (1.65) were reasonably similar, suggesting a psychophysiological link between these variables. Similar power functions for the relation between blood [Hla] and RPE have been reported by Borg, Ljunggren, and Ceci (1985). In addition, Ekblom and Goldbarg (1971) observed that for a given blood [Hla], RPE did not differ between arm and leg exercise, between cycle and treadmill exercise, and between pre- and postexercise training. This evidence suggests that blood [Hla] mediates the intensity of exertional perceptions under a variety of exercise conditions.

Differential Mediating Effect: Blood pH and [Hla]

It is apparent that considerable experimental evidence both supports and refutes blood [Hla] as a physiological mediator for exertional perceptions. These divergent findings can be explained by separating the sensory effects of blood [Hla] from those of blood pH. Inducing metabolic alkalosis via $NaHCO_3$ ingestion provides a mechanism to perturb both blood [Hla] and pH during high-intensity exercise (Robertson et al. 1988). As both [Hla] and pH are higher under alkalosis than under placebo conditions (Jones et al. 1977; Sutton, Jones, and Toews 1981), their separate effects on peripheral exertional perceptions can be studied simultaneously. That is, the intensity of exertional perceptions in active limbs should vary directly with blood [Hla] and inversely with blood pH, assuming both variables mediate the effort sense. As noted in a previous section, peripheral ratings of perceived exertion are attenuated in the presence of alkalotic shifts in blood pH. However, under induced alkalosis the normal inverse relation between blood pH and [Hla] is altered physiologically. The relatively more alkaline environment following $NaHCO_3$ ingestion prolongs glycolytic production of ATP for myofibril contraction, resulting in more complete use of muscle glycogen stores and greater production of [Hla] (Jones et al. 1977; Sutton, Jones, and Toews 1981; Kostka and Cafarelli 1982). As a result, [Hla] is inversely related to peripheral exertional perceptions arising from exercising limbs under conditions of induced alkalosis (fig. 6.7). During high-intensity dynamic exercise, the perception of exertion in peripheral skeletal muscle is mediated by blood pH shifts but is independent of blood [Hla] (Robertson et al. 1988).

What, if any, is the role of blood [Hla] in studying physiological correlates of perceived exertion? A partial answer to this question is found in the strong, positive relation between power output and both rated perceptions of exertion and blood [Hla] during dynamic exercise. Borg, Ljunggren, and Ceci (1985); Borg, Hassmen, and Lagerstrom (1987); and Noble et al. (1983) report that RPE and [Hla] vary as a curvilinear function of power output when cycle ergometer exercise intensity is progressively incremented. It follows that RPE and blood [Hla] are related to each other when power output increases progressively (Borg, Ljunggren, and Ceci 1985; Borg, Hassmen, and Lagerstrom 1987). However, such a relation does not necessarily imply causality. Rather, both RPE and blood

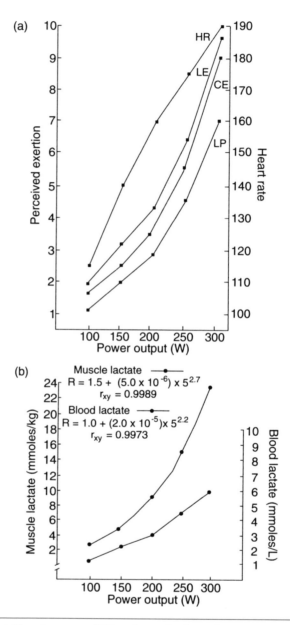

Figure 6.6 (a) Mean heart rate (HR) and perceived exertion responses (LE = leg effort, CE = cardiorespiratory effort, LP = leg pain) plotted as a function of power output (W). (b) Muscle lactate and blood lactate expressed as a function of power output. The exponent of the power function for blood lactate is approximately quadratic (2.2), while the muscle lactate exponent is approximately cubic (2.7).
Reprinted from Noble et al. 1983.

134

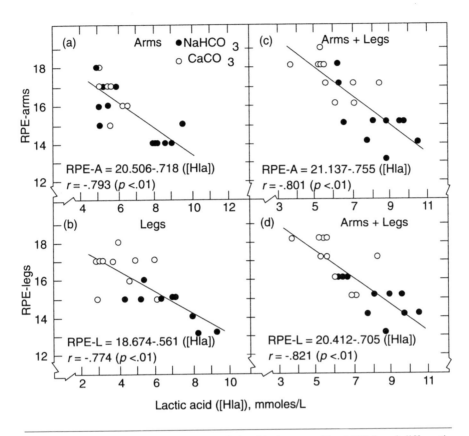

Figure 6.7   Regression analysis of the relationship between blood [Hla] and differenti-ated ratings of perceived exertion (RPE) during separate and combined arm and leg exercise at 80% $\dot{V}O_2$max.
Reprinted from Robertson et al. 1988.

[Hla] serve as specific cases of a more generalized psychophysiological response that reflects the relative intensity of exercise (Borg, Hassmen, and Lagerstrom 1987). The clinical application of exertional perceptions during high-intensity exercise can then be undertaken without assuming a causal link between lactate appearance in blood and peripheral perceptual responsiveness. Each variable is an independent but corresponding marker of exercise intensity. As an example, the equations presented in figure 6.8 (Borg, Hassmen, and Lagerstrom 1987) use the relative [Hla] and HR at varying exercise intensities to predict RPE during both arm and leg ergometry.[1] The clinical utility of these prediction equations

[1]The relative [Hla] and HR are calculated as percentages of the response range for each variable (Borg, Hassmen, and Lagerstrom 1987).

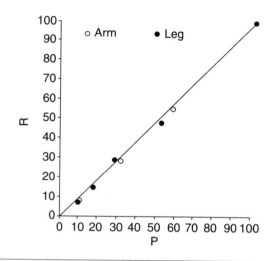

Figure 6.8   A graphic presentation of the relationship between relative values (relative to the variation range and in percent) of ratings of perceived exertion (R) on the CR scale and the mean of heart rate and blood lactate concentration (P). ● R = −0.47 + 0.993P (0.999); ○ R = −1.15 + 1.004P (0.999).
Reprinted from Borg, Hassmen, and Lagerstrom 1987.

is based on the direct relation between blood [Hla] and RPE at exercise intensities that exceed the blood lactate inflection point (Borg, Ljunggren, and Ceci 1985).

The correlation between lactate appearance in blood and perceptual responsiveness holds at higher (Noble et al. 1983) but not lower (Johansson 1986) exercise intensities owing to limited anaerobic glycolysis at lower metabolic rates. This suggests that the interrelations among power output, blood [Hla], and RPE may not take on practical value as a means of evaluating exercise intensity until a metabolic threshold, such as the lactate inflection point, is exceeded (DeMello et al. 1987; Johansson 1986; Robertson et al. 1986). The lactate inflection point serves as a metabolic marker for the exercise intensity above which metabolic acidosis begins to influence the intensity of exertional perceptions in active skeletal muscle (Robertson et al. 1986; DeMello et al. 1987; Haskvitz et al. 1992; Seip et al. 1991; Hetzler et al. 1991).

Muscle Lactic Acid

Experimental study of a possible link between muscle [Hla] and exertional perceptions is limited to two investigations, the results of which are inconsistent. Löllgen, Graham, and Sjogaard (1980) found muscle lactate to be independent of pedal frequency when cycle ergometer power output was held constant. In contrast, RPE evinced a parabolic relation with pedal frequency, being lowest at 60 and 80 rpm and highest at 40 and 100 rpm. These findings refute muscle lactate production or accumulation as a mediator for exertional perceptions. On the other hand, Noble et al. (1983) report that RPE-L and the concentration of lactate in muscle and blood increase as positively accelerating functions of power output during progressive cycle exercise. These data suggest that the gradient for diffusion of lactic acid from muscle to blood is linked to the perceived intensity of exertion. However, RPE appeared to be more closely related to blood than muscle [Hla]. It was concluded that blood [Hla] may be more important than muscle [Hla] in mediating the intensity of exertional perceptions. Owing to the extremely limited availability of experimental evidence, the foregoing conclusions regarding the role of muscle [Hla] in mediating exertional perceptions must be interpreted cautiously.

Summary of Metabolic Acidosis Findings

Metabolic acidosis appears to mediate the intensity of exertional perceptions in skeletal muscle during high-intensity exercise. Experimental evidence indicates that blood pH is more important than blood [Hla] in mediating peripheral perceptual signals. However, sufficient evidence is not available to draw conclusions regarding the possible role of muscle [Hla] in mediating the intensity of perceived exertion during dynamic exercise.

Muscle Fiber Type

The contractile properties of slow- and fast-twitch muscle fibers may differentially mediate the intensity of peripheral exertional perceptions. Noble et al. (1983) and Ljunggren, Ceci, and Karlsson (1987) found that rated perceptions of exertion during cycle ergometer exercise were influenced by the relative distribution of slow- and fast-twitch muscle fibers. On the other hand, Löllgen, Graham, and Sjogaard (1980) found no such relation for the same type of exercise. Nevertheless, a causal relation between exertional perceptions and muscle fiber type is theoretically attractive (Noble et al. 1983). It is possible that the contractile properties of skeletal muscle are linked to exertional perceptions through a cascade of metabolic and neuromotor events. Noble et al. (1983) report that exertional signals arising from the legs during cycling are more intense for subjects with a greater fast-twitch than slow-twitch fiber distribution in the vastus lateralis muscle. In this same experiment, lactate production during exercise was positively related ($r = .85$) to the percentage of fast-twitch fibers. This response is generally consistent with Tesch, Sjodin, and Karlsson's (1978) observation that [Hla] and [H^+] are greater in fast-twitch than in slow-twitch muscle fibers during high-intensity exercise. As intracellular [H^+] increases, the number of calcium ions available to bind with troponin decreases, inhibiting muscle contraction. Therefore, the onset of muscular fatigue secondary to metabolic acidosis occurs sooner in muscles rich in fast-twitch as opposed to slow-twitch fibers (Noble et al. 1983). In the presence of muscular fatigue, force production can only be maintained if motor unit recruitment and firing frequency are increased. A greater level of motor unit activation requires concomitant increases in central motor outflow commands (as evidenced by an increased EMG). It is the greater level of these motor commands that triggers the comparatively more intense exertional signals associated with fast-twitch muscle fibers.

Muscle Blood Flow

The effect of muscle blood flow in mediating the intensity of exertional perceptions has been studied during both isometric and isotonic contractions. When forearm blood flow is occluded by auscultation, the magnitude of exertional sensations during handgrip exercise intensifies as compared with a nonoccluded limb (Cain and Stevens 1973; Stevens and Krimsley 1977). An extension of these laboratory findings suggests that nutritive blood flow to muscle is an important mediator of exertional sensations during high-intensity exercise. That is, under exercise conditions where the level of muscular tension is a high percentage of maximal voluntary contraction, portions of the vascular bed are mechanically occluded. Peripheral vascular resistance is correspondingly elevated, reducing tissue perfusion. A reduction in nutritive blood flow causes fatigue in metabolically active muscle and intensifies peripheral exertional signals.

The interruption of blood flow to metabolically active muscle appears to mediate the intensity of exertional sensations during the later but not earlier part of an exercise performance (Cain and Stevens 1973; Stevens and Krimsley 1977). At the initiation of muscular contraction, tissue stores of phosphagen can be readily accessed, negating the importance of blood-borne energy substrate pools. After approximately 30 s of repeated contractions, intramuscular phosphagen stores are depleted. The need for circulatory replacement of energy substrates and delivery of oxygen becomes critical to the continuation of exercise. Under these conditions, an interruption of nutritive blood flow results in a greater reliance on anaerobic glycolysis for energy production. Muscle fibers begin to fatigue secondary to metabolic acidosis. Exertional signals arising from these muscles begin to intensify in conjunction with the onset and progression of fatigue.

Energy Substrates

During prolonged submaximal exercise, the blood levels of glucose and free fatty acids (FFA) are thought to mediate the intensity of exertional perceptions (Robertson et al. 1990; Burgess et al. 1991; Nieman et al. 1987; Dohm et al. 1986). However, caution must be taken when interpreting laboratory experiments that have examined the perceptual mediating effect of these energy substrates. Under some exercise conditions the blood levels of glucose and FFA change as approximate reciprocals of one another. This makes it difficult to examine each substrate's independent effect in mediating the perceived intensity of exertion.

The most desirable experimental procedure is to manipulate each substrate separately. As an example, experimental paradigms that employ carbohydrate (CHO) supplementation prior to or during exercise are ideally suited to study the perceptual mediating effect of blood glucose. Experimental paradigms that use preexercise caffeine ingestion are helpful in studying the effects of FFA oxidation on exertional perceptions.

Blood Glucose

The level of blood glucose during exercise is a key metabolic factor in determining submaximal endurance capacity (Coyle et al. 1986). As blood glucose declines, there is an increased reliance on muscle glycogen to fuel CHO metabolism. Over time, the depletion of CHO fuel sources triggers muscular fatigue, causing the termination of endurance exercise. Horstman et al. (1979) have shown that the termination point for endurance exercise is also dependent on the subjective tolerance of exertional fatigue and discomfort. These somewhat separate lines of research suggest that the subjective decision to terminate prolonged exercise is linked to physiological factors that regulate CHO metabolism. Both perceptual and physiological fatigue begin and progress in concert, pointing to a causal relation between variables. It is possible that during endurance exercise of 60 min or more, the level of blood glucose mediates the intensity of peripheral exertional perceptions arising from active skeletal muscle.

Evidence from laboratory experiments involving CHO supplementation is suggestive but not totally supportive of blood glucose as a physiological mediator for exertional perceptions. (Robertson et al. 1990, Coyle et al. 1986; Coggan and Coyle 1987; Miyashita, Onodera, and Tabata 1986). Robertson et al. (1990) manipulated CHO metabolism and exertional perceptions by having subjects consume a diet enriched with dihydroxyacetone and pyruvate over a seven-day period. Immediately following completion of the seven-day diet, arm ergometer exercise was performed at an intensity equivalent to 60% $\dot{V}O_2$peak. Arm endurance performance was terminated at the point of exhaustion. After 60 min of exercise, rated perception of exertion was higher and the blood level of glucose lower in the placebo than in the CHO supplementation trial (fig. 6.9). In addition, endurance time to exhaustion was inversely related ($r = -.789$) to the RPE-Arms obtained after 60 min of arm exercise (fig. 6.10). These findings confirmed a link between CHO substrate depletion and exertional perceptions in setting the limits of endurance performance. It appears that the decline in blood glucose during the later stages of endurance exercise initiates fatigue and in turn intensifies perceptions of exertion arising from involved muscles. Similar conclusions regarding the importance of blood glucose in mediating exertional perceptions have been reported by Coggan and Coyle (1987) for repeated bouts of exhaustive exercise and by Burgess et al. (1991) for prolonged cycle exercise.

The decline in blood glucose during prolonged exercise may also mediate the perceived intensity of exertional signals by altering central nervous system (CNS) functions (Coggan and Coyle 1987; Nieman et al. 1987). Glucose is an important

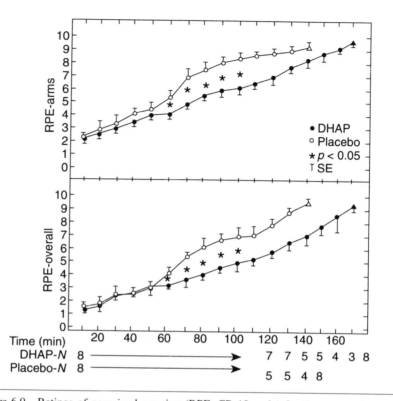

Figure 6.9   Ratings of perceived exertion (RPE, CR-10 scale) for the arms and overall body during prolonged arm exercise. Values are means (±*SE*) for the dihydroxy-acetone/pyruvate (DHAP ●) and placebo (○) trials. * indicates that for a given time point means are significantly different between trials ($p < .05$). Dashed lines signify that data were not statistically analyzed for mean differences. Triangles indicate the average RPE at termination of exercise for the DHAP (▲) and placebo (△) trials and do not represent a real-time average. N = the number of subjects for which data were obtained at a given time point.
Reprinted from Robertson et al. 1990.

energy substrate for the CNS. During prolonged submaximal exercise, hypoglycemia may cause CNS dysfunction, altering the final common pathway for sensory-motor signals. In turn, the perception of physical exertion is intensified.

A number of investigations have found that the intensity of peripheral exertional perceptions during prolonged exercise are independent of alterations in blood glucose levels (Foster, Costill, and Fink 1979; Ivy et al. 1979; Felig et al. 1982; Okano et al. 1988). Differences between these investigations and those described earlier may in part be due to experimental variations in the glucose dose or its schedule of supplementation. Such variations cause blood glucose to peak at different times during the experimental procedure. The effect of blood glucose in mediating exertional perceptions would be expected to show similar variations.

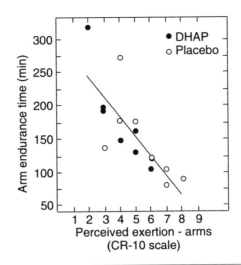

Figure 6.10   Relationship between endurance time (ET) and ratings of perceived exertion of the arms (RPE-A) following 60 min of continuous arm exercise. Data are pooled from the dihydroxyacetone/pyruvate (DHAP ●) and placebo (○) trials. ET = 303.2 − 30.0 (RPE-A); $r = -.789$; $p < .05$; *SE* = 41.4.
Reprinted from Robertson et al. 1990.

Free Fatty Acids and Glycerol

The results of laboratory experiments are neither consistent nor strongly supportive of plasma FFA and glycerol as mediators of exertional perceptions during long-term exercise. Several of these experiments have examined the effect of caffeine ingestion on perceived exertion and on lipid metabolism during submaximal endurance exercise (Casal and Leon 1985; Ivy et al. 1979). Caffeine-induced increases in plasma FFA and glycerol did not affect the intensity of exertional perceptions during prolonged exercise. In contrast, Costill, Dalsky, and Fink (1978) found that lipid metabolism during endurance exercise increased following caffeine ingestion and was associated with less intense perceptions of exertion and fatigue. However, this apparent relation between exertional perceptions and lipid metabolism may be confounded by the use of caffeine as an experimental forcing function. Caffeine lowers the threshold for muscle fiber recruitment and nerve transmission. The subsequent alterations in muscle fiber contractility may attenuate the intensity of exertional perceptions independent of a direct metabolic influence (Costill, Dalsky, and Fink 1978; Casal and Leon 1985).

What then is the role of lipid metabolism in mediating the intensity of exertional perceptions? Coyle et al. (1986) reported that during a submaximal endurance performance, RPE increased as exercise progressed. Over the same time period, plasma FFA increased in conjunction with a steady decline in blood glucose. It appears that the intensity of exertional perceptions is linked to alterations in CHO, not to lipid metabolism. This conclusion is also supported by several investigations that used a fasting paradigm to manipulate exertional perceptions and fat metabolism during dynamic exercise (Nieman et al. 1987; Dohm et al. 1986). The absence of a link between exertional perceptions and lipolysis is not surprising. Under most exercise conditions, blood-borne pools of FFA are abundant and are rarely depleted to levels that directly trigger fatigue. Rather, lipid metabolism is indirectly related to perceived exertion through its CHO-sparing effect. A comparatively greater rate of lipid metabolism decreases reliance on energy derived from CHO pools, prolonging exercise and attenuating associated perceptions of exertion.

Summary of Energy Substrate Findings

The level of blood glucose appears to be an important physiological mediator for peripheral exertional perceptions. In contrast, plasma FFA and glycerol are not influential in determining the intensity of perceived exertion. It is significant that CHO metabolism is a principle energy source for exercise intensities above but not below the lactate inflection point. As such, blood glucose functions as a metabolic mediator only at higher exercise intensities. Energy substrates do not appear to have a direct influence on perceptions of exertion at lower exercise intensities, where metabolic functions seldom produce fatigue in peripheral skeletal muscle.

Nonspecific Mediators

Physiological mediators that are not directly linked to peripheral or respiratory-metabolic perceptual signals are termed *nonspecific*. This class of mediators consists of such processes as hormonal regulation, temperature regulation, and pain reactivity. Nonspecific mediators exert a generalized or systemic influence on the intensity of exertional perceptions. For the most part, experimental evidence supports the perceptual role of nonspecific mediators. However, the neurophysiological pathway for their mediating effect is not uniform. Some nonspecific mediators influence exertional perceptions via regulation of energy metabolism (e.g., catecholamines), while others exert a perceptual influence through neuronal pathways (e.g., exercise-induced pain). It also appears that some nonspecific mediators are consequences of the performance environment as well as muscular exertion. For example, nonspecific perceptual signals reflecting body temperature regulation are influenced by both internal physiological events and external environmental factors. The following sections discuss those physiological mediators that seem to fit best in the nonspecific classification. Where appropriate, these nonspecific mediators will be juxtaposed with peripheral and respiratory-metabolic mediators.

Hormonal Regulation

Hormonal regulation is a nonspecific mediator of perceived exertion. Catecholamines and beta-endorphins are two types of hormone whose roles in perceived exertion have been investigated.

Catecholamine Secretion

During exercise, the hypothalamus activates adrenal-medullary secretion of norepinephrine and epinephrine. These catecholamines (CATs) regulate the body's reaction to a variety of stressors, including exercise (Frankenhaeuser et al. 1969, Docktor and Sharkey 1971). The concentration of CATs in plasma increases as a positive function of increasing exercise intensity (Howley 1976). However, norepinephrine appears to be comparatively more responsive to elevations in metabolic rate than does epinephrine (Skrinar, Ingram, and Pandolf 1983). Because RPE also increases as a positive function of exercise stress, it has been proposed that CATs are nonspecific mediators for exertional perceptions.

Evidence supporting CATs as hormonal mediators for perceived exertion is suggestive but not totally consistent. During multistage treadmill testing, central perceived exertion (RPE-C) correlates positively with both norepinephrine ($r = .63$) and epinephrine ($r = .54$) (fig. 6.11; Skrinar, Ingram, and Pandolf 1983). In addition, Docktor and Sharkey (1971) found that both RPE and vanillylmandelic acid (a urinary index of CAT secretion) were attenuated at a fixed submaximal power output following a five-week exercise training program. These data suggest that CAT production may mediate the intensity of perceived exertion. In contrast, several investigations have shown that the intensity of exertional perceptions was independent of CAT levels when the hormonal response to exercise was manipulated by CHO supplementation (Felig et al. 1982) and by alterations in exercise mode (Horstman et al. 1979; Coast, Cox, and Welch 1986).

The lack of general agreement regarding the perceptual mediating effect of adrenal-medullary CAT secretion may be attributable to variations in experimental paradigms and methodology. It appears that CATs mediate exertional perceptions at higher (i.e., $\geq 70\%$ $\dot{V}O_2$max) but not lower exercise intensities (Carton and Rhodes 1985). Frankenhaeuser et al. (1969) noted that at a comparatively high exercise intensity corresponding to an RPE of 17 (i.e., "laborious"), epinephrine was 84% and norepinephrine 42% greater than the preexercise level. On the other hand, CAT levels changed very little at lower power outputs even though RPE increased with progressive increments in exercise intensity. These findings suggest an intensity threshold for the perceptual mediating effect of CATs. Possibly, this threshold occurs around the lactate inflection point and coincides with the relatively greater reliance on CHO metabolism that accompanies high-intensity exercise. Experimental paradigms that do not employ power outputs above this threshold may erroneously dismiss a causal link between exertional perceptions and CAT secretion.

Two separate mechanisms explain the perceptual mediating effect of CAT secretion. The first mechanism is metabolic in origin, while the second is psychological. One of the primary functions of CAT secretion during prolonged exercise is to regulate the level of blood glucose. CAT secretion is minimal at lower power outputs but increases markedly as exercise intensity exceeds 50% to 70% $\dot{V}O_2$max (Carton and Rhodes 1985). Sympathetic activation of CAT secretion parallels the fall in blood glucose or muscle glycogen that occurs during high-intensity endurance exercise (Felig et al. 1982). Increased levels of circulating

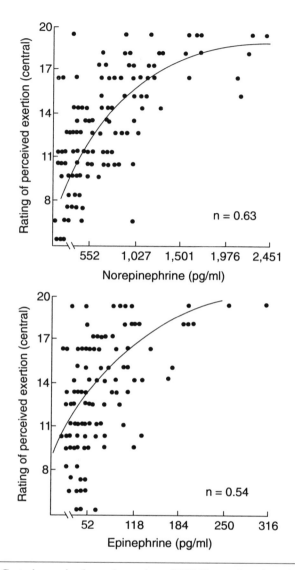

Figure 6.11   Central perceived exertion ratings (RPE-C) as a function of plasma norepinephrine ($F_{1,127}$ = 5.22, $p < .05$) and epinephrine ($F_{1,127}$ = 3.80, $p < .10$).
Reprinted from Skrinar, Ingram, and Pandolf 1983.

CATs stimulate muscle and liver glycogenolysis in order to offset a decline in
CHO energy substrates. Therefore, CATs likely mediate the intensity of exertional
perceptions through metabolic pathways, directly reflecting a decline in both
blood glucose and muscle glycogen.

CATs also mediate the intensity of perceived exertion through a psychological
mechanism (Frankenhaeuser et al. 1969; Docktor and Sharkey 1971). While both

norepinephrine and epinephrine are secreted in response to exercise stress, they differ in some of their regulatory functions. Plasma levels of norepinephrine during muscular exercise are primarily linked to metabolic processes. The circulating level of epinephrine appears to have psychological outcomes. Epinephrine is secreted in response to the emotional stress and unpleasant sensations that accompany high-intensity exercise. Therefore, the perceptual mediating effect of CAT secretion may be as much psychological as metabolic in origin, especially at higher power outputs, where exercise is emotionally stressful to some individuals.

Beta-Endorphins

The hypothesized link between exertional perceptions and plasma beta-endorphin levels is attractive but has not been extensively examined. Beta-endorphins are endogenous ligands with morphinelike properties (Farrell et al. 1982). They are released from the corticotrophs of the anterior pituitary as part of a generalized hormonal response to a variety of stressors, including exercise. The morphinelike action of beta-endorphins exerts an analgesic effect during high-intensity exercise. Because of this analgesic effect, it is hypothesized that beta-endorphins mediate the intensity of exertional perceptions, especially those associated with pain and discomfort during heavy exercise.

The role of beta-endorphins as a nonspecific hormonal mediator of exertional perceptions has received very little direct experimental attention. Farrell et al. (1982) observed that RPE was lowest under exercise conditions where plasma beta-endorphins were highest, suggesting a link between these variables. However, support for this conclusion requires direct manipulation of beta-endorphin responses using an opiate-receptor blocking agent such as naloxone. More extensive laboratory experiments of this type are needed to examine the role of beta-endorphins as a perceptual mediator during exercise.

It is noteworthy that the beta-endorphin concentration in plasma (where the hormone is typically measured in exercise studies) does not necessarily reflect the concentration in the central nervous system. Therefore, it may be difficult to identify the perceptual mediating role of beta-endorphins if their sensory effect is differentially influenced by concentrations in cerebrospinal fluid and systemic circulation. The findings of Droste et al. (1991) seem to support this conclusion. They reported that RPE did not correlate with exercise-induced increases in beta-endorphins. Similarly, Kraemer et al. (1992) reported that neither proenkephalin peptited F nor RPE differed between hypnotic and waking control conditions, suggesting that endogenous opioids are not mediators of the effort sense. However, it is possible that the subjects used in this investigation were only moderately responsive to hypnotic suggestion, partially negating the experimental forcing function.

Temperature Regulation

Exertional perceptions during dynamic exercise intensify as ambient temperature increases (Pandolf et al. 1972; Skinner et al. 1973). This suggests that the perceived intensity of exertion is influenced by physiological processes that regulate body temperature during exercise. Nonspecific physiological mediators involving thermal regulation include (1) body core temperature (Tc), (2) skin temperature (Ts), (3) sweat production, and (4) skin conductance. It is also possible that exertional responses are mediated by thermal sensation and comfort.

Body Core Temperature

Body core temperature and rated perceptions of exertion increase as metabolic heat production increases during dynamic muscle contractions. However, experimental evidence does not support a causal relation between physiological factors that regulate Tc and the intensity of exertional perceptions. The correlation between Tc and RPE is consistently low ($r = .14$ to .20) and not statistically significant (Kamon, Pandolf, and Cafarelli 1974; Toner, Drolet, and Pandolf 1986). In addition, no correspondence is noted between Tc and RPE during exercise involving hot (Knuttgen et al. 1982; Pivarnik and Senay 1986), neutral (Davies and Sargeant 1979), and cold (Toner, Drolet, and Pandolf 1986) environments; arm and leg ergometry (Pivarnik, Grafner, and Elkins 1988; Toner, Drolet, and Pandolf 1986); eccentric muscle training (Knuttgen et al. 1982); thermal acclimation (Pivarnik and Senay 1986); and varying stages of the menstrual cycle (Stephenson, Kolka, and Wilderson 1982). As an example, Pivarnik, Grafner, and Elkins (1988) found Tc did not differ between exercise trials in hot (33° C) and thermoneutral (23° C) environments, while the overall rating of perceived exertion was higher under heat stress. These data indicate that Tc does not influence the intensity of exertional sensations during dynamic exercise.

What, then, accounts for the parallel increase in Tc and perceived exertion during graded exercise testing? Core temperature is driven by the relative metabolic rate rather than ambient temperature (Nadel 1980). Similarly, RPE is positively related to the relative metabolic demand. Therefore, the increase in relative metabolic rate that occurs with increasing power output is accompanied by parallel increases in Tc and RPE. The apparent relation between Tc and RPE is really a function of their shared relation with the relative metabolic rate.

Skin Temperature

Skin temperature at rest and during exercise is affected by ambient temperature and thus is an index of thermal strain. Correlational evidence that links Ts with the intensity of exertional perceptions during exercise in hot and cold environments is both limited and inconsistent. Using a stepwise regression analysis, Noble et al. (1973) found that Ts accounted for a significant amount of variance in RPE for the overall body under hot environmental conditions. In contrast, Toner, Drolet, and Pandolf (1986) did not find a significant correlation between Ts and RPE during arm and leg exercise in cold water.

Experimental evidence derived from investigations in which environmental temperature has been manipulated generally supports Ts as a mediator of exertional perceptions under both hot and cold conditions (Knuttgen et al. 1982;

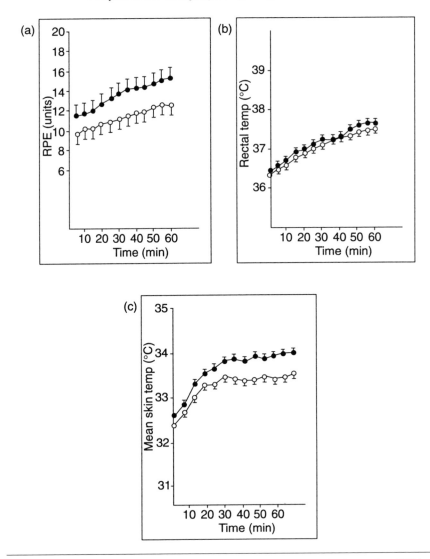

Figure 6.12   Mean (with standard error bars) (*a*) ratings of perceived exertion (RPE), (*b*) rectal temperatures, and (*c*) skin temperatures during the exercise tasks both before (●) and after (○) endurance training–heat acclimation.
Reprinted from Pivarnik and Senay 1986.

Bergh et al. 1986; Noble et al. 1973; Pivarnik, Grafner, and Elkins 1988; Pivarnik and Senay 1986). As an example, figure 6.12 shows that both RPE overall and T*s* were attenuated during arm and leg exercise in hot ambient conditions following a four-week endurance training–heat acclimation program (Pivarnik and Senay 1986). Under thermal stress, skin temperature mediated the intensity of the nonspecific exertional signal. Core temperature, on the other hand, did not differ between experimental conditions, negating its role as a perceptual signal mediator.

Skin temperature responses to thermal stress are influenced by sweat production and both skin blood flow and volume (Knuttgen et al. 1982). Therefore, the physiological processes that regulate sweating and peripheral vascular resistance may also mediate the perceived intensity of exertion when exercise is performed in abnormally hot or cold ambient temperatures.

Thermal Sensation and Comfort

Exertional perceptions during exercise in hot and cold ambient conditions may be influenced by interrelated processes involving thermal sensation and thermal comfort. Thermal sensation is measured by a seven-point category scale with responses ranging from cold (1) to hot (7). Thermal comfort is measured by a four-point category scale having a response range of comfortable (1) to very uncomfortable (4). If the strictest psychophysical definition is applied, thermal comfort is not considered a sensory continuum in that it does not involve a physical stimulus or a sense organ (Gagge, Stolwijk, and Saltin 1969). Nevertheless, thermal sensation and thermal comfort are related to a number of physiological indices of thermal strain. Therefore, both of these thermal measures may also influence exertional perceptions during exercise in hot and cold ambient conditions.

Thermal sensation is related to skin ($r = .73$) and ambient ($r = .72$) temperature but is independent of metabolic rate, muscle temperature, and rectal temperature (Gagge, Stolwijk, and Saltin 1969; Kamon, Pandolf, and Cafarelli 1974; Pandolf et al. 1972; Toner, Drolet, and Pandolf 1986). Sensory mechanisms in the skin are responsible for the regulation of thermal sensation (Gagge, Stolwijk, and Saltin 1969). Because skin temperature reflects ambient temperature, these factors act together to shape thermal sensation. As noted previously, Ts is an important mediator of exertional perceptions. Possibly, thermal sensation is a catalyst for the link between Ts and perceived exertion during exercise in hot environments. However, it is not known whether the relation between thermal sensation and perceived exertion holds under cold conditions. Toner, Drolet, and Pandolf (1986) did not find a correlation between thermal sensation and RPE during cold-water immersion. In this instance, the thermal stress of cold water did not appear to influence perceptual responses.

Thermal comfort is related to skin sweat ($r = .66$) and to conductance (i.e., blood flow; $r = .56$) but is independent of metabolic rate and of muscle, skin, core, and ambient temperature (Gagge, Stolwijk, and Saltin 1969; Kamon, Pandolf, and Cafarelli 1974; Marcus and Redman 1979). Therefore, thermal comfort is determined by effector mechanisms that regulate sweating and peripheral vascular tone (Gagge, Stolwijk, and Saltin 1969). It is possible that the degree of thermal comfort-discomfort that is experienced during exercise under hot conditions mediates exertional perceptions. This perceptual mediating effect may mirror the extent to which the appearance of sweat and vasodilation (i.e., skin redness) are considered an uncomfortable index of thermal stress.

Thermal Mechanisms

Temperature regulatory processes mediate the intensity of exertional perceptions through one or both of the following physiological pathways. First, fluctuations in ambient temperature perturb certain physiological responses to exercise. Temperature-induced alterations in these physiological processes in turn mediate the intensity of exertional perceptions. As an example, exposure to hot environments accentuates ventilatory drive during exercise. The greater ventilation for a given oxygen uptake under hot conditions intensifies respiratory-metabolic signals of perceived exertion (Noble et al. 1973). In this instance, temperature regulation plays an indirect role in mediating exertional perceptions.

In the second pathway, exposure to hot ambient temperatures causes thermal strain, as indicated by the onset of sweating or changes in Ts. These thermal responses exert a direct mediating effect on exertional perceptions.

Thermal Comfort Zone

Exertional perceptions are not likely influenced by temperature regulation within the thermal comfort zone (Gagge, Stolwijk, and Saltin 1969). The lower boundary of the comfort zone is defined as the exercise intensity and air temperature at which skin sweat is zero. The upper boundary is marked by a skin sweat rate equivalent to evaporative heat loss of 150 kcal/(m · h). This corresponds to approximately 65% skin wetness and to an exercise intensity that does not exceed 50% $\dot{V}O_2$max. Within the comfort zone, changes in Ts and sweating are comparatively small. Therefore, it is likely that the physiological responses to thermal strain do not mediate exertional perceptions until exercise intensity and air temperature exceed the upper boundary of the comfort zone.

Exercise-Induced Pain

Sensations of pain, especially in the limbs and chest, are a common experience during high-intensity exercise or when exercise is undertaken for prolonged periods of time. It is not entirely clear if and how perceptions of exertion are influenced by exercise-induced pain (Droste et al. 1991). Borg, Ljunggren, and Ceci (1985) reported that RPE and ratings of pain intensity in the legs were strongly correlated ($r = .91$). Both variables increased as a positively accelerating function of power output during multistage cycle exercise.

The physiological basis of pain sensation during exercise is not completely known but appears to involve localized muscular ischemia (Coldwell and Smith 1966). During the static phase of muscle contraction, mechanical pressure exceeds systolic pressure, interrupting nutritive blood flow to exercising body regions. The resulting ischemia is associated with exercise-induced pain, which is especially pronounced when muscle contractions are intense.

The appearance of lactate in blood has been suggested as a precursor for exercise-induced pain (Borg, Ljunggren, and Ceci 1985). During dynamic exercise, ratings of pain intensity (using the CR-10 scale) are positively correlated with venous blood [Hla] ($r = .76$). However, Ljunggren, Ceci, and Karlsson (1987) reported that pain sensation did not differ between groups of subjects who exhibited varying levels of blood lactate during a 15-min cycle exercise performance. These latter data question the role of blood [Hla] in mediating the intensity of exercise-induced pain. Likely, the apparent relation between pain sensation and [Hla] reported by Borg, Ljunggren, and Ceci (1985) is not causal but rather a function of each variable's shared relation with power output. As power output increases, both blood [Hla] and the intensity of pain sensation increase.

Because data are comparatively limited, it is difficult to determine the extent to which pain plays a role in signaling exertional sensations. Pain may operate independently or in concert with other physiological mediators to set the perceived intensity of exertion. Whatever its mode of action, the influence of pain on exercise-related sensations is more pronounced at high power outputs. At low power outputs it is hard to determine exactly what constitutes pain and whether it can be distinguished from reports of generalized exertional discomfort (Borg, Ljunggren, and Ceci 1985).

Summary

Physiological mediators of peripheral exertional perceptions during dynamic exercise involve metabolic acidosis, muscle fiber type, regional blood perfusion, and energy substrate availability. Experimental and correlational investigations support blood pH as a potent mediator of exertional perceptions, especially at exercise intensities that equal or exceed the lactate threshold. It is assumed that muscle pH plays a similar role in mediating exertional perceptions. However, additional evidence is needed to support this assumption. Correlational investigations strongly suggest that blood and muscle [Hla] are mediators of peripheral exertional signals. In contrast, when [Hla] is experimentally perturbed, corresponding changes in RPE are not observed. These experimental findings question the role of [Hla] in mediating perceptual intensity.

The intensity of the peripheral perceptual signal appears to be more intense when the skeletal muscle involved in the exercise has a comparatively high concentration of fast-twitch fibers. Blood flow to exercising muscle determines the availability of energy substrates for exercise metabolism. Inadequate perfusion of tissue limits metabolism, inducing fatigue and intensifying the peripheral perceptual signal.

Blood-borne glucose pools are important mediators of the peripheral perceptual signal. As blood glucose is depleted during the middle to later stages of submaximal endurance exercise, muscle fatigues, causing an increase in perceptual signal strength. In contrast, differential rates of lipid mobilization and metabolism do not independently influence the intensity of the peripheral perceptual signal.

Nonspecific mediators of exertional perceptions include hormonal secretion, temperature regulation, and exercise-induced pain. Elevated catecholamine levels appear to mediate perceptual signal strength through both metabolic and psychological pathways. Evidence regarding the perceptual mediating role of beta-endorphin concentration in cerebrospinal fluid is presently only suggestive. Skin temperature—but not core temperature—appears to systematically influence nonspecific exertional perceptions. In addition, both thermal sensation and comfort may act as perceptual mediators. Finally, exercise-induced pain and discomfort interact with both peripheral and respiratory-metabolic mediators to intensify exertional perceptions.

References

Allen, P.D., and K.B. Pandolf. 1977. Perceived exertion associated with breathing hyperoxic mixtures during submaximal work. *Med. Sci. Sports* 9:122-27.

Allen, W.K., D.R. Seals, B.F. Hurley, A.A. Ehsani, and J.M. Hagberg. 1985. Lactate threshold and distance-running performance in young and older endurance athletes. *J. Appl. Physiol.* 58:1281-84.

Bergh, U., U. Danielsson, L. Wennberg, and B Sjödin. 1986. Blood lactate and perceived exertion during heat stress. *Acta Physiol. Scand.* 126:617-18.

Borg, G., P. Hassmen, and M. Lagerstrom. 1987. Perceived exertion related to heart rate and blood lactate during arm and leg exercise. *Eur. J. Appl. Physiol.* 56:679-85.

Borg, G., G. Ljunggren, and R. Ceci. 1985. The increase of perceived exertion, aches and pains in the legs, heart rate and blood lactate during exercise on a bicycle ergometer. *Eur. J. Appl. Physiol. Occup. Physiol.* 54:343-49.

Burgess, M.L., R.J. Robertson, J.M. Davis, and J.M. Norris. 1991. RPE, blood glucose, and carbohydrate oxidation during exercise: Effects of glucose feedings. *Med. Sci. Sports Exerc.* 23:353-59.

Cafarelli, E. 1977. Peripheral and central inputs to the effort sense during cycling exercise. *Eur. J. Appl. Physiol.* 37:181-89.

Cain, W.S., and J.C. Stevens. 1973. Constant effort contractions related to the electromyogram. *Med. Sci. Sports* 5:121-27.

Carton, R.L., and E.C. Rhodes. 1985. A critical review of the literature on rating scales for perceived exertion. *Sports Med.* 2:198-222.

Casal, D.C., and A.S. Leon. 1985. Failure of caffeine to affect substrate utilization during prolonged running. *Med. Sci. Sports Exerc.* 17:174-79.

Coast, J.R., R.H. Cox, and H.G. Welch. 1986. Optimal pedalling rate in prolonged bouts of cycle ergometry. *Med. Sci. Sports Exerc.* 18:225-30.

Coggan, A.R., and E.F. Coyle. 1987. Reversal of fatigue during prolonged exercise by carbohydrate infusion or ingestion. *J. Appl. Physiol.* 63:1-8.

Coldwell, L.S., and R.P. Smith. 1966. Pain and endurance of isometric muscle contractions. *J. Engineer. Psychol.* 5:25-32.

Costill, D.L., G.P. Dalsky, and W.J. Fink. 1978. Effects of caffeine ingestion on metabolism and exercise performance. *Med. Sci. Sports* 10:155-58.

Coyle, E.F., A.R. Coggan, M.K. Hemmert, and J.L. Ivy. 1986. Muscle glycogen utilization during prolonged strenuous exercise when fed carbohydrate. *J. Appl. Physiol.* 61:165-72.

Davies, C.T., and A.J. Sargeant. 1979. The effects of atropine and practolol on the perception of exertion during treadmill exercise. *Ergonomics* 22:1141-46.

DeMello, J.J., K.J. Cureton, R.E. Boineau, and M.M. Singh. 1987. Ratings of perceived exertion at the lactate threshold in trained and untrained men and women. *Med. Sci. Sports Exerc.* 19:354-62.

Docktor, R., and B. Sharkey. 1971. Note on some physiological and subjective reactions to exercise and training. *Percept. Motor Skills* 32:233-34.

Dohm, G.L., R.T. Beeker, R.G. Israel, and E.B. Tapscott. 1986. Metabolic responses to exercise after fasting. *J. Appl. Physiol.* 61:1363-68.

Droste, C., M.W. Greenlee, M. Schreck, and H. Roskamm. 1991. Experimental pain thresholds and plasma beta-endorphins levels during exercise. *Med. Sci. Sports Exerc.* 23:334-41.

Edwards, R.H.T., A. Melcher, C.M. Hesser, O. Wigebtz, and L.G. Ekelund. 1972. Physiological correlates of perceived exertion in continuous and intermittent exercise with the same average power output. *Eur. J. Clin. Invest.* 2:108-14.

Ekblom, B., and A.N. Goldbarg. 1971. The influence of physical training and other factors on the subjective rating of perceived exertion. *Acta Physiol. Scand.* 83:399-406.

Essig, D., D.L. Costill, and P.J. Van Handel. 1980. Effects of caffeine ingestion on utilization of muscle glycogen and lipid during leg ergometer cycling. *Int. J. Sports Med.* 1:86-90.

Farrell, P.A., W.K. Gates, M.G. Maksud, and W.P. Morgan. 1982. Increases in plasma β-endorphin/β-lipotropin immunoreactivity after treadmill running in humans. *J. Appl. Physiol. Respir. Environ. Exerc. Physiol.* 52:1245-49.

Felig, P., A. Cherif, A. Minagawa, and J. Wahren. 1982. Hypoglycemia during prolonged exercise in normal men. *New Engl. J. Med.* 306:895-900.

Foster, C., D.L. Costill, and W.J. Fink. 1979. Effects of pre-exercise feedings on endurance performance. *Med. Sci. Sports* 11:1-5.

Frankenhaeuser, M., B. Post, B. Nordheden, and H. Sjoeberg. 1969. Physiological and subjective reactions to different physical work loads. *Percept. Motor Skills* 28:343-49.

Gagge, A.P., A.J. Stolwijk, and B. Saltin. 1969. Comfort and thermal sensations and associated physiological responses during exercise at various ambient temperatures. *Environ. Res.* 2:209-29.

Gamberale, F. 1972. Perception of exertion, heart rate, oxygen uptake and blood lactate in different work operations. *Ergonomics* 15:545-54.

Haskvitz, E.M., R.L. Seip, J.Y. Weltman, A.D. Rogol, and A. Weltman. 1992. The effect of training intensity on ratings of perceived exertion. *Int. J. Sports Med.* 13:377-83.

Hetzler, R.K., R.L. Seip, S.H. Boutcher, E. Pierce, D. Snead, and A. Weltman. 1991. Effect of exercise modality on ratings of perceived exertion at various lactate concentrations. *Med. Sci. Sports Exerc.* 23:88-92.

Horstman, D.H., W.P. Morgan, A. Cymerman, and J. Stokes. 1979. Perception of effort during constant work to self-imposed exhaustion. *Percept. Motor Skills* 48:1111-26.

Howley, E.K. 1976. The effect of different intensities of exercise on the excretion of epinephrine and norepinephrine. *Med. Sci. Sports* 8:219-22.

Ivy, J.L., D.L. Costill, W.J. Fink, and R.W. Lower. 1979. Influence of caffeine and carbohydrate feedings on endurance performance. *Med. Sci. Sports* 11.1:6-11.

Johansson, S.E. 1986. Perceived exertion, heart rate and blood lactate during prolonged exercise on a bicycle ergometer. In *Perception of exertion in physical work,* ed. G. Borg and D. Ottoson, 199-206.

Jones, N.L., J.R. Sutton, R. Taylor, and C.J. Toews. 1977. Effect of pH on cardiorespiratory and metabolic responses to exercise. *J. Appl. Physiol.* 43:959-64.

Kamon, E., K. Pandolf, and E. Cafarelli. 1974. The relationship between perceptual information and physiological responses to exercise in the heat. *J. Human Ergol.* 3:45-54.

Knuttgen, H.G., E.R. Nadel, K.B. Pandolf, and J.F. Patton. 1982. Effects of training with eccentric muscle contractions on exercise performance, energy expenditure and body temperature. *Int. J. Sports Med.* 3:13-17.

Kostka, C.E., and E. Cafarelli. 1982. Effect of pH on sensation and vastus lateralis electromyogram during cycling exercises. *J. Appl. Physiol.* 52:1181-85.

Kraemer, W.J., R.V. Lewis, N.T. Triplett, L.P. Koziris, S. Heyman, B.J. Noble. 1992. Effects of hypnosis on plasma proenkephalin peptide F and perceptual and cardiovascular responses during submaximal exercise. *Eur. J. of Appl. Physiol. Occup. Physiol.* 65(6):573-8.

Ljunggren, G., R. Ceci, and J. Karlsson. 1987. Prolonged exercise at a constant load on a bicycle ergometer: Ratings of perceived exertion and leg aches and pain as well as measurements of blood lactate accumulation and heart rate. *Int. J. Sports Med.* 8:109-16.

Löllgen, H., T. Graham, and G. Sjogaard. 1980. Muscle metabolites, force, and perceived exertion bicycling at varying pedal rates. *Med. Sci. Sports Exerc.* 12:345-51.

Marcus, P., and P. Redman. 1979. Effect of exercise on thermal comfort during hypothermia. *Physiol. Behav.* 22:831-35.

McCloskey, D.I., S. Gandevia, E.K. Porter, and J.G. Colebatch. 1983. Muscle sense and effort: Motor commands and judgements about muscular contractions. *Adv. Neurol.* 39:151-67.

Miyashita, M., K. Onodera, and I. Tabata. 1986. How Borg's RPE-scale has been applied to Japanese. In *Perceptual exertion in physical work,* ed. G. Borg and D. Ottoson, 27-34. London: Macmillan.

Moffatt, R.J., and B.A. Stamford. 1978. Effects of pedalling rate changes on maximal oxygen uptake and perceived effort during bicycle ergometer work. *Med. Sci. Sports* 10:27-31.

Morgan, W.P., and M.L. Pollock. 1977. Psychologic characterization of the elite distance runner. *Ann. N.Y. Acad. Sci.* 301:382-403.

Nadel, E.R. 1980. Circulatory and thermal regulations during exercise. *Fed. Proc.* 39:1491-97.

Nieman, D.C., K.A. Carlson, M.E. Brandstater, R.T. Naegele, and J.W. Blankenship. 1987. Running endurance in 27-h-fasted humans. *J. Appl. Physiol.* 63:2502-9.

Noble, B.J., G. Borg, I. Jacobs, R. Ceci, and P. Kaiser. 1983. A category-ratio perceived exertion scale: Relationship to blood and muscle lactates and heart rate. *Med. Sci. Sports Exerc.* 15:523-29.

Noble, B.J., K.F. Metz, K.B. Pandolf, and E. Cafarelli. 1973. Perceptual responses to exercise: A multiple regression study. *Med. Sci. Sports* 5:104-9.

Okano, G., H. Takeda, I. Morita, M. Katoh, Z. Mu, and S. Miyake. 1988. Effect of pre-exercise fructose ingestion on endurance performance in fed men. *Med. Sci. Sports Exerc.* 20:105-9.

Pandolf, K.B. 1983. Advances in the study and application of perceived exertion. *Exerc. Sport Sci. Rev.* 11:118-58.

————. 1986. Local and central factor contributions in the perception of effort during physical exercise. In *Perception of exertion in physical work,* ed. G. Borg and D. Ottoson, 97-110. London: Macmillan.

Pandolf, K.B., E. Cafarelli, B.J. Noble, and K.F. Metz. 1972. Perceptual responses during prolonged work. *Percept. Motor Skills* 35:975-85.

Pederson, P.K., and H.G. Welch. 1977. Oxygen breathing, selected physiological variables and perception of effort during submaximal exercise. In *Physical work and effort,* ed. G. Borg, 385-400. New York: Pergamon Press.

Pivarnik, J.M., T.R. Grafner, and E.S. Elkins. 1988. Metabolic, thermoregulatory, and psychophysiological responses during arm and leg exercise. *Med. Sci. Sports Exerc.* 20:1-5.

Pivarnik, J.M., and L.C. Senay. 1986. Effect of endurance training and heat acclimation on perceived exertion during exercise. *J. Cardiopul. Rehab.* 6:499-504.

Poulus, A.J., H.J. Docter, and H.G. Westra. 1974. Acid-base balance and subjective feelings of fatigue during physical exercise. *Eur. J. Appl. Physiol.* 33:207-13.

Robertson, R.J., J.E. Falkel, A.L. Drash, A.M. Swank, K.F. Metz, S.A. Spungen, and J.R. LeBoeuf. 1986. Effect of blood pH on peripheral and central signals of perceived exertion. *Med. Sci. Sports Exerc.* 18:114-22.

Robertson, R.J., R. Gilcher, K.F. Metz, C. Casperson, T. Allison, R. Abbott, G. Skrinar, J. Krause, and P. Nixon. 1988. Effect of simulated altitude erythrocythemia in women on hemoglobin flow rate during exercise. *J. Appl. Physiol.* 64:1674-79.

Robertson, R.J., R.L. Gillespie, J. McCarthy, and K.D. Rose. 1979a. Differentiated perceptions of exertion: Part I. Mode of integration of regional signals. *Percept. Motor Skills* 49:683-89.

———. 1979b. Differentiated perceptions of exertion: Part II. Relationship to local and central physiological responses. *Percept. Motor Skills* 49:691-97.

Robertson, R.J., F.L. Goss, T.E. Auble, R. Spina, D. Cassinelli, E. Glickman, R. Galbreath, and K. Metz. 1990. Cross-modal exercise prescription at absolute and relative oxygen uptake using perceived exertion. *Med. Sci. Sports Exerc.* 22:653-59.

Robertson, R.J., P.A. Nixon, C.J. Casperson, K.F. Metz, R.A. Abbott, and F.L. Goss. 1992. Abatement of exertional perceptions following high intensity exercise: Physiological mediators. *Med. Sci. Sports Exerc.* 24:346-53.

Robertson, R.J., R.T. Stanko, F.L. Goss, R.J. Spina, J.J. Reilly, and K.D. Greenawalt. 1990. Blood glucose extraction as a mediator of perceived exertion during prolonged exercise. *Eur. J. Appl. Physiol.* 61:100-105.

Sargeant, A.J., and C.T. Davies. 1973. Perceived exertion during rhythmic exercise involving different muscle masses. *J. Human Ergol.* 2:3-11.

Seip, R.L., D. Snead, E.F. Pierce, P. Stein, and A. Weltman. 1991. Perceptual responses and blood lactate concentration: Effect of training state. *Med. Sci. Sports Exerc.* 23:80-87.

Skinner, J.S., R. Hustler, V. Bersteinova, and E.R. Buskirk. 1973. Perception of effort during different types of exercise and under different environmental conditions. *Med. Sci. Sports* 5:110-55.

Skrinar, G.S., S.P. Ingram, and K.B. Pandolf. 1983. Effect of endurance training on perceived exertion and stress hormones in women. *Percept. Motor Skills* 57:1239-50.

Stamford, B.A., and B.J. Noble. 1974. Metabolic cost and perception of effort during bicycle ergometer work performance. *Med. Sci. Sports* 6:226-31.

Stephenson, L.A., M.A. Kolka, and J.E. Wilderson. 1982. Perceived exertion and anaerobic threshold during the menstrual cycle. *Med. Sci. Sports Exerc.* 14:218-22.

Stevens, J.C., and A. Krimsley. 1977. Build-up of fatigue in static work: Role of blood flow. In *Physical work and effort,* ed. G. Borg, 145-56. New York: Pergamon Press.

Sutton, J.R., N.L. Jones, and C.J. Toews. 1981. Effect of pH on muscle glycolysis during exercise. *Clin. Sci.* (London) 61:331-38.

Tesch, P., B. Sjodin, and J. Karlsson. 1978. Relationship between lactate accumulation, LDD activity, LDH activity, LDH isoenzyme and fiber type distribution in human skeletal muscle. *Acta Physiol. Scand.* 103:40-46.

Toner, M.M., L.L. Drolet, and K.B. Pandolf. 1986. Perceptual and physiological responses during exercise in cool and cold water. *Percept. Motor Skills* 62:211-20.

Young, A.J., A. Cymerman, and K.B. Pandolf. 1982. Differentiated ratings of perceived exertion are influenced by high altitude exposures. *Med. Sci. Sports Exerc.* 14:223-28.

7

CHAPTER

Final Common Neurophysiological Pathway for Exertional Perceptions

The final common pathway for peripheral and respiratory-metabolic signals of exertion involves both a central feedforward and a combined feedforward-feedback neurophysiological mechanism (Cafarelli 1982).[1] These sensory mechanisms are depicted in figure 7.1 (Cafarelli 1982). In a feedforward mechanism, a copy of efferent commands from the central motor cortex is simultaneously transmitted to the sensory cortex for interpretation and conscious expression as exertional perception. A feedback mechanism transmits signals from peripheral receptors in muscle, joints, tendons, and skin to the sensory cortex. These afferent sensory signals feedback information about the magnitude of intramuscular tension and cutaneous pressure. A functional interaction exists between the feedforward and feedback loops. Such a combined mechanism provides a precise adjustment of the sensory response according to the level of force production in contracting muscle (McCloskey et al. 1983; Cafarelli and Bigland-Ritchie 1979). This chapter explores the role of both the feedforward and the combined feedforward-feedback pathways in signaling peripheral and respiratory-metabolic perceptions of exertion.

---

[1] It should be noted that neurophysiological signals for nonspecific exertional perceptions most likely involve these same sensory pathways. However, a clear understanding of the final common pathway for nonspecific exertional signals has yet to be identified.

157

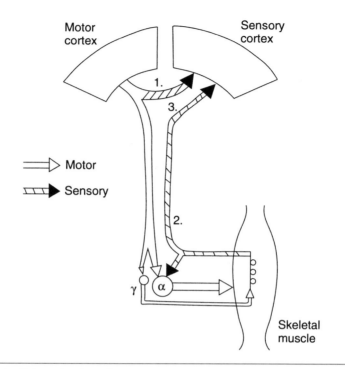

Figure 7.1   Schematic of possible mechanisms for generating muscle sensations. Reprinted from Cafarelli 1982.

Sensory Pathway for Peripheral Exertional Signals

Feedforward Mechanism

The neurophysiological link between exertional perceptions and central motor commands has been demonstrated experimentally for both dynamic and static muscular contractions (McCloskey et al. 1983). Many of these experiments relied on the simultaneous measurement of sensory and motor responses. Electromyography (EMG) indicates the level of excitatory input to muscle, providing an indirect measure of the magnitude of efferent motor commands (Cafarelli and Bigland-Ritchie 1979; Cain and Stevens 1973; Kostka and Cafarelli 1982). Assuming that the neurophysiological pathway for exertional perceptions has its origin in efferent activity, sensory intensity should increase with increases in the amplitude of muscle EMG during exercise (McCloskey et al. 1983; Jones and Hunter 1983a).

As an example, let us consider an experiment by Cafarelli and Bigland-Ritchie (1979), wherein EMG was measured during contralateral matching of muscle contractions. This procedure requires that the subject match force sensations between contracting muscle groups that are located in opposite (i.e., contralateral) limbs (fig. 7.2). The subject is instructed to contract the *right* adductor pollicis (the reference muscle) to achieve a predetermined target tension. The *left* adductor pollicis (the indicator muscle) is simultaneously contracted to achieve a level of force sensation that matches that perceived for the reference muscle (Cafarelli 1982; fig. 7.3a). The tension produced by the indicator muscle is a measure of the level of force sensation that is perceived in the reference muscle. Under these control conditions, force sensation (i.e., developed tension) and EMG are the same between contralateral muscle groups (fig. 7.3c). Next, the reference muscle is functionally weakened by shortening its precontraction length. This is done by decreasing the angle between the thumb and index finger of the reference hand prior to the onset of contraction. The subject is again instructed to contract the reference muscle until the target tension is achieved while simultaneously contracting the indicator muscle to attain a matching level of force sensation. During contraction the tension produced by the indicator muscle is greater than the reference muscle (Cafarelli 1982; fig. 7.3b). This means that the intensity of force sensation for the reference contraction increased when the muscle was weakened. However, despite differences in tension between muscle groups, EMG was the same for reference and indicator muscles (Cafarelli 1982; fig. 7.3c). The neurophysiological signal upon which subjects matched the sense of force between the reference and indicator muscle originated in central motor outflow commands. Under these experimental conditions, peripheral sensory feedback reflecting the level of muscular tension did not influence force sensation. A feedforward mechanism reflecting the magnitude of centrally generated motor commands produced the sense of force (Cafarelli 1982; Cafarelli and Bigland-Ritchie 1979; Jones and Hunter 1983a).

Support for a feedforward mechanism in evaluating force sensations has also been shown when sensory feedback is altered by high- and low-frequency vibration of muscle tendons (McCloskey et al. 1983), neuromotor blockade with curare (Cafarelli 1982), paraplegia (Hobbs and Gandevia 1985), and neuromuscular disease (Bar-Or and Reed 1986). The latter experiment by Bar-Or and Reed (1986) involving pediatric patients with neuromuscular disease serves as an example of such research. Exertional sensations during dynamic exercise were determined for patients with dystrophic, atrophic, and spastic limbs. Afferent sensory signals, particularly during exercise, are altered in these patients, while the pathway for central motor outflow commands is not. Therefore, exertional perceptions (RPE) at a relative power output do not differ between patients with and without neuromuscular disease. These data further suggest that exertional sensations are signaled by a feedforward rather than a feedback mechanism. The reader is referred to research reviews by Cafarelli (1982), McCloskey (1978), and McCloskey et al. (1983) for a more detailed explanation of the final common neurophysiological pathway for exertional sensations.

In order to understand the role of central motor commands in signaling exertional perceptions, it is necessary to examine how efferent transmissions are

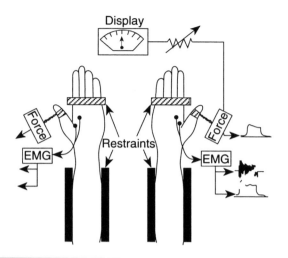

Figure 7.2   Diagram of matching technique used to study muscle sensation in humans. The meter labeled *display* has a variable resistance, is visible to the subject, and is driven by the output of the strain-gauge dynamometer. Recordings of force and EMG can be made simultaneously from both muscles.
Reprinted from Cafarelli 1982.

monitored by the sensory cortex. The most likely explanation is that an advance copy of the central motor outflow command is sent to the sensory cortex through corollary discharges (McCloskey 1978; McCloskey et al. 1983; Jones and Hunter 1983a; Cafarelli 1982). That is, when a supraspinal motor command is discharged, it proceeds caudally through the neuromotor pathway to activate muscle. Simultaneously, a copy of this efferent signal moves rostrally via corollary pathways that terminate in the sensory cortex (McCloskey 1978; McCloskey et al. 1983). These corollary pathways are thought to originate above the spinal motoneurons, branching from corticifugal motor efferent fibers (McCloskey 1978). The corollary signals enter the sensory cortex, evoking perceptions of muscular exertion consistent with the amplitude of the original efferent motor commands (McCloskey et al. 1983).

Combined Feedforward-Feedback Mechanism

In the beginning of this chapter it was noted that a feedback mechanism involving afferent transmissions from peripheral sensory receptors might combine with a feedforward mechanism to signal exertional sensations. Let us briefly examine the evidence that supports such a combined sensory pathway. Peripheral sensory receptors feed back information about the magnitude of developed intramuscular tension, contraction velocity, and joint position. This peripheral afferent feedback

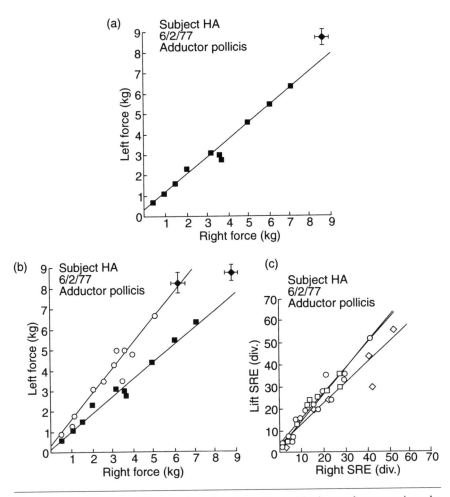

Figure 7.3   Adductor pollicis matching functions. Control both muscles approximately same MVC. Reference muscle is shortened (weakened). (c) Smoothed, rectified electromyogram (SRE) amplitudes obtained from contractions shown in (*a*) and (*b*). Note that EMG (central drive) is not systematically influenced by changing length in this muscle.

originates in (1) primary endings of muscle spindles that detect changes in fiber length, (2) Golgi tendon organs that monitor changes in intramuscular tension, and (3) mechanoreceptors in tendons, joints, and skin (McCloskey et al. 1983; Cafarelli 1982; Jones and Hunter 1983b). The majority of experimental evidence indicates that signals arising from peripheral receptors do not independently influence perceptions of exertion; that is, the sense of muscular exertion and muscular tension are largely independent perceptual domains (McCloskey et al. 1983; Gandevia and McCloskey 1977). What is therefore the role, if any, of peripheral afferent feedback in signaling exertional perceptions? Cafarelli and Bigland-Ritchie (1979) propose a dual-input model that describes an interaction between feedback and feedforward sensorimotor mechanisms. The feedback and feedforward sensory pathways are simultaneously activated at the onset of muscle contraction. An increase in central motor excitation of muscle is accompanied by an increase in peripheral feedback from muscle spindles, ancillary muscles, joints, and skin. The original central motor command is compared to peripheral kinesthetic feedback, the effect of which is to scale the intensity of exertional perceptions according to the size and strength of the contracting muscle (Matthews 1977; Cafarelli and Bigland-Ritchie 1979; McCloskey 1978; McCloskey et al. 1983; Gandevia and McCloskey 1977). The conscious expression of exertional perception can then be more precisely adjusted to account for specific peripheral events that influence force, frequency, and duration of muscular contraction.

Muscle Contractile Pattern and Central Motor Commands

The magnitude of central motor drive during dynamic exercise is directly related to the level of tension (force) produced and to the frequency of muscular contraction. It follows that the intensity of peripheral perceptions of exertion should correspond directly with changes in skeletal muscle contractile patterns, i.e., force and frequency(Stevens and Cain 1970; Edwards et al. 1972). Increases in either of these contractile patterns require a greater level of motor unit recruitment and firing frequency. These changes in muscle fiber activation are the direct result of an increased level of central motor outflow commands. Corollary copies of the efferent motor signals also increase in magnitude, intensifying exertional perceptions. In support of this hypothesis, Cafarelli (1977, 1978) observed that both EMG and exertional perceptions increase in correspondence with an increase in muscular force and contraction frequency. Because EMG is a marker of central motor outflow, it would appear that alterations in muscle contractile patterns are linked to corollary discharges that signal exertional perceptions.

The relation between exertional perceptions and muscle contractile patterns can be seen in research paradigms where power output is held constant while pedaling rate varies from a slow (40 rev/min[-1]) to fast (120 rev/min[-1]) cadence (Stamford and Noble 1974; Pandolf and Noble 1973; Robertson et al. 1979; Edwards et al. 1972). At a given power output, force production is high at a slow cadence and low at a fast cadence. The sensory effects of variations in both the level of force production and in the frequency of contraction can then be evaluated in the same experiment. When using such paradigms, an inverse relation has been found between exertional perception and force production. That is, the intensity of exertional perception is greatest when resistance on the cycle ergometer is high and pedal frequency is low (Löllgen et al. 1975; Pandolf and Noble 1973; Henriksson, Knuttgen, and Bonde-Peterson 1972). On first inspection this suggests that the level of force production may be more important than contraction frequency in signaling perceptions of exertion. However, contraction frequency also appears to play an important sensory role during exercise (Edwards et al. 1972). Löllgen et al. (1975) observed that, for a given power output, RPE was positively correlated with pedaling frequency in athletic ($r = .932$ to $.989$) and nonathletic ($r = .712$ to $.762$) groups. Several investigations report a parabolic relation (fig. 7.4) between pedaling frequency and exertional perceptions (Löllgen, Graham, and Sjogaard 1980; Coast, Cox, and Welch 1986). In these experiments, exertional perceptions are more intense at slower (40 rev/min^{-1}) and at faster (100 rev/min^{-1}) pedaling rates than at intermediate rates (60-80 rev/min^{-1}). Apparently, exertional perceptions are linked to pedaling frequency at the higher cadence and to force production at the lower cadence. When examined collectively, these data indicate that exertional perceptions during dynamic exercise are equally influenced by the absolute level of force production and by the frequency of muscle contraction (Löllgen, Graham, and Sjogaard 1980).

It is possible that force and frequency of muscular contraction operate in a time-dependent manner to signal exertional perceptions (Cafarelli 1977, 1978). During exercise of short duration (< 15 s), the absolute force produced by a

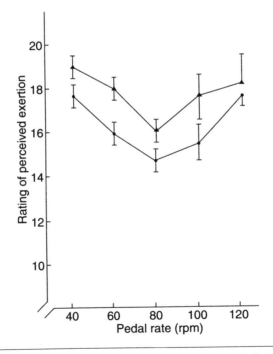

Figure 7.4   RPE vs. pedaling rate. Curves represent separate sampling periods. Points are mean ± *SE*. RPE values were different between pedal rates for each sampling time. ● = 10 min of exercise; ▲ = 20 min of exercise.
Reprinted from Coast, Cox, and Welch 1986.

muscle contraction is the principal factor in signaling exertional perceptions. When exercise duration is greater than 15 s, contraction frequency also begins to influence the sensory intensity of exertion. Therefore, force and frequency of muscle contraction operate sequentially in time to signal exertional perceptions.

The intensity of exertional perceptions also appears to be differentially influenced by the type (i.e., concentric or eccentric) of muscle contraction. At a given power output, effort sensation is greater when muscle develops tension by concentric (i.e., fiber shortening) than by eccentric (i.e., fiber stretching) contraction (Henriksson, Knuttgen, and Bonde-Peterson 1972). The explanation for this sensory response may involve a difference between the number of muscle fibers activated during concentric and eccentric contractions. For the same level of tension, more muscle fibers are innervated during concentric than during eccentric contractions. This suggests the level of central motor outflow required to develop a given level of tension is greater for concentric contractions. Corollary discharge signals to the sensory cortex are correspondingly greater, resulting in more intense exertional perceptions during concentric than during eccentric contractions.

Sensory Pathway for Respiratory-Metabolic Signals of Exertion

Inspiratory Muscle Tension and Effort Sensations

During exercise, ventilatory drive and alveolar ventilation increase in order to meet tissue oxidative requirements (i.e., oxygen uptake) and to buffer metabolic acidosis (i.e., carbon dioxide excretion). Both static and dynamic inspiratory muscle tension must increase to produce a greater pulmonary ventilation (Killian 1986). As inspiratory muscle tension increases, so does the magnitude of respiratory effort sensation. The intensity of respiratory effort is related to those factors that directly influence inspiratory muscle contractile properties: (1) the pattern of tension development, (2) functional weakening of the inspiratory muscles, and (3) inspiratory muscle fatigue (Jones 1984; El-Manshawi et al. 1986; Killian, Bucens, and Campbell 1982; Killian and Campbell 1983; Killian et al. 1984; Killian 1986).

Pattern of Tension Development

As ventilatory drive increases, inspiratory muscle tension also increases in order to overcome elastic and airway resistance (Killian and Campbell 1983). The magnitude of respiratory effort sensation increases as a direct function of developed inspiratory muscle tension and of the subsequent shift in intrathoracic subatmospheric pressure (Gandevia 1982; El-Manshawi and Killian 1986; fig. 7.5). However, respiratory effort is not only a function of the peak inspiratory

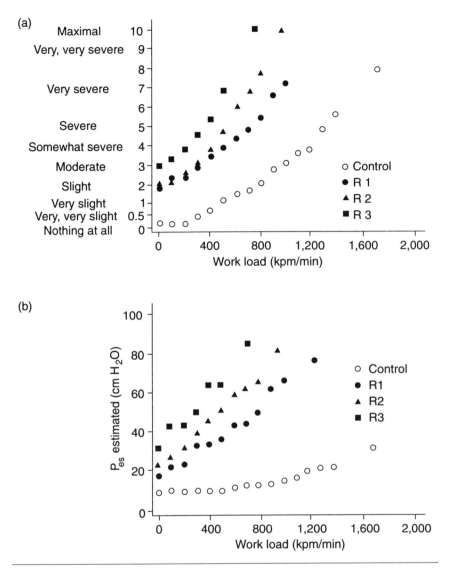

Figure 7.5 (*a*) Rating of breathlessness in control unloaded study (C) and with re-sistive loading (R1, R2, R3) at each workload in incremental exercise. (*b*) Estimated peak esophageal pressure (P_{es}) in C and with resistive loading (R1, R2, R3). Group mean data.

Reprinted from El-Manshawi and Killian 1986.

muscle tension achieved, but also of the pattern by which tension is developed (Killian 1985). Most important among the factors that influence the pattern of inspiratory muscle tension development are the velocity of shortening, frequency of contraction, and the duty cycle (Killian 1986). To a lesser extent, tidal volume, flow rate, and the degree of muscle shortening also determine breathing patterns. The perceived magnitude of respiratory effort increases in direct correspondence with increases in each of the factors that determine the pattern of tension development in inspiratory muscle (Bakers and Tenney 1970; Killian 1986; El-Manshawi et al. 1986). When considered as an aggregate, these factors account for 71% of the variance in perceived respiratory effort (El-Manshawi et al. 1986).

Functional Weakening of Inspiratory Muscle

During exercise, the operating length of inspiratory muscle is shortened, causing a functional weakening (Jones 1984; Killian 1985). Inspiratory muscle weakening is evinced by a reduction in tension-generating capacity (MIP) and is the direct result of the larger tidal volume and flow rate required to meet an increased ventilatory drive (Jones 1984).[2] MIP decreases by 7% for each L/s increase in flow and by 15% for each 10% of the total lung capacity that is accounted for by an increased tidal volume (Jones 1984). Because inspiratory muscles are functionally weakened during exercise, the magnitude of respiratory effort for a given level of tension (i.e., peak inspiratory pressure) is significantly greater than for the generation of comparable tension under isometric conditions (Jones 1984; Killian et al. 1984; El-Manshawi et al. 1986). That is, as muscles weaken, a given level of tension represents a relatively greater percentage of the maximum tension that can be developed. The respiratory effort required to generate a given level of inspiratory muscle tension is correspondingly increased (Jones 1984; El-Manshawi et al. 1986).

Inspiratory Muscle Fatigue

The perceived magnitude of respiratory effort increases as inspiratory muscles fatigue at higher levels of pulmonary ventilation. This sensory response is independent of the changes in respiratory effort that occur when inspiratory pressure (i.e., developed tension) is increased or when inspiratory muscles are weakened due to shortening of their operational length. However, in the absence of lung disease, inspiratory muscle fatigue may not occur, even during peak exercise. Under most circumstances, exercise is terminated due to peripheral muscle fatigue, which normally develops prior to the onset of respiratory muscle fatigue (Killian 1985). While inspiratory muscle fatigue influences respiratory effort, its

---

[2]In a laboratory or clinical setting, the tension-generating capacity of respiratory muscles (i.e., strength) is measured by the maximum intrathoracic subatmospheric pressure (MIP, Torr) generated against an occluded airway during peak inspiration (Killian 1986).

sensory input during exercise is not as important as that of developed tension and functional muscular weakening.

Neurophysiological Pathway

The final common pathway for the respiratory-metabolic signal of exertion is thought to involve a conscious awareness of central motor outflow commands. A competing hypothesis proposes that respiratory effort is mediated by sensory feedback from receptors in the respiratory musculature. Of these two possible neurophysiological pathways, experimental evidence is strongest in support of a link between sensory signals of respiratory exertion and the magnitude of centrally generated motor efferent commands. As an example, Killian et al. (1984) examined the sensory response when lung volume and airway impedance (i.e., elastic loading) were varied while tidal volume and duty cycle were held constant. The perceived magnitude of effort increased with increases in both lung volume (i.e., functional muscular weakening) and elastic impedance (i.e., greater developed tension). In contrast, the magnitude of perceived tension increased with increasing elastic loads but was unaffected when inspiratory muscles were functionally weakened by increasing lung volume. It appears that the final common pathway for the perception of respiratory effort is clearly distinct from the pathway that signals the perceived magnitude of muscular tension. This distinction is significant in that the perceived magnitude of tension in respiratory muscle is mediated by peripheral receptors, most likely the primary endings of muscle spindles (Altose, DiMarco, and Strohl 1981). Effort sensation is not responsive to such afferent feedback (Killian et al. 1984). Rather, signals of respiratory effort arise from a conscious awareness of centrally mediated motor commands.

A greater number of motor commands must be discharged centrally when inspiratory muscle tension is increased to meet an increased ventilatory drive or to compensate for muscular weakening and fatigue. The neurophysiological signal for respiratory effort is transmitted by corollary discharges that diverge from these descending motor commands (Killian et al. 1984; Gandevia, Killian, and Campbell 1981; McCloskey et al. 1983). The greater the number of central corollary discharge signals, the more intense are sensations of respiratory effort (Gandevia, Killian, and Campbell 1981; McCloskey 1978; El-Manshawi et al. 1986). In contrast, afferent neuronal feedback from muscle spindle primaries, stretch receptors (lungs), and joint receptors (chest wall) subserves an awareness of outgoing motor commands. These muscle afferent signals reflect the level of force production and are not consciously perceived as effort. However, peripheral afferents may help to scale and calibrate central motor outflow commands (Killian et al. 1984; Killian 1986; McCloskey et al. 1983; Gandevia, Killian, and Campbell 1981). The afferent signals are integrated centrally with information derived from efferent motor commands. Such sensory integration of feedforward and feedback mechanisms provides a fine-tuning adjustment of the exertional signal according to contractile requirements of the respiratory muscle (McCloskey et al. 1983;

Killian and Campbell 1983). In this manner, the respiratory-metabolic and peripheral exertional signals share a final common neurophysiological pathway.

Summary

The final common neurophysiological pathway for peripheral and respiratory-metabolic signals of perceived exertion involves a combined feedforward-feedback mechanism. During exercise, increases in motor unit recruitment and firing frequency in both peripheral and respiratory skeletal muscle require an increase in central motor feedforward commands. Corollary discharges diverge from the descending motor commands, terminating in the sensory cortex. The greater the magnitude of the corollary signals, the more intense are the perceptions of physical exertion. Afferent feedback signals help to scale and calibrate central motor outflow commands. The resulting sensory integration of feedforward and feedback mechanisms provides a fine-tuning adjustment of the exertional signal.

References

Altose, M.D., A.F. DiMarco, and K.P. Strohl. 1981. The sensation of respiratory muscle force. *Am. Rev. Respir. Dis.* 126:807-11.

Bakers, J.H., and S.M. Tenney. 1970. The perception of some sensations associated with breathing. *Respir. Physiol.* 10:85-92.

Bar-Or, O., and S.L. Reed. 1986. Ratings of perceived exertion in adolescents with neuromuscular disease. In *The perception of exertion in physical work*, ed. G. Borg and D. Ottoson, 137-48. London: Macmillan.

Cafarelli, E. 1977. Peripheral and central inputs to the effort sense during cycling exercise. *Eur. J. Appl. Physiol.* 37:181-89.

———. 1978. Effect of contraction frequency on effort sensations during cycling at a constant resistance. *Med. Sci. Sports* 10:270-75.

———. 1982. Peripheral contributions to the perception of effort. *Med. Sci. Sports Exerc.* 14:382-89.

Cafarelli, E., and B. Bigland-Ritchie. 1979. Sensation of static force in muscles of different length. *Exper. Neurol.* 65:511-25.

Cain, W.S., and J.C. Stevens. 1973. Constant effort contractions related to the electromyogram. *Med. Sci. Sports* 5:121-27.

Coast, J.R., R.H. Cox, and H.G. Welch. 1986. Optimal pedalling rate in prolonged bouts of cycle ergometry. *Med. Sci. Sports Exerc.* 18:225-30.

Edwards, R.H.T., A. Melcher, C.M. Hesser, O. Wigebtz, and L.G. Ekelund. 1972. Physiological correlates of perceived exertion in continuous and intermittent exercise with the same average power output. *Eur. J. Clin. Invest.* 2:108-14.

El-Manshawi, A., K.J. Killian, E. Summers, and N.L. Jones. 1986. Breathlessness during exercise with and without resistive loading. *J. Appl. Physiol.* 61:896-905.

Gandevia, S.C. 1982. The perception of motor commands or effort during muscular paralysis. *Brain* 105:151-59.

Gandevia, S.C., K.J. Killian, and E.J. Campbell. 1981. The effect of respiratory muscle fatigue on respiratory sensations. *Clin. Sci.* 60:463-66.

Gandevia, S.C., and D.I. McCloskey. 1977. Sensations of heaviness. *Brain* 100:345-54.

Henriksson, J., H.G. Knuttgen, and F. Bonde-Peterson. 1972. Perceived exertion during exercise with concentric and eccentric muscle contractions. *Ergonomics* 15:537-44.

Hobbs, S.F., and S.C. Gandevia. 1985. Cardiovascular responses and the sense of effort during attempts to contract paralyzed muscles: Role of the spinal cord. *Neurosci. Letters* 57:85-90.

Jones, L.A., and I.W. Hunter. 1983a. Force and EMG correlates of constant effort contractions. *Eur. J. Appl. Physiol. Occup. Physiol.* 51:75-83.

————. 1983b. Perceived force in fatiguing isometric contractions. *Percept. Psychophys.* 33:369-74.

Jones, N.L. 1984. Dyspnea in exercise. *Med. Sci. Sports Exerc.* 16:14-19.

Killian, K.J. 1985. The objective measurement of breathlessness. *Chest* 88 (Suppl.): 84S-90S.

————. 1986. Breathlessness—The sense of respiratory muscle effort. In *Perception of exertion in physical work,* ed. G. Borg and D. Ottoson, 71-82. London: Macmillan.

Killian, K.J., D. Bucens, and E. Campbell. 1982. Effect of breathing patterns on the perceived magnitude of added loads to breathing. *J. Appl. Physiol.* 52:578-84.

Killian, K.J., and E.J. Campbell. 1983. Dyspnea and exercise. *Ann. Rev. Physiol.* 45:465-79.

Killian, K.J., S.C. Gandevia, E. Summers, and E.J.M. Campbell. 1984. Effect of increased lung volume on perception of breathlessness, effort, and tension. *J. Appl. Physiol. Respir. Environ. Exerc. Physiol.* 57:686-91.

Kostka, C.E., and E. Cafarelli. 1982. Effect of pH on sensation and vastus lateralis electromyogram during cycling exercises. *J. Appl. Physiol.* 52:1181-85.

Löllgen, H., T. Graham, and G. Sjogaard. 1980. Muscle metabolites, force, and perceived exertion bicycling at varying pedal rates. *Med. Sci. Sports Exerc.* 12:345-51.

Löllgen, J., H.V. Ulmer, R. Gross, G. Wilbert, and G. von Neiding. 1975. Methodical aspects of perceived exertion rating and its relation to pedalling rate and rotating mass. *Eur. J. Appl. Physiol.* 35:205-15.

Matthews, B. 1977. Muscle afferents and kinaesthesia. *Br. Med. Bull.* 33:137-42.

McCloskey, D.I. 1978. Kinesthetic sensibility. *Physiol. Rev.* 58:763-820.

McCloskey, D.I., S. Gandevia, E.K. Porter, and J.G. Colebatch. 1983. Muscle sense and effort: Motor commands and judgements about muscular contractions. *Adv. Neurol.* 39:151-67.

Pandolf, K.B., and B.J. Noble. 1973. The effect of pedalling speed and resistance changes on perceived exertion for equivalent power outputs on the bicycle ergometer. *Med. Sci. Sports* 5:132-36.

Robertson, R.J., R.L. Gillespie, J. McCarthy, and K.D. Rose. 1979. Differentiated perceptions of exertion: Part I. Mode of integration of regional signals. *Percept. Motor Skills* 49:683-89.

Stamford, B.A., and B.J. Noble. 1974. Metabolic cost and perception of effort during bicycle ergometer work performance. *Med. Sci. Sports* 6:226-31.

Stevens, J.C., and W.S. Cain. 1970. Effort in isometric muscular contractions related to force level and duration. *Percept. Psychophys.* 8:240-44.

8

CHAPTER

The Influence of Psychological Factors on the Setting of Perceived Exertion: Psychophysiological Modeling

A growing number of reports emanating from the sport psychology literature support the notion that psychological factors, both *situational* and *dispositional,* play a role in the setting of perceptual self-reports. Of course, this is not a new notion. Morgan, as early as 1973, pointed out the fact that a dispositional factor such as personality could modulate exercise perceptions. More recent reports by Rejeski (1981), Hardy, Hall, and Prestholdt (1986), and Boutcher, Fleischer-Curtian, and Gines (1988), to name only a few, support Morgan's notion. It is, indeed, physiocentric to believe that the only perceptual inputs arise from physiological sources (Rejeski 1981). Further, it seems utterly reasonable to think of exercise perceptions emanating from a variety of psychological, physiological, and social sources.

Definition of Terms

Since the terminology used in this chapter may be unfamiliar to some readers, the following terms are defined as an aid to better understanding of the subject matter.

Attentional focus — manipulation of sensory cues, internal or external, to control conscious awareness.

Coactor — one who plays the role of a paired subject so as to manipulate the experimental social environment of a principle subject, for example, one paired as a competitor.

Competitive cognitive strategy — a cognitive strategy that concentrates on somatic sensory stimulation and competitive behavior (*association*) or suppresses somatic stimulation by directing thinking toward other subjects (*dissociation*), for example, recalling favorite music during an exercise performance.

Dispositional factors — those factors embedded in one's temperament that might affect the process of perception, for example, personality.

Locus of control — a dispositional factor that identifies the way an individual assesses the attribution of outcomes. *Internal locus* refers to one who believes behavior influences outcomes. *External locus* refers to one who attributes outcomes to outside forces.

Personality — the totality of qualities and traits that are peculiar to a particular individual. Personality can be broadly subdivided into two attitudes: *extrovert,* an individual interested in others or in the environment as opposed to or to the exclusion of self, and *introvert,* one whose thoughts and feelings are directed toward oneself.

Self-efficacy — belief or conviction that one has the capability to successfully engage in a course of action.

Sex-role typology — degrees of gender, feminine and masculine, can be identified (or typed) in both men and women. For example, a man can be more or less masculine. *Feminine* and *masculine* refer to gender principles rather than sex characteristics per se. Moreover, sex-role typology should not be confused with sexual orientation or preference.

Self-presentation — the degree to which one values presenting oneself in a socially desirable manner.

Situational factors — those factors embedded in the environmental context (e.g., social influence) rather than one's personal characteristics.

Social influence — alteration of one's behavior, feelings, or attitudes by what others say or do.

Stimulus-intensity modulation — the process by which one regulates sensory input. Some individuals have been found to amplify input (*augmentors*), while others attenuate their estimate of input (*reducers*).

Review of Literature

Physiological inputs can account for 50% to 80% of the variance in perceptual ratings in a thermally neutral environment (Noble et al. 1973). The variation in accountability in this experiment was a function of exercise duration, with greater explained variance at 15 min of bicycle exercise than at 5 and 30 min. These authors, all exercise physiologists, explicitly stated their working assumption as follows: "Responses to exertion (RPE) are made from sensations which result from physiological processes." It should be obvious, however, to even the most casual observer that physiological exclusivity with respect to the origin of perceptual ratings is not a tenable position. The rather unilateral approach to the establishment of perceptual theory taken by physiologists has caused one sport psychologist to comment that seeking salience only on the physiological side "has led to an incomplete, if not misleading characterization of RPE" (Rejeski 1981).

Growing experimental data shows clearly that interindividual differences in perceptual response are commonly observed when physiological response is held constant (Morgan 1976; Robertson et al. 1977; Rejeski & Ribisl 1980; Hardy et al. 1986; Prestholdt 1986; Boutcher and Trenski 1990). The genesis of these differences is psychosocial. We agree with Rejeski (1981) that unless social and psychological inputs are considered in future modeling of exercise perceptual response we will be unable to fully unravel the riddles of human perception.

The goal of this chapter is to review the papers that provide the underpinnings of support for psychological influence in the setting of exertional responses. The review will describe those studies that have examined the influence of both situational and dispositional factors. In addition, a psychophysiological model will be proposed.

Influence of Situational Factors on Perceived Exertion

Situational factors can affect the perception of exertion. Such factors include hypnotic suggestion, expected duration of exercise, expected performance level, and the social influence of a coactor or the experimenter. It appears psychological factors are more important at light and moderate exercise intensities, although additional research is needed to determine the extent to which the effect of such factors is situation specific.

Hypnosis

Perhaps the first exercise psychologist to posit psychological factors as an explanation for individual differences in perceived exertion was William P. Morgan. In 1973, he reported the results of several experiments dealing with perceived exertion. In one of these experiments he found that subjects increased RPE when hypnotic suggestion indicated they were riding up a steep hill. Further investigation (Morgan et al. 1976) confirmed this result and found that the suggestion alone was accompanied by significant increases in pulmonary ventilation. However, a recent attempt to replicate this experiment (Kraemer et al. 1992) could not confirm earlier results.

Expected Duration

Over the past 10 to 15 years, Jack Rejeski has made significant contributions to our understanding of the psychological underpinnings of perceived exertion. His initial paper (Rejeski and Ribisl 1980) hypothesized that RPE has "cognitive as well as perceptual foundations." He and his coauthor posited that one's expectancy of exercise duration could modify ratings of exertion. When subjects were told they were riding a 30 min trial subsequent to a 20 min trial, RPE was depressed even though exercise was terminated after 20 min. This result occurred despite the fact that physiological variables did not change. It was suggested that subjects either attempted to dissociate physiological feedback or that their ratings were affected by the duration goal.

Expected Performance

When subjects received full performance feedback—that is, distance covered in the previous 3-min segment of a 45-min test—the actual performance in a subsequent test segment closely paralleled expected performance (Zohar and Spitz 1981). Subjects were instructed to pedal the bicycle as fast as they could throughout, keeping in mind the need to preserve energy for the full 45-min test. Ratings of exertion were not significantly correlated with expected performance because, as time progressed, expected performance remained relatively unchanged while RPE gradually increased. Similar results were observed when partial feedback was provided. However, in a no-feedback condition, expected performance declined as RPE increased ($r = -.91$). In other words, with no feedback subjects "hedged their bets" by continuing to decrease their expectations even though actual performance remained relatively unchanged. Because actual performance stayed up, RPE rose due to the length of the test. RPE increased linearly in the no-feedback trial compared with steady-state responses in the other conditions. HR plateaued at approximately 160 bpm after 5 min in all trials. The authors concluded that "physiological sources other than heart rate have become the source of exertion perceptions." However, since actual performance seemed to be higher in the no-feedback condition, it is likely that metabolic cost was also higher, making the heart rate data questionable.

Self-Presentation

Self-presentation theory suggests that "in social situations, individuals typically attempt to present themselves in a socially desirable manner by appearing attractive, competent, and honest" (Baumeister 1982). Presentation of self can take a specific form, audience pleasing, or a general form, self-construction. In both forms, there is an attempt to present oneself favorably, but in the former the attempt is specific to the values of a particular audience. Self-construction is the motive to impress others in general. Those designated as high self-constructors rate RPE significantly lower than low self-constructors at low exercise intensities (Boutcher, Fleischer-Curtian, and Gines 1988).

It is thought that the self-presentation effect is dependent on the intensity of social information. For example, in cases where low-intensity social information is available, it is hypothesized that RPE is lower than when exercising alone. On the other hand, when social information is high, self-presentation theory predicts that RPE is the same whether the exerciser is alone or in the presence of others. The work of Hardy, Hall, and Prestholdt (1986) illustrates this point. Subjects were asked to ride a bicycle for 15 min at 50% $\dot{V}O_2$max under two conditions, alone and in the presence of a coactor. With half the subjects the coactor provided low-intensity information; that is, the coactor rode at 25% $\dot{V}O_2$max. The other half rode with a coactor exhibiting high-intensity information, that is, riding at 75% $\dot{V}O_2$max. Under the low-intensity condition, subjects rated the exercise significantly lower. With high-intensity information there was no significant difference. The authors concluded that RPE may be influenced by manipulating the saliency of social cues.

In a companion experiment (Hardy, Hall, and Prestholdt 1986), subjects rode alone and in the presence of a coactor performing at the same exercise intensities (25%, 50%, and 75% $\dot{V}O_2$max). With the coactor, RPE was significantly lower at 25% and 50% but not at 75%. Again, social influence appeared to mediate RPE. Additionally, the results suggest a curvilinear relationship between physiological and psychological inputs to RPE. Social influence appears to be most salient at light and moderate exercise intensities. At high intensities, when physiological cues are most powerful, social influence is less salient. This apparent curvilinear relationship will be discussed in detail later.

Social influence may be less salient for highly trained athletes (Sylva, Boyd, and Mangum 1990). Male and female track athletes rode a bicycle alone and in the presence of a male coactor and a female coactor. Neither coactor gender nor social influence affected RPE response in this highly trained sample. The authors suggested that these results may be specific to this sample; however, the 60 and 41 ml/kg/min aerobic power of these subjects belies the authors' description as ''elite.''

In a related study, Rejeski and Sanford (1984) investigated the role of social modeling on perception of exertion. They hypothesized that the presence of an intolerant social model would lead to higher perceptual ratings in feminine-typed females. Subjects were shown a film in which the experimental task, bicycle ergometer exercise, was modeled by a woman who was ''optimistic, energetic, and relaxed'' (tolerant model) or by one who showed signs of difficulty with the exercise task (intolerant model). Indeed, those who viewed the intolerant model rated the exertion as higher. Again, manipulation of the social environment modulated the perceptual response.

The gender and race of the experimenter may influence perceived exertion under certain specific circumstances. Males were found to rate exertion higher in the presence of a female experimenter during heavy exercise (Boutcher, Fleischer-Curtian, and Gines 1988). Black subjects reported higher exertional ratings with black testers than with white testers (Bubb et al. 1985). Further, black males and females both rated exertion lower than white counterparts during light exercise in the presence of a white tester.

Attentional Focus

It is likely that internal and external sensory cues compete with one another prior to the setting of exertional ratings. Once exertional symptoms reach awareness, it may be possible for cues from one source to dampen the effect of the other. Several investigations have hypothesized that promotion of external attentional focus will decrease awareness of internal sensations.

Pennebaker and Lightner (1980) reported the results of two experiments in which this hypothesis was tested. In the first experiment beginning joggers walked on a treadmill for 10 min (3.4 mph and 12°) under three conditions. In one condition subjects listened to street sounds to provide an external attentional focus. In another condition they listened to their own breathing to maintain an internal focus. The third condition offered no attentional manipulation. Fatigue was monitored on a 100-point scale. Fatigue was experienced as greater during the breathing condition, confirming the hypothesis that an external attentional focus would decrease symptoms. In the second experiment subjects were instructed to jog or walk at a comfortable pace over two 1,800-m courses. One course was a cross-country trail, and the other consisted of nine laps around a 200-m open field. The design was predicated on the presumption that the cross-country trail offered a greater external attentional focus. The authors asserted that, because fatigue was equivalent in the two conditions and because the subjects ran the cross-country course with a significantly faster pace, the external environment reduced internal sensation.

Fillingim and Fine (1986) questioned the success of Pennebaker and Lightner's design in the second experiment. Pennebaker and Lightner assumed that the attentional focus on the cross-country trail was external without having an empirical confirmation. In addition, when Pennebaker and Lightner asked subjects to listen to their own breathing, they were, in fact, receiving external not internal information. Thus, Fillingim and Fine designed an experiment to correct these design deficiencies. The subjects, a group of active joggers, were instructed to jog for 1 m as fast as possible without experiencing discomfort. In one condition they listened to a tape with the instruction to count the number of times they heard the word *dog* (word-cue condition). In another condition subjects were asked to focus their attention on their breathing and the beating of their heart (breathing condition). Symptoms were rated on a 1-to-7 scale following each condition. "Exercise-relevant symptoms under the word-cue condition were significantly ($p < .05$) lower than under the breathing and control conditions" (Fillingim and Fine 1986). Since there were no differences between conditions for exercise-irrelevant symptoms, the authors posited that the attention manipulation was task specific. Again, with improved experimental procedures, the hypothesis that an external attentional focus can reduce internal symptomatology was confirmed.

Johnson and Siegel (1987) compared two different methods of delivering external information. Using an active method, subjects were required to solve a constant flow of math problems. Listening to asynchronous music was termed a passive method. Perceived exertion was significantly lower with the active method compared to the passive or a control condition. The music condition (passive) was not different from the control condition. If we assume that subjects focused on internal sensations during the control condition, it can be said that the general hypothesis was again confirmed. Music did not prove to be a potent distracter.

Visual and auditory deprivation has been used to force an internal attentional focus (Boutcher and Trenske 1990). A deprivation condition was compared to a music and to a control condition at light (60%), moderate (75%), and high (85%) exercise intensities. There were no differences in RPE at the high exercise intensity. Music produced a significantly lower RPE compared with the deprivation condition at the light intensity, confirming the distracting effect of an external focus. The authors suggested that the music condition "may have generated positive emotional states rather than acting as a distractor." The result for the moderate intensity is somewhat confusing. Here, the only significant difference was a lower RPE response to the deprivation condition compared to the control. Thus, an internal focus resulted in lower RPE.

Boutcher and Trenske (1990) suggest that their data support the view that the greatest influence from psychological factors is observed at light and moderate intensities rather than high intensities, where greater salience is provided by physiological inputs. The origin of this observation has been attributed to Rejeski and Ribisl (1980). In their work a significant effect was found with subjects running at 85% $\dot{V}O_2$max. These authors concluded that the positive effect of the situational context utilized—expected duration—is "limited to moderate-work levels." This cautionary statement has been taken as support for the nonlinear relationship between psychological and physiological inputs previously mentioned. Such a conclusion is questionable because the so-called moderate work level was not compared to other work levels and because 85% $\dot{V}O_2$max is more appropriately designated as high rather than moderate (Boutcher and Trenske 1990). Real support for the nonlinear response comes from the work of Hardy, Hall, and Prestholdt (1986). In their work, evidence for the influence of social context—a coactor—was found only at 25% (light) and 50% (moderate) but not at 75% $\dot{V}O_2$max (high). Although we believe the general concept has merit, the designations of light, moderate, and high exercise intensity are confusing. For example, Rejeski and Ribisl (1980) found an effect at 85% $\dot{V}O_2$max but called the exercise moderate. However, Hardy, Hall, and Prestholdt (1986) found no effect at 75% $\dot{V}O_2$max and called the exercise high. Moreover, the presence of a female experimenter had an effect on males only during heavy exercise (85%

$\dot{V}O_2$max; Boutcher, Fleischer-Curtian, and Gines 1988). It may be that we are dealing with both an exercise-intensity effect and also an effect related to the specificity of the situational context.

Several investigations have not been able to support a change in RPE with manipulation of attentional focus. Wrisberg et al. (1988) provided internal focus by having subjects watch themselves in a mirror and listen to their own breathing. A film was used to provide an external focus. The exercise RPE was recorded only at the termination of the maximal exercise task. No intercondition differences were observed for RPE. This is an example of an exercise situation in which the physiological stress is so high (maximum) that there is little likelihood that the situational manipulation would have an effect. The result appears to support the nonlinear relationship between psychological and physiological inputs. We would have a much better picture of the relationship had RPE data been collected throughout the exercise conditions.

Fillingim, Roth, and Haley (1989) exercised subjects for 10 min at a very low bicycle exercise intensity (300 kpm). Subjects were exercised under distraction (slides) and no-distraction conditions. No significant differences in RPE were observed. Since the RPE at the end of the 10 min of exercise was about 14, one would have to conclude that the exercise was experienced as moderate in intensity. In this case the nonlinear response hypothesis does not seem to be supported. The authors suggest that the response might be related to the fact that the subject sample was largely unfit. However, the Hardy, Hall, and Prestholdt (1986) experiment that serves as the prototype for the nonlinear response also used unfit subjects. Certainly the interaction of fitness level with exercise intensity and situational method needs to be studied.

Copeland and Franks (1991) claim to have found evidence for a depression in RPE during a maximal exercise test through the use of music. However, this conclusion was based on a 0.10 alpha level ($p = .08$). Because of the emotional impact of music, it may not be an appropriate distracter of attentional focus.

Franks and Myers (1984) could not find an influence on RPE using question asking as a distracter during a maximal exercise test. Since only three questions were asked in each stage, the distraction must have been minor at best. Moreover, a more robust test of the hypothesis would have included RPE recorded at several exercise intensities.

It seems clear that perceived exertion can be modulated by altering attentional focus. The extent to which this response is affected by exercise intensity is still murky.

Summary of Findings on the Influence of Situational Factors

At this juncture it should be obvious that manipulation of one's attention as well as social environment can have a profound affect on perception of exertion. If an exercise task is made to appear difficult, through hypnotic suggestion (Morgan 1973; Morgan et al. 1976) or by negative social modeling (Rejeski and Sanford 1984), exertional perceptions increase. Moreover, exertional sensations can be dampened when subjects expect longer duration exercise (Rejeski and Ribisl 1980), are in the presence of a coactor during light and moderate exercise (Hardy, Hall, and Prestholdt 1986), are male and are in the presence of a female experimenter during heavy exercise (Boutcher, Fleischer-Curtian, and Gines 1988), or are distracted from an internal sensation focus by street sounds (Pennebaker and Lightner 1980) or by math computations (Johnson and Siegel 1987).

Certain experimental situations have been ineffective as modulators of perceived exertion. For example, when highly trained (but not elite) athletes exercised in the presence of a coactor (Sylva, Boyd, and Mangum 1990), when untrained subjects exercised at a high intensity in the presence of a coactor (Hardy, Hall, and Prestholdt 1986), and when slides were used as a distracter (Fillingim, Roth, and Haley 1989), no alterations of RPE were observed. Visual and auditory distracters may vary in their effectiveness. Film did not alter RPE in one study (Wrisberg et al. 1988), but reports were only made at maximal exercise when few, if any, psychosocial interventions appear to be effective. Music did not alter perception in two studies (Johnson and Siegel 1987; Copeland and Franks 1991), but, again, in one of those studies (Copeland and Franks 1991) ratings were only made at the termination of maximal exercise. In the one study in which music had an effect (Boutcher and Trenske 1990), it lowered RPE only at the light exercise intensity. The authors suggested that music may affect perception because of its emotional impact rather than because it acts as a distracter of internal attentional focus.

Several authors (Hardy, Hall, and Prestholdt 1986; Boutcher and Trenske 1990) have pointed to the apparent nonlinear relationship between psychological and physiological factors as they affect ratings of perceived exertion. That is to say, physiological factors have more saliency at high exercise intensities, whereas psychological factors have greater import at light and moderate intensities. Inconsistencies in results and in determining what constitutes moderate- and high-intensity exercise point to the need for more precise definitions and to the possibility that the nonlinearity is situation specific.

Further investigation is indicated to determine the extent to which fitness level interacts with situational factors in the setting of perceived exertion. While Hardy, Hall, and Prestholdt (1986) found the presence of a coactor depressed perceived exertion in a group of untrained subjects, a similar result was not observed in a trained sample (Sylva, Boyd, and Mangum 1990).

Influence of Dispositional Factors on Perceived Exertion

An individual's disposition, or psychological traits, may also affect perceived exertion. Dispositional factors that have been investigated include style of stimulus intensity modulation (augmentation or reduction), external or internal locus of control, sex-role type, associative or dissociative cognitive style, one's judgments of self-efficacy, and other personality traits.

Stimulus Intensity Modulation

Sparse attention was given to psychological factors impacting perceived exertion in the 1970s. Robertson et al. (1977) were among the first to do so. They hypothesized that individuals classified as augmentors of sensory input by the kinesthetic aftereffect test would be less tolerant of pain and therefore would rate perceived exertion higher than those classified as reducers of sensory input. Subjects rode a bicycle at 450, 750, and 1,050 kpm/min, with perceived exertion recorded at each exercise level. A significant main effects F test indicated that augmentors rated the exertion higher than reducers. Coupled with a nonsignificant interaction between modulation style and exercise level, the authors assumed that the effect was consistent across the exercise levels. Further calculation of the Robertson et al. data indicates that their subjects were exercising at roughly 47%, 63%, and 86% of predicted $\dot{V}O_2$max. If their assumption of effect consistency across exercise levels and our percent calculations are correct, the hypothesis of nonlinearity of psychological and physiological factors may not be supported. That is to say, the data of this study indicate a relative linearity across exercise intensities. Again, as with situational factors, linearity may be specific to the experimental condition.

Locus of Control

''People with an internal locus of control tend to believe their behavior influences outcomes. External locus of control people tend to attribute outcome to outside forces such as fate, chance and other people'' (Kohl and Shea 1988). Therefore, it may be hypothesized that those people disposed to locate control externally would rate exertion higher when they are exposed to a situation in which exercise intensity is manipulated to indicate they are working harder than they really are. In an experiment designed to test this hypothesis, Kohl and Shea (1988) were unable to find a difference between subjects with external and with internal loci. In another experiment in this report, exercise duration was manipulated so that 6 min of exercise was visually monitored as only 5 min. The result indicated an opposite outcome to that predicted by locus of control theory. Subjects with an internal locus of control were more affected by contextual cues (duration) than were subjects with an external locus. Although the results of this experiment were negative, the potential viability of the locus of control hypothesis makes it ripe for further experimental harvesting.

Sex-Role Typology

Sex-role typology should have an affect on the manner in which one experiences exertion. It has been hypothesized that feminine-typed women would rate exertion higher than those typed as masculine or androgynous (Hochstetler, Rejeski, and

Best 1985). Eleven women of each type ran on a treadmill for 30 min at 70% $\dot{V}O_2$max. No significant differences were observed between the masculine and androgynous groups. However, as hypothesized, the feminine-typed women rated the exertion higher than the other two groups. Subsequently, a similar study was conducted in which feminine-, androgynous-, and masculine-typed males were compared (Rejeski et al. 1985). Subjects rode a bicycle ergometer 6 min at 85% estimated $\dot{V}O_2$max. During the last minute of the ride, feminine-typed males rated the exertion higher than both androgynous and masculine men. Thus, the hypothesis was confirmed in males.

Cognitive Style

Morgan and Pollock (1977) identified two divergent mental strategies that differentiate elite marathoners from recreational long-distance runners. Marathoners were said to use an association strategy whereby attention is paid to internal sensory cues. Recreational runners utilized a dissociation strategy in which they deflected internal bodily signals with various forms of distractive thinking. This concept was broadened by Schomer (1986), who hypothesized that the associative strategy was more related to the intensity of training than the status of the runner; that is, as one increases training intensity, the proportion of associative thinking also increases. Highly experienced marathoners were compared with minimally experienced marathoners as well as beginning marathoners. More experience was associated with higher intensity training and, therefore, higher perceived exertion levels while training. A strong positive relationship was observed between the proportion of associative thinking and perceived exertion while training. This result was partially confirmed by Jones and Cale (1989). As perceived effort increased in the course of a 10.5-mi run, subjects engaged in more associative thinking. These results may shed some light on the somewhat opaque findings discussed in the previous section with regard to the interaction of exercise intensity and attentional focus. More highly trained and fatigued exercisers may shift to a more internally focused cognitive style, making psychological interventions less salient.

Self-Efficacy

It would seem that what we sometimes speak of as self-esteem or self-confidence in our ability to succeed at a task would be related to perception of exertion. A person with more confidence would likely rate exertion less effortful. Bandura (1977) organized this idea into a well-developed construct called self-efficacy. "Broadly defined, self-efficacy cognitions concern the beliefs or convictions that one has in one's capabilities to successfully engage in a course of action sufficient to satisfy the situational demands" (McCauley and Courneya 1992). Self-efficacy is not a function of one's skills but of one's judgments about one's skills. It would be predicted that a person with high self-efficacy would "approach more challenging tasks, put forth more effort, and persist longer in the face of obstacles, barriers, and aversive or stressful stimuli" (McCauley and Courneya 1992). In an exercise context, it would be hypothesized that highly self-efficacious subjects would rate effort lower than those with less self-efficacy. In the only study to test this hypothesis, 88 male and female subjects rode a bicycle ergometer to 70% of HR max (McCauley and Courneya 1992). Since this construct is task specific, self-efficacy was determined by measuring each subject's perception of his or her ability to ride a bicycle for various amounts of time. The experimental hypothesis was supported, even though the contribution of self-efficacy to perceived exertion was found to be rather modest (3.1%). The authors suggest that the contribution would most likely increase at a higher exercise intensity. This hypothesis requires empirical testing, but considerable other research predicts that higher exercise levels (>70%) would be accompanied with greater attention to internal symptomatology, which could very well dampen the effect of self-efficacious judgments.

Personality

C.G. Jung published his extensive study of human personality in 1921. This work, entitled *Psychological Types*, defined the characteristics of the introverted and extroverted personalities. The extrovert is oriented to objects outside of himself or herself. On the other hand, the introvert directs attention primarily to the subject, the self, rather than to external objects. Because of the extrovert's external orientation, pain tolerance is thought to be higher. Since personality as a construct is so general, it has been difficult to measure and, therefore, its utility as an explanation of human behavior has been limited.

Judging by the number of publications, however, no other psychological factor has received as much attention as the relationship between perceived exertion and personality. Morgan (1973) had university students, who were identified as introverts or extroverts using the Eysenck Personality Inventory (EPI), ride a bicycle ergometer at several exercise intensities. He observed correlations of −.62, −.69, and −.71 at 900, 1,200, and 1,500 kpm/min, respectively. This confirmed the hypothesis that university-aged extroverts suppress painful stimuli; that is, the higher the extroversion, the lower the RPE at each exercise level. Using the Junior Eysenck Personality Inventory (JEPI), no significant correlations could be found in a group of 16-year-old boys, however (Williams and Eston 1986).

During the 1970s Friedman and Rosenman (1974) noticed that a certain behavior style seemed to be more prone to heart disease. Hard driving, time conscious, fatigue suppressing individuals, termed type A, were found to have a higher incidence of heart disease than an equally productive but more passive personality style, called type B. Type A individuals are said to constantly strive to exert mastery over their environment. Carver, Coleman, and Glass (1976) used the student version of the Jenkins Activity Survey (JAS) to measure the presence of the coronary-prone personality pattern in college students. As predicted, fatigue ratings were found to be lower in the type A subjects. The authors suggested that if type A subjects acknowledged their fatigue, it would interfere with their striving for task mastery.

Three other studies have utilized the Jenkins Activity Survey to assess type A and B personality styles. While one study (DeMeersman 1988) found that type As rated their exertion lower while exercising at 60% $\dot{V}O_2$max, two other studies could not confirm the relationship between RPE and type A personality. Rejeski, Morley, and Miller (1983) failed to find a significant correlation between type A orientation and RPE during a maximal exercise test in coronary patients. Likewise, Hardy, McMurray, and Roberts (1989) found no difference in the way As and Bs perceive effort while working at 40%, 60%, and 80% $\dot{V}O_2$max. Dishman et al. (1991) have posited that the conflicting results in previous investigations may be due to the use of different exercise protocols, varying measures of perceived effort, and the fact that measurement of type A and B personality with the JAS format does not exceed chance, at least in middle-aged subjects. Future research using more precise measurements of personality seems to be indicated.

Summary of Findings on the Influence of Dispositional Factors

Dispositional factors are by definition more permanent psychological traits. Although it is difficult to say definitively whether dispositional factors are based in genetics, development, or a combination of both, they are more or less immutable psychological characteristics. They may interact with situational factors, but they are not in themselves subject to change with contextual alterations. One can be classified, for example, as an augmentor or reducer of stimulus intensity. Reducers were found to rate exertion lower across a wide spectrum of exercise intensities. Although locus of control as an influence on exertional perceptions is a promising hypothesis, subjects with an internal locus were not found to rate exertion higher than externally oriented subjects. Both males and females typed as feminine rated exertion higher than those typed as androgynous or masculine. Although cognitive mental strategies might be thought of as dispositional, experimental results discussed in this section indicate that the association strategy is subject to change with training and fatigue. As subjects become more highly trained or fatigued, they use a higher proportion of associative thinking. Those with high self-efficacy rate perceived exertion lower than those characterized as low in self-efficacy. It has been difficult to establish personality as an important factor in the setting of perceived exertion partly because of methodological problems. Studies using the Eysenck Personality Inventory have shown a definite relationship. However, those incorporating the Jenkins Activity Survey (JAS) have shown mixed results. The JAS is known to be no better than chance in its ability to discriminate type A from type B personalities.

Psychophysiological Modeling

Much of the physiological modeling to date has its origin in the 1976 Kinsman and Weiser model, later adapted by Pandolf (1978). The basic premise of all models developed by exercise physiologists has embraced the Kinsman and Weiser (1976) assumption that "symptoms have their genesis in known or as yet unidentified physiological changes occurring during work, i.e., within the physiological substrata." These substrata are said to produce groupings of "conceptually clear, discrete symptoms which increase together" during bicycle exercise (Kinsman, Weiser, and Stamper 1973). The model postulates three levels of organization for physiological symptoms leading to the perceptual report: subordinate, ordinate, and superordinate (see fig. 4.2). The symptom groupings arising from the physiological substrata form the subordinate level and contain cues directly related to bicycle fatigue, an ordinate level category. The subordinate groupings are cardiopulmonary fatigue symptoms, also called central cues; leg fatigue, also called local (or peripheral) cues; and general fatigue, containing feelings of tiredness not localized to specific physioanatomical loci. Bicycle fatigue, which encompasses these three discrete symptom groupings, provides a primary input into the perceptual self-report (superordinate level). Two other primary inputs to the self-report, motivation and task aversion, are more psychological in tone but are also said to be derived from the physiological substrata, each with discrete symptom groupings.

Our scientific curiosity implores us to ask whether indeed psychological inputs must only have their genesis in the physiological substrata. Of course, exercise sensations begin as physiological entities. But perceptions about the exercise experience need not arise from sensation alone. They can also arise from the psychological disposition of the exerciser and the situational context within which exertion takes place. It seems clear from the experimental results presented in this chapter that psychological inputs arise from separate sources, situational and dispositional, and become integrated with physiological inputs.

Influence of Psychological Factors
on the Preconscious Level

The source of specific inputs aside, some kind of integration of diverse cues (bicycle fatigue, motivation, and task aversion) is implied prior to the final setting of the self-report in the Kinsman and Weiser model. A variety of inputs are organized, assessed, and, in the case of an undifferentiated report (overall rating), reduced to a single sensory intensity estimate.

However, it is notable that the Kinsman and Weiser model omits the possibility of psychological factors having their influence at a preconscious level. The argument has been put forward that perceived exertion is an active process rather than the passive process indicated in physiological modeling (Rejeski 1985). "The passive approach attempts to explain much of perception and attention by measurement and understanding of stimulus characteristics," that is, the underlying physiological cues. Physiological modeling rests on the assumption of a direct connection between sensation and perceptual response. That would mean that sensory cues would not be amenable to mediation by psychological factors preconsciously, prior to sensory awareness. Thus, most previous models (Kinsman and Weiser 1974; Pandolf, Burse, and Goldman 1975; Robertson 1982; Cafarelli 1982) put forward by exercise physiologists have been sequential models that characterize perceived exertion as an additive not a parallel process. That is to say, psychological factors, if considered at all, enter or modulate the process after the individual experiences the sensation.

Rejeski (1985) posits perception of effort as an active process, utilizing the pain perception model of Leventhal and Everhart (1979; fig. 8.1). Psychological variables alter sensory cues prior to reaching the cerebral cortex. To support this position, Rejeski (1985) argues that "similar peripheral physiological changes in two individuals do not necessarily result in similar percepts." The Leventhal and Everhart information processing model proposes four stages in the processing of sensory stimulation. The stages are: encoding, elaboration, perception, and attention selection and signal amplification. In the first stage, sensory stimuli are encoded into neural signals. The second stage involves elaboration of the neural signal, the preconscious processing stage. Presumably during this stage at least some psychological factors become integrated with the sensory stimuli. Rejeski (1985) has suggested, and we agree, that the hypnosis studies of Morgan et al. (1976) illustrate the assumption that psychological factors can preconsciously elaborate the sensory signal. Sensory information enters the perceptual field, thus consciousness, during stage three. Low temperature becomes cold, tactile stimulation becomes touch, muscular contraction becomes exertion, and so forth. During the final stage, the signal enters attention channels. Here attention becomes focused and the signal is amplified. The model distinguishes between perception and focal awareness. "Whereas perception refers to all the processed material to which one can attend, focal awareness represents that segment of potential stimuli to which one does attend" (Rejeski 1985). The work on attentional focus, discussed earlier, would be an illustration of this stage in action. For example, Johnson and Siegel (1987) found that when subjects' attention was manipulated by mathematical computations, perceived exertion was lower than in a control condition; that is, awareness was shifted from inner sensations to an external focus. This would also be the level where the effect of exercise intensity would play its part. For example, a contextual variable that may be salient at a moderate intensity may drop out of awareness at a high intensity; that is, physiological symptomatology would become the prime focus of awareness.

186

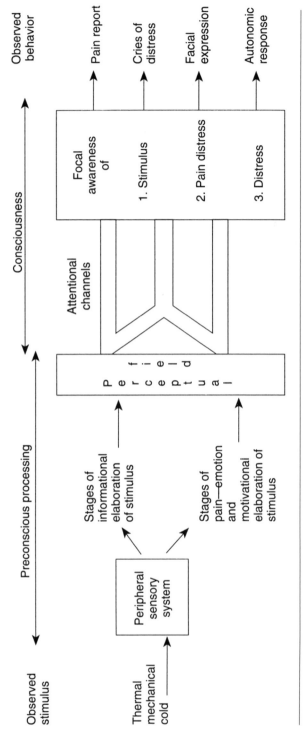

Figure 8.1   Parallel processing of information, pain, and distress
Reprinted from Leventhal and Everhart 1979.

The Noble (1977) and Noble et al. (1986) models (figs. 8.2 and 8.3) hypothesized an integration of sensory signals with various psychological factors such as personality (Morgan 1973) and stimulus intensity modulation (Robertson et al. 1977). These models are conceptually psychophysiological. They assume that certain physiological cues, such as pulmonary ventilation, can be directly perceived, while others, such as oxygen consumption, cannot. Depending on the nature of the sensory stimulus, the signal is more or less amenable to conscious attention. Thus, the possibility of both preconscious and conscious attention to sensations was posited. The Noble and Noble et al. models used the term *filter* as a symbolic analogue to illustrate a possible mechanism of integration of sensory cues with various psychological factors. Although it was not specifically stated, it was implied that a psychological factor like personality could modulate the physiological signal preconsciously. An extrovert, for example, does not consciously think about this trait and make judgments accordingly. The extrovert's tendency to reduce pain stimuli unconsciously filters the sensory signal. Filter here is meant in the electronic sense, that is to say, literally to remove or attenuate components of undesired frequency or undue prominence. Perhaps *modulator* would be a better term because that's exactly what is meant. The so-called filter blends, dampens, or amplifies the more or less pure sensory signal by entering the psychological factor into the perceptual mix. The final perceptual process by which individuals set the self-report was thought to be largely a conscious one. However, it is quite possible for largely unconscious processes to impact the selection of perceptual intensity after the signal reaches the cortex. The role of the unconscious in the setting of exertional perceptions is discussed in more detail in the next chapter.

Summary

The psychophysiological process governing perceived exertion is a complex one, and we are a long way from understanding it completely. Empirical data is not extensive enough to propose a definitive model at this time, but we would be remiss if we did not propose a working model from which future research might be generated. We can begin with some assumptions. First, it is clear to us that both physiological and psychological factors affect perceptual ratings. Second, the relative contribution of each component may be dependent on corollary factors such as exercise intensity, training level, and accumulated fatigue. Third, the so-called psychological factors consist of two subcategories: situational and dispositional. Fourth, physiological and psychological factors affect perceptual ratings independently and in concert. A few examples will illustrate this final assumption. It should be remembered that each exerciser brings his or her own preexisting psychological traits and physiological capacities to the exercise setting. Let us say that we have two

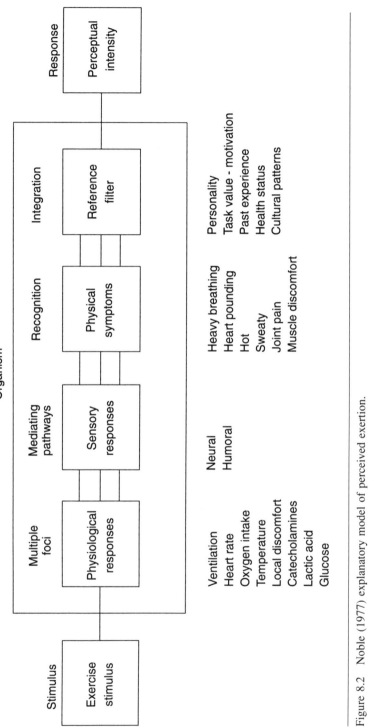

Figure 8.2 Noble (1977) explanatory model of perceived exertion.

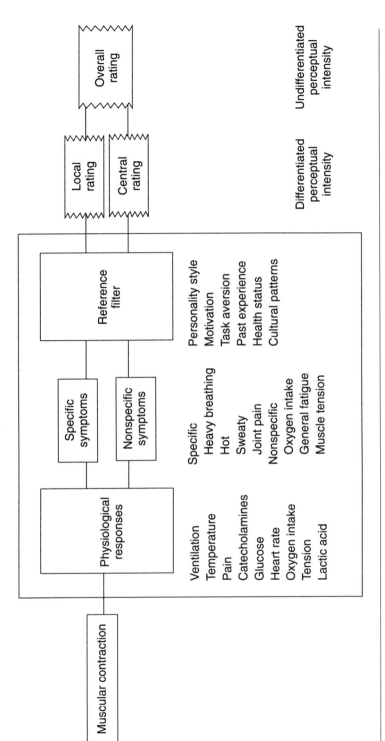

Figure 8.3 Noble et al. (1986) explanatory model of perceived exertion.
Reprinted from Borg and Ottoson 1986.

exercise trials in which physiological factors are held constant. The metabolic demand of the exercise is relativized to adjust for each person's aerobic capacity ($\dot{V}O_2$max). In addition, the psychosocial setting and subject disposition would have to be tightly controlled. Then, if a single psychological variable is manipulated, say attentional focus, the expected change in perceived exertion would be independently caused by the psychological variable. In contrast, if psychological variables and metabolic demands are held constant and a single physiological variable is manipulated, say pulmonary ventilation, we could attribute the RPE change solely to the physiological manipulation. Further, if both components were manipulated by altering attentional focus and pulmonary ventilation, one would say that physiological and psychological variables were integrated in order for the perceptual rating to be set. In a realistic setting, the latter case would describe most human exercise perceptions.

The proposed model can be seen in figure 8.4. Exercise provides the sensory stimulation from which the perceptual self-report will eventually be made. As in the Leventhal and Everhart (1979) model, sensory cues are encoded into neural signals. These signals can be amplified or dampened depending on one's dispositional characteristics, for example, self-efficacy. It is likely that most dispositional factors are integrated preconsciously. On the other hand, situational factors may be integrated with the sensory signal both consciously and preconsciously. Take the manipulation of self-presentation as an example. The presence of a female experimenter while a male subject is exercising at high intensity could influence RPE consciously or preconsciously. The signal may be further modulated by focal awareness. Again, Leventhal and Everhart's (1979) model is instructive. There can be several possible sources of attention, with focal awareness—specific attention—of a particular channel(s) dependent on the context, that is, situational factors. In addition, such factors as exercise intensity, training status, and accumulated fatigue most likely exert their influence by altering focal awareness. Rejeski (1981) has suggested in what he calls an integrative model (fig. 8.5) that psychological factors are more salient at light and moderate exercise intensities than at high intensities. At high intensities, and longer durations, it is likely that attention is focused on the noxious exercise sensations, which dominate focal awareness, with little opportunity for psychological factors to gain saliency. The final setting of perceived exertion is proportional to the intensity of the sensation during high-intensity exercise, while at lower exercise intensities the rating is adjusted depending on the psychological factors exerting influence at the time.

Again, we would like to suggest a certain cautious enthusiasm for the role of exercise intensity and duration in the psychological modulation of exertional perceptions. While the nonlinear relationship between psychological and physiological inputs based on exercise intensity and duration are attractive, we believe considerable more research is called for.

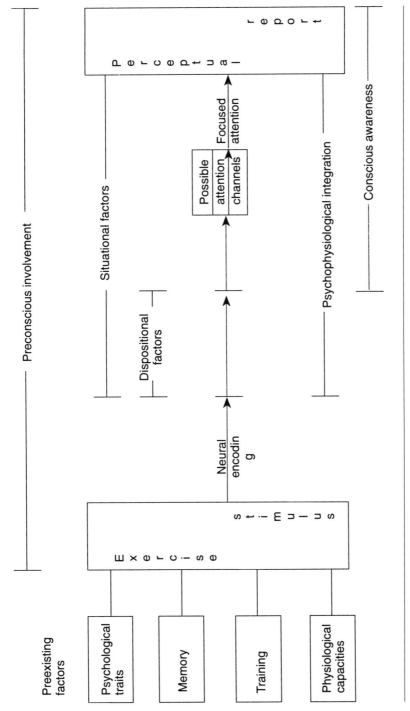

Figure 8.4　Psychophysiological model of perceived exertion.

191

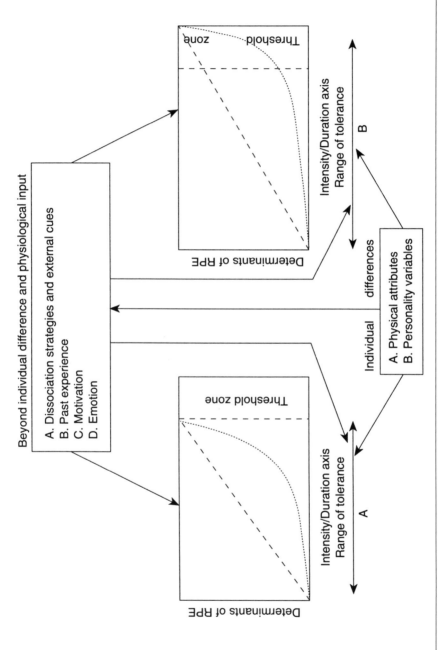

Figure 8.5 RPE: A social psychophysiological integration.
Reprinted from Rejeski 1981.

References

Bandura, A. 1977. Self-efficacy: Toward a unifying theory of behavioral change. *Psychol. Rev.* 84:191-215.

Baumeister, R.F. 1982. A self-presentational view of social phenomena. *Psychol. Bull.* 91:3-26.

Boutcher, S.H., L.A. Fleischer-Curtian, and S.D. Gines. 1988. The effects of self-presentation on perceived exertion. *J. Sport Exerc. Psychol.* 10:270-80.

Boutcher, S.H., and M. Trenske. 1990. The effects of sensory deprivation and music on perceived exertion and affect during exercise. *J. Sport Exerc. Psychol.* 12:167-76.

Bubb, W.J., B.C. Myers, R.P. Claytor, D.L. Varnum, L. Watts, and B.D. Franks. 1985. Experimenter effects in exercise tolerance testing: The race and gender of the tester and the tester/subject relationship. *Res. Q. Exerc. Sport* 56:370-77.

Cafarelli, E. 1982. Peripheral contributions to the perception of effort. *Med. Sci. Sports* 14:382-89.

Carver, C.S., A.E. Coleman, and D.C. Glass. 1976. The coronary-prone behavior pattern and the suppression of fatigue on a treadmill test. *J. Personality Soc. Psychol.* 33:460-66.

Copeland, B.L., and B.D. Franks. 1991. Effects of types and intensities of background music on treadmill endurance. *J. Sports Med. Phys. Fitness* 31:100-103.

DeMeersman, R.E. 1988. Personality, effort perception and cardiovascular reactivity. *Neuropsychobiol.* 19:192-94.

Dishman, R.K., R.E. Graham, R.G. Holly, and J.G. Tieman. 1991. Estimates of type A behavior do not predict perceived exertion during graded exercise. *Med. Sci. Sports Exerc.* 23:1276-82.

Fillingim, R.B., and M.A. Fine. 1986. The effects of internal versus external information processing on symptom perception in an exercise setting. *Health Psychol.* 5:115-23.

Fillingim, R.B., D.L. Roth, and W.E. Haley. 1989. The effects of distraction on the perception of exercise-induced symptoms. *J. Psychosom. Res.* 33:241-48.

Franks, B.D., and B.C. Myers. 1984. Effects of talking on exercise tolerance. *Res. Q. Exerc. Sport* 55:237-41.

Friedman, M., and R.H. Rosenman. 1974. *Type A behavior and your heart*. New York: Knopf.

Hardy, C.J., R.G. McMurray, and S. Roberts. 1989. A/B types and psychophysiological responses to exercise stress. *J. Sport Exerc. Psychol.* 11:141-51.

Hardy, C. J., E.G. Hall, and P.H. Prestholdt. (1986). The mediational role of social influence in the perception of exertion. *J. Sport Exerc. Psychol.* 8: 88-104.

Hochstetler, S.A., W.J. Rejeski, and D.L. Best. 1985. The influence of sex-role orientation on ratings of perceived exertion. *Sex Roles* 12:825-35.

Johnson, J., and D. Siegel. 1987. Active vs. passive attentional manipulation and multidimensional perceptions of exercise intensity. *Can. J. Sport Sci.* 12:41-45.

Jones, J.G., and A. Cale. 1989. Changes in mood and cognitive functioning during long distance running—An exploratory investigation. *Phys. Ed. Rev.* 12:78-83.

Jung, C.G. 1921. *Psychological types.* Princeton, NJ: Princeton University Press.

Kinsman, R.A., and P.C. Weiser. 1976. Subjective symptomatology during work and fatigue. In *Psychological aspects and physiological correlates of work and fatigue,* ed. E. Simonson and P.C. Weiser, 336-405. Springfield, IL: Charles C Thomas.

Kinsman, R.A., P.C. Weiser, and D.A. Stamper. 1973. Multidimensional analysis of subjective symptomatology during prolonged strenuous exercise. *Ergonomics* 16:211-26.

Kohl, R.M., and C.H. Shea. 1988. Perceived exertion: Influences of locus of control and expected work intensity and duration. *J. Human Move. Stud.* 15:225-72.

Kraemer, W.J., R.V. Lewis, N.T. Triplett, L.P. Koziris, S. Heyman, and B.J. Noble. 1992. Effects of hypnosis on plasma proenkephalin peptide F and perceptual and cardiovascular responses during submaximal exercise. *Eur. J. Appl. Physiol.* 65:573-78.

Leventhal, H., and D. Everhart. 1979. Emotion, pain and physical illness. In *Emotions in personality and psychopathology,* ed. C.E. Izard, 263-99. New York: Plenum Press.

McCauley, E., and K.S. Courneya. 1992. Self-efficacy relationships with affective and exertion responses to exercise. *J. Appl. Soc. Psychol.* 22:312-26.

Morgan, W.P. 1973. Psychological factors influencing perceived exertion. *Med. Sci. Sports* 5:97-103.

Morgan, W.P., K. Hirota, G.A. Weitz, and B. Balke. 1976. Hypnotic perturbation of perceived exertion: Ventilatory consequences. *Am. J. Clin. Hypn.* 18:182-90.

Morgan, W.P., and M.L. Pollock. 1977. Psychological characteristics of elite runners. *Ann. N.Y. Acad. Sci.* 301:382-403.

Noble, B.J. 1977. Physiological basis of perceived exertion: A tentative explanatory model. Paper presented at the Annual Meeting of American Alliance of Health, Physical Education and Recreation, Seattle, WA.

Noble, B.J., W.J. Kraemer, J.G. Allen, J.S. Plank, and L.A. Woodard. 1986. The integration of physiological cues in effort perception: Stimulus strength vs. relative contribution. In *The perception of exertion in physical work,* ed. G. Borg and D. Ottoson, 83-96. London: Macmillan.

Noble, B. J., K.F. Metz, K.B. Pandolf, and E. Cafarelli. 1973. Perceptual responses to exercise: A multiple regression study. *Med. Sci. Sports* 5:104-9.

Pandolf, K.B. 1978. Influence of local and central factors in dominating rated perceived exertion during physical work. *Percept. Motor Skills* 46:683-98.

Pandolf, K.B., R.L. Burse, and R.F. Goldman. 1975. Differentiated ratings of perceived exertion during physical conditioning of older individuals using leg-load weighting. *Percept. Motor Skills* 40:563-74.

Pennebaker, J.W., and J.M. Lightner. 1980. Competition of internal and external information in an exercise setting. *J. Personality Soc. Psychol.* 39:165-74.

Rejeski, W.J. 1981. The perception of exertion: A social psychophysiological integration. *J. Sport Psychol.* 4:305-20.

———. 1985. Perceived exertion: An active or passive process? *J. Sport Psychol.* 7:371-78.

Rejeski, W.J., D. Best, P. Griffith, and E. Kinney. 1985. Feminine males in exercise: Is the inappropriateness of activity the cause of dysfunction in gross-gender behavior? Unpublished manuscript.

Rejeski, W.J., D. Morley, and H. Miller. 1983. Cardiac rehabilitation: Coronary-prone behavior as a moderatory of graded exercise. *J. Cardiac Rehab.* 3:339-46.

Rejeski, W.J., and P.M. Ribisl. 1980. Expected task duration and perceived effort: An attributional analysis. *J. Sport Psychol.* 2:227-36.

Rejeski, W.J., and B. Sanford. 1984. Feminine-typed females: The role of affective schema in the perception of exercise intensity. *J. Sport Psychol.* 6:197-207.

Robertson, R.J. 1982. Central signals of perceived exertion during dynamic exercise. *Med. Sci. Sports Exerc.* 14:390-96.

Robertson, R.J., R.L. Gillespie, E. Hiatt, and K.D. Rose. 1977. Perceived exertion and stimulus intensity modulation. *Percept. Motor Skills* 45:211-18.

Schomer, H. 1986. Mental strategies and the perception of effort of marathon runners. *Int. J. Sport Psychol.* 17:41-59.

Sylva, M., R. Boyd, and M. Mangum. 1990. Effects of social influence and sex on rating of perceived exertion in exercising elite athletes. *Percept. Motor Skills* 70:591-94.

Williams, J.G., and R.G. Eston. 1986. Does personality influence the perception of effort? The results from a study of secondary schoolboys. *Phys. Ed. Rev.* 9:94-99.

Wrisberg, C.A., B.D. Franks, M.W. Birdwell, and D.M. High. 1988. Physiological and psychological responses to exercise with an induced attentional focus. *Percept. Motor Skills* 66:603-16.

Zohar, D., and G. Spitz. 1981. Expected performance and perceived exertion in a prolonged physical task. *Percept. Motor Skills* 52:975-84.

9

CHAPTER

The Role of the Unconscious in Effort Perception

Why the unconscious? Isn't such a concept antithetical to modern science, the concepts of which are the very foundation of this book? Webster tells us that the word *unconscious* means freedom from self-awareness and not marked by conscious thought, sensation, or feeling. How can perception pertain to a concept unrelated to sensing and feeling?

From a point of view of strictly scientific measurement, if it cannot be sensed, it cannot be quantified. If something cannot be quantified, it exists outside the realm of scientific inquiry. But for knowledge to be complete, one must not leave any stone unturned in the search for truth, even when that search takes us down a philosophical path that is somewhat foreign to us. Our study of effort perception thus far has not put forward hypotheses wherein psychic processes outside of human awareness might be related to perceptual variance. Nonetheless, an extensive body of knowledge, begun with Freud's psychoanalytic theories, shows a powerful effect on human attitudes and behavior emanating from unconscious processes. Such theories have been mostly applicable to clinical psychological practice but may inform our future search for perceptual truth.

This chapter is somewhat of a departure from those previously and subsequently presented. Its theme is philosophical rather than experimental. The material herein is offered in the spirit of intellectual inclusiveness. Borg himself has advocated an attitude of comprehensiveness from the very beginning, a spirit of multidisciplinary inquiry.

The Unconscious and the Concept of Threshold

Threshold is a common term in both physiology and psychology. We speak of a threshold as the point at which a stimulus is of sufficient intensity to begin to produce an effect, such as an electrophysiological threshold. Likewise, the term *limen* has been used in psychology to designate the point at which a sensory stimulus can be perceived. The *difference limen*, for example, has been discussed in chapter 2. The threshold of consciousness, in Freudian terms, may be said to be located in the preconscious, where elements not currently conscious can become so by the will of attention. Truly unconscious material, of course, cannot be accessed merely by effort of attention.

Thus, it can be said that the concept of threshold in both physiology and psychology recognizes an unconscious component. Even in physiology we don't reject the presence or the significance of a process just because it is below threshold. What is below threshold, such as cellular and subcellular mechanisms, is unconscious to us. In fact, one might characterize the modern study of physiology as an attempt to unlock the secrets of the physiological unconscious.

During situations charged with great emotionality, it is possible, for short periods of time at least, to suppress incoming stimuli in the service of achieving an important goal. For example, athletes have been known to continue playing with injuries that normally would be incapacitating. Likewise, lifesaving rescues have been accomplished by individuals overcoming seemingly impossible odds. In these cases, where the demands of the context are appropriate, normally suprathreshold stimuli are temporarily relegated to the unconscious. We can say in these cases that perception has been altered.

What role do unconscious processes play in the setting of human perceptual responses? First, it will be useful to examine the analogue of the unconscious psyche in human physiology.

Unconscious Physiology

Most physiological function occurs involuntarily on an unconscious level. We don't have to ask our hearts to beat, our lungs to inflate, our muscles to maintain posture. On the other hand, it is possible to override some involuntary functions with our will. Therefore, we can say that the physical self has an unconscious plane in the same sense the psyche has an unconscious. Each of these unconscious planes acts adaptively, sometimes in a complementary fashion (e.g., adrenal response to flight, fright, fight), at other times compensating (e.g., antagonistic contraction in muscle), as the need dictates.

It is axiomatic to say that human physiology is capable of adaptation. Suppression as a characteristic physiological response, on the other hand, is not commonly discussed but represents a real capability. The suppression of sensory input is illustrative of the adaptive capability in the nervous system. It is well known that humans "suppress the perception of sensory information until attention is drawn to it" (Ross 1978). For example, we suppress the sensation of touch from our clothing unless something calls our attention to it. Similarly, ventilatory cues are suppressed during long term aerobic exercise following a period of initial awareness.

Movement proprioception is another example of a physiological process that operates unconsciously. Proprioception involves feedback of parallel processes, tension, and stretch. When muscle increases its tension, the proprioceptive mechanism provides the feedback loop that automatically initiates inhibition. Feedback from a stretched muscle, conversely, initiates contraction. Thus, when an arm is held out from the body for a period of time, these parallel feedback loops provide continuous unconscious information concerning limb movement. If the arm relaxes, muscles contract to bring it up. Contracting muscles that may raise the arm unnecessarily result in an inhibition of this function. This is all accomplished without conscious control. However, if a heavy weight were placed in the hand, the conscious mind would override the unconscious neuromotor signals to evoke the continuous muscle contraction necessary to overcome the new force.

Unconscious response is the hallmark of the autonomic nervous system (ANS). Organic function is actively supported by both the sympathetic (largely facilitatory) and parasympathetic (largely inhibitory) branches of the ANS. The naming of these branches was based on the apparent "sympathy" that one organ showed for another under certain conditions. The secretion of norepinephrine by the sympathetic nerve fibers in the heart acts to accelerate cardiac contraction. In contrast, the vagus, a parasympathetic nerve, secretes acetylcholine at its nerve endings to decrease cardiac function. The highly developed conscious control of the yogi and the effects that accompany biofeedback training are said to intervene upon unconscious autonomic functions in ways that have not been favored by evolutionary development; that is, the conscious mind can be trained to override otherwise unconsciously controlled processes such as heart rate and blood pressure.

The evolutionary development of both psychological and physiological response has provided humans with a wonderfully efficient adaptation system. Information provided to us, be it psychic or physical, can be selectively suppressed if consciousness is not mandatory. It has been advantageous to secrete adrenaline automatically during flight, for instance. Considerable time and energy is then made available for conscious attention to the external world. However, subconsciousness is not without its dark side. In psychology, we know that psychic repression can lead to insidious disorders. Posttraumatic stress disorder is an example of a process in which previous trauma is reexperienced following a period of repression. On the physiological side, suppression of sensory input can lead to lack of awareness of dangerous stimuli during exercise. Any attempt to block perception of pain could lead to "pushing through" when termination would be more salutary. In both cases it would be wise to become judiciously aware of repressed material. The unconscious appears to function in human physiological systems as well as in the psychic realm. At this point it would be good for us to look more comprehensively at what is known about the unconscious psyche.

The Unconscious Psyche: Freud and Jung

Twentieth-century psychology has been dominated by two schools of thought: behaviorism and psychoanalysis. Both schools were established out of the mechanistic tradition of modern science. Behaviorism was built upon the advances in anatomy and physiology forged in the 19th century. Similarly, psychoanalysis grew from the biological model of science developed in medicine. Differences between the two schools can be seen in their view of the unconscious and conscious domains.

Unlike behaviorism, psychoanalysis concerned itself with an introspective view of consciousness. Freud divided the psyche into a conscious component, awareness, and an unconscious component, consisting of repressed personal material. Freud is credited with discovering the unconscious. Probing the deeply rooted dynamics of the unconscious is the basis of psychoanalytic technique, which has also been appropriately called depth psychology. Attainment of mental health, according to psychoanalytic theory, is a matter of increasing consciousness by helping the unconscious to reveal its repressed sources of motivation.

Behaviorism, a branch of psychology based upon manipulation of behavior through appropriate conditioning paradigms, has little need for constructs of unconsciousness or consciousness. John Watson, founder of behaviorism, wrote, "Psychology, as the behaviorist views it, is a purely objective, experimental branch of natural science which needs consciousness as little as do the sciences of chemistry and physics" (Capra 1982). Nonetheless, the scientific studies that led to psychoanalytic theory were informed by knowledge of the unconscious and affected 20th-century thought well beyond the confines of psychology.

Freud's groundbreaking work with the unconscious was greatly extended by Carl Gustav Jung, Swiss physician and pioneer experimentalist in depth psychology. Unlike Freud, the traditional biomedical empiricist, Jung utilized a systems approach more characteristic of modern-day physics (Capra 1982). The unconscious, to Freud, was strictly personal and represented a *tabula rasa* (blank slate) developed concomitantly with one's individual life. Building on Freud's work, Jung thought that the conscious mind "grows out of an unconscious psyche which is older than it" (Capra 1982), that is, an unconscious that is not personal. Retaining the concept of the personal unconscious, Jung discovered a deeper layer, the collective unconscious.

The crux of our interest here is the process by which the unconscious mind might affect our conscious perception. Of course, psychoanalytic theory postulates that such is the case. One way to examine how such a process might work is through Jung's study of word association. Jung developed a test that was an early precursor to the lie detector test. In this test subjects were presented with a series of words. The elapsed time between the presentation of the stimulus word and the subject's association was recorded. Jung found that extended response times were related to unconscious psychological complexes. Complexes consist of emotion-laden groupings of unconscious ideas. Typical examples of complexes are mother, father, inferiority, money, power, and so on. A stimulus word like *baby* may trigger a mother complex, delaying response because of unconscious interference. When a complex is engaged, heart rate and respiration are usually accelerated.

Discussion of Jung's association experiments is not intended to suggest its use in contemporary studies of perception, but to illustrate the impact of the unconscious on human response. An example is in order. Let us hypothesize a subject with a mother complex having a specific manifestation—namely, the subject's unconscious attempts to free him- or herself from mother dominance—resulting in behavior in which unusual physical risks are commonly taken. Such a subject (remember here that we are not speaking of empirical findings) may exaggerate the degree of difficulty of a physical challenge. One would think that such a person might dampen perceptual response in an attempt to show personal mastery in the face of high-intensity exercise.

Another example from Jung's scientific studies may prove instructive. Jung was the first to identify the personality types we refer to as extroversion and introversion. He suggested that "when orientation by the object predominates in such a way that decisions and actions are determined not by subjective views but by objective conditions, we speak of an extroverted attitude" (Jung 1971). The extroverted attitude "never expects to find any absolute factors in his own inner life, since the only ones he knows are outside himself" (Jung 1971). "The introvert is distinguished from the extrovert by the fact that he does not, like the latter, orient himself by the object and by objective data, but by subjective factors" (Jung 1971).

How might effort be perceived from the perspective of personality typology? It would be reasonable to assume that extroverts may devalue internal signals, whereas introverts, more aware of the inner subjective life, might amplify disturbances of the internal environment. Personality typology, an unconscious characteristic, provides us with a convenient system upon which to base hypotheses about conscious perceptual traits. Indeed, we discussed data in the previous chapter that supports this contention (Morgan 1973).

As we set perceptions, the psychological filter through which effort sensations must pass is extremely complex. This complexity demands that we consider flexible theories that would capture unconscious influences in our scientific models.

The Unconscious in Human Movement

If we consciously recognized the presence of the unconscious in our movement behavior, it would not be unconscious. Nevertheless, we move effectively because we are supported, at least partially, by unconscious processes. *Optimal experience* (Csikszentmihalyi 1990) during movement is illustrative of the unconscious working behind the scenes. Optimal experience might be called the experience of a wholeness in movement, with all the parts fitting together in an unusual synchrony. Joseph Campbell (1988), quintessential mythologist, spoke of a personal optimal experience:

"When I was running at Columbia, I ran a couple of races that were just beautiful. During the second race, I knew I was going to win even though there was no reason for me to know this, because I was touched off as an anchor in the relay with the leading runner thirty yards ahead of me. But I just knew, and it was my peak experience. Nobody could beat me that day. That's being in full form and really knowing it. I don't think I have ever done anything in my life as competently as I ran those two races—it was the experience of really being at my full and doing a perfect job."

Such a state can feel incredible, even out of control. However, there *has* been control—in fact, extraordinary control—by the unconscious self. Such experiences are difficult, if not impossible, to duplicate in the laboratory. Thus, scientific scrutiny of the phenomenon is limited, but anecdotal evidence is quite convincing.

The *Inner Game of Tennis,* written by Tim Gallwey (1974), was a heavily discussed book in the 1970s. Unlike most learning texts before and since, Gallwey did not address himself to the skills and strategy of tennis per se. Instead, as the title implies, he considered the inner life of the player and asked the question, What effect does internal dialogue have on performance? He used the metaphor of the *inner critic,* the voice that critiques technique following each point. He suggested that allowing the inner critic to access the conscious mind disrupted learned and unconsciously controlled movement patterns. Feedback from the inner critic is often technical and always judgmental. Bringing the technical details of physical skill into conscious awareness, according to Gallwey, is counterproductive. After learning the skill, the imprint of the movement pattern is stored in unconscious memory. The secret to good tennis performance is leaving the movement to the unconscious, while the conscious psyche concentrates on monitoring environmental demands, that is, position and speed of the ball. High cognitive loading should only be characteristic of early learning of motor skills.

We owe the identification of the three stages of motor skill learning to the work of Fitts and Posner (1967). Early learning is termed the *cognitive phase* and is marked by the need to think about movement as the instructional process is integrated. After the learner knows how to perform the required movement(s), the intermediate or *associative phase* of learning is entered. Fitts and Posner (1967) named the final stage of learning (of interest for this discussion) the *autonomous phase.* In this stage the skilled learner utilizes minimal conscious control, leaving the movement patterns to unconscious control. Thus, one's conscious awareness can more productively attend to strategic issues. The nature of the autonomous phase of the Fitts and Posner model, like Gallwey's hypothesis, suggests that cognitive intervention (consciousness) can serve as an interference for the skilled performer.

Repetitious practice of a motor skill can result in reduced performance. Following a period of rest, the performance is not only restored but often increased. This phenomenon is called *reminiscence.* Reminiscence is often observed during the first play of the season in games such as tennis and golf. Serves and drives can be accurate and powerful in contrast to those displayed at the end of the previous season, for example. Decreased past performance can be ascribed to fatigue, boredom, or staleness, and reminiscence to the removal of such factors. Returning after a period of rest can result in the performer coming back relaxed and expecting less of him- or herself. The restored performance is reminiscent of a previously attained skill level. The phenomenon could also be explained on the basis of the removal of cognitive overload. Relaxed physically and motivationally, the performer lets the unconscious take control. Literally, reminiscence means recalling past experiences or events, that is, recalling that which was known but forgotten for some reason. The reason may be related to allowing conscious cognition to interfere with that which is already known by the unconscious.

Posture, walking, and bicycle riding are other common examples of activities that are performed unconsciously. Unconscious control allows humans to transact higher-level activities simultaneously. For example, one can type at the same time sentences are created. The skilled typist moves fingers without conscious control and can thus direct consciousness to creativity or transcription.

A common tendency is to relegate scientific explanation to conscious factors alone. Physiologists often attribute causation in effort perceptions to various physiological factors alone. It can be a trap to give credence only to those variables that we think are under conscious control and devalue or dismiss variables under unconscious control. We may think that because we are dealing with a perceptual self-report, the subject must be monitoring only those variables within the conscious range. The previous examples remind us that unconscious processes can be quite effectively monitored, even though they may not be consciously perceived. Certain factors are within our awareness, even though they are not conscious. The physiologist should not use conscious awareness as a limiting definition for inclusion of causative factors in the perceptual process. For instance, just because we do not consciously perceive energy metabolism, as reflected in oxygen consumption, does not mean we do not perceive it.

Of course, the same caution can be directed toward psychological research. Psychologists are accustomed to studying phenomenon they cannot directly observe. We cannot see a percept, for example. That should not limit their approach to those factors that appear to be under conscious control. In fact, it should encourage the inclusion of unconscious processes.

The study of perceived exertion has been, from the very beginning, an eclectic science embracing both psychology and physiology. If we wish to understand perception on a very practical level, effective model building will require continued multidisciplinary cooperation and, further, integrative thinking. Omission of the unconscious from these models will keep our goal of completeness always out of reach.

"Who" Directs Perception?

An interesting aspect of effort perception is that it involves intrinsic sensing, a sensing of the self. It is not the mind/body system directly sensing the world in which it lives (exteroception), but the mind/body system sensing *itself* (proprioception). We usually think of the human organism as having a complex system of sense organs that serve it by monitoring its interface with the external world, that is, sensation. Perception is the higher-level process by which we interpret these extrinsic stimuli for the purpose of self-preservation, that is, providing the basis for choice of action. Equally important is the sensing and interpretation of intrinsic stimuli, whether those stimuli arise from interaction with the external world, as in sensing physical effort, or, more directly, from rather spontaneous organic activity, as in sensing hunger or thirst.

Sensing effort is sensing the self as it responds to the demands of the external world. At birth the infant experiences itself as being one with the external world. Thus, there appears to be no difference between inner and outer reality. As the child differentiates, however, the self becomes the subject while other people and things become the object. It seems as if we live *in* the world but are not *of* the world. That is, the world seems to be external to us, an object, the other. The external world is that which needs to be acted on or responded to.

Psychologically it is possible to split off the subject from the object. The mind (subject) can be separated from the body (object). It is as if the body were part of the external world or, at the most, the vehicle that carries the mind through the world. The brilliant 17th-century mathematician Rene Descartes, founder of the scientific method, rejected all unsubstantiated knowledge, including knowledge about the body. The only thing he could not doubt was the mind; thus, he made the ultimate mind/body splitting statement, *Cogito, ergo sum* (I think, therefore I exist). The body was thought of as an object.

Charles Sherrington (1900), the British physiologist, posed the question, Can the mind sense effort independently of the nervous system? Is the mind independent of physiology, the body? His question, an astute one, reflects an ambiguity in mind/body splitting. Carl Jung felt no such ambiguity. He reasoned that "since psyche and matter are contained in one and the same world, and moreover are in continuous contact with one another . . . . it is not only possible but fairly probable, even, that psyche and matter are two different aspects of the same thing" (Jacobi 1973). In fact, according to his notion, mind and body, the perceiver and the perceived, are part of a complex, dependent, integrated system, not separate but whole.

Descartes' statement did not denigrate the body but certainly established the mind as the dominant component. He thought of the mind as the director of existence. Descartes might have said, the thinking self is the one that is looking, the one that is aware.

One can think of the role of the mind in the perception of effort in much the same way as we think of an outside observer, perhaps a teacher or movement therapist, monitoring our effort. It is possible for the teacher or therapist to directly observe sweating, facial grimacing, gait alterations, and heavy breathing and deduce intense perceptual effort. That is to say, "another" can observe and estimate our effort. As we perceive our own effort, it can seem as if "another" was watching. It is probable that Sherrington's question concerning the independence of mind and nervous system may have probed this ambiguity of human awareness.

According to both Freud and Jung the ego is the "I" that becomes aware. Awareness is the domain of the conscious mind, or of the conscious mind/body, a phrase that more appropriately reflects Jung's more inclusive, integrative construct of psyche and matter. The ego is the center of that awareness, the center of the conscious mind/body. To be conscious is to be aware of one's own existence, sensations, thoughts, and surroundings. Not to be aware is to be in the realm of the unconscious. Sensory systems provide information about our existence. Perception interprets sensory input for the purpose of successful integration of psyche and matter, mind and body.

We might postulate that the ego is the director of this "movie" we call existence, living awareness. Its job is to protect the system. The genius of survival is having an ego that can make successful interpretations and develop appropriate adaptive responses. However, the movie analogy may not hold up completely, because a director usually does not play a part in the movie. Is the ego the director or only the main character?

We must not exclude the unconscious psyche. It should be clear that the conscious mind does not act alone. We need only to recall experiences like finishing all or portions of a long run without memory or awareness of it. Return to full consciousness occurs *ex post facto*. Obviously, the appropriate twists and turns of the road have been negotiated and, so far as we know, local laws have been obeyed. It is as if even the "I" has not been the runner. "Another" has directed the successful relocation to the starting place.

The conscious mind is only the visible tip of the iceberg in the human psyche. Below consciousness with its central "eye," the ego, below the surface of awareness is the realm of the unconscious. The unconscious, another portion of the human psyche, can be viewed as containing several levels of material, beginning with the personal unconscious that consists of forgotten or repressed information. A deeper level of the unconscious psyche has been described by Jung and consists of a collective, or archetypal, stratum containing impersonal material available to all humans. To gain a physiological perspective we might compare the collective unconscious to primitive and autonomic biological instincts. Unconscious material, whether at the personal or collective level, is not readily accessible to conscious awareness. Only under special conditions, dreaming for example, can the unconscious be revealed and only then in symbolic rather than concrete terms.

Returning to our search for a director or, as some philosophers have described it, the search for the "little man inside the little man," it seems a plausible hypothesis to look to the unconscious. Psychoanalytic theory posits the unconscious as the seat of much of our conscious motivation. According to Jungian theory, the center of the unconscious, and indeed of the entire psyche, is the Self. The Self is said to be superordinate to the conscious ego (Jacobi 1973). The Self can only be experienced, not scientifically observed. It may be that during periods of conscious awareness the ego serves as a director, the one who watches. Perhaps during situations in which "altered awareness" is experienced we can posit the unconscious as the director. More likely both the conscious and unconscious portions of the psyche act in concert to observe and control our interaction with the external world.

Perceptual Ratings and Unconscious Projection

Psychoanalytic theory holds that unconscious contents are projected onto persons or things in the external world. Since the material is unconscious, the projection is unknown to the subject. The material is in the "shadow," that is, the part of you cast by the absence of light, thus not conscious. Projection means mistaking for reality something that is only an image in the mind. Shadow material can be either positive or negative; thus, so can the projection (Jung 1971).

An illustration of projection related to effort perception can be taken from the experience of a child unflinchingly taught to withstand physical hardship as a sign of personal character strength. As an adult, although this modus operandi is not consciously called upon during intense physical effort, it can be unconsciously projected onto the situation. In such an example, the projection may cause the individual to rate the effort as less intense than might be expected. Our attempts to discover attributions for perceptions of effort have not considered examining the effects of unconscious processes like projection. Such examinations are fraught with methodological complexities but are certainly open to qualitative inquiry.

Exercise Intensity, Perceptual Ratings, and the Unconscious

Evidence has been presented in earlier chapters that indicates that the roles of respiratory-metabolic and peripheral factors in effort perception vary with exercise intensity. It is likely that conscious and unconscious influences respond in a similar fashion. It can be hypothesized that consciousness becomes more critical with increasing exercise intensity. This does not mean that unconscious factors do not play an important role during high-intensity exercise, but that successful performance and safety requires conscious attention to the demands of the task. This idea is related to cognitive association (Morgan 1981), in which directed thinking dominates exercise attentional focus.

A Conceptual Framework of Effort Perception

The purpose of this chapter has been to discuss the hypothesis that the unconscious psyche plays a role in the setting of effort perceptions. The discussion has been largely theoretical rather than data based. Psychoanalytic theory, developed and therapeutically validated over the past century, as well as wide-ranging behavioral and physiological studies provide a sufficient base for constructing productive psychophysiological hypotheses containing both conscious and unconscious psychic components. The following diagram provides a sample framework from which future experimental hypotheses might be formed.

	Conscious	*Unconscious*
Psychology	Affect assessment	Self-efficacy; mood states
Physiology	Suprathreshold sensation	Cellular and subcellular mechanisms

Perceived self-efficacy (Bandura and Adams 1977) is a psychological construct, widely used in the past decade, that shows promise, at least in part, for explaining effort perception. Those who perceive themselves as performing successfully in an exercise task may well rate effort intensity to be lower. While we commonly say ''perceiving themselves,'' with at least an implicit reference to consciousness, we cannot truly classify self-efficacy as having a conscious connection to the rating choice. It is quite possible that a conscious awareness of success or failure exists, but it is unlikely that a rational causative linkage is established between that awareness and the rating. The psychic origin of the percept does not remove the viability of self-efficacy as a factor in setting perceptual intensity.

Moods have a definite emotional tone and are initiated by unconscious sources. A mood state is not willed into existence. Certainly one might expect a depressed subject to rate effort differently than one uninfluenced by depression. In both the self-efficacy and mood states examples, unconscious mechanisms may well influence ratings of perceived effort.

It is likely that we could make a case for the unconscious as a powerful contributor to most psychological constructs involving choice contingencies. However, some constructs are clearly more conscious than others. Affect assessment, for example, unequivocally forces a conscious choice. It appears that positive or negative affect is an important construct to be used in conjunction with perceived effort as we attempt to unravel the attributions that can be assigned to human psychophysiological response to fatigue (Hardy and Rejeski 1989).

Possible physiological mechanisms have been discussed to a great extent in previous chapters. Many hypotheses are yet to be examined. A final reminder may be appropriate. Most of the physiological processes that we associate with the perception of effort occur more or less unconsciously, including heart rate, oxygen consumption, blood pressure, and even lactate production. As exercise intensity grows, so does the possibility that sensation will receive more conscious attention, especially to those variables readily available to consciousness, such as pulmonary ventilation and regionalized pain. This certainly does not mean that many cellular and subcellular variables have not been contributing their share to the setting of exertional ratings even during light exercise. They may have been operating at subthreshold levels or suppressed in the service of the performance goal. For example, in our early studies CO_2 production appeared as an important correlate with perceived exertion during prolonged submaximal exercise (Noble et al. 1973). Certainly, CO_2 production is not directly accessed by consciousness. The more comprehensive, integrated answers are still beyond our consciousness.

Summary

This chapter honors inclusiveness. It invites exercise scientists to view physical effort from a broad perspective, to cast a wide net in the search for perceptual understanding. Philosophical and clinical theory is embraced in the search. The main theme of the chapter surrounds the hypothesis that the unconscious plays a role in the setting of effort perceptions. Sensory suppression, proprioception, and autonomic response are used as examples of involuntary mechanisms that represent unconscious physiological activity. The theories of Sigmund Freud and Carl Jung, especially Jung's association experiments and personality construct, illustrate the potential role of unconscious psychological factors in the perception of reality. Czikszentmihalyi's idea that *optimal experience*, or altered states of consciousness, can be achieved in sport and Gallwey's concept of disruptive inner dialogue while playing tennis both represent ways in which the unconscious may work in a movement context. The chapter takes up a philosophical argument of long standing, that is, whether a nonphysiological contruct like the mind can be thought of as acting independently of physiological response. Finally, a conceptual framework is presented as a guide to future experimental hypotheses and theory building that comprehensively includes conscious and unconscious factors as well as physiological and psychological response.

References

Bandura, A., and N. Adams. 1977. Analysis of self-efficacy theory of behavioral change. *Cognitive Ther. Res.* 1 (4): 287-310.

Capra, F. 1982. *The turning point: Science, society and the rising culture.* New York: Simon and Schuster.

Campbell, J. 1988. *The power of myth.* New York: Doubleday.

Csikszentmihalyi, M. 1990. *Flow: The psychology of optimal experience.* New York: Harper and Row.

Fitts, P.M. and M.I. Posner. 1967. *Human performance.* Pacific Grove, CA: Brooks/Cole.

Gallwey, T. 1974. *The Inner Game of Tennis.* New York: Random House.

Hardy, C., and W. Rejeski. 1989. Not what, but how one feels: The measurement of affect during exercise. *J. Sport Exerc. Psychol.* 11:304-17.

Jacobi, J. 1973. *The psychology of C.G. Jung.* New Haven, CT: Yale University Press.

———. 1971. *Psychological types.* Princeton, NJ: Princeton University Press.

Morgan, W. 1973. Psychological factors influencing perceived exertion. *Med. Sci. Sports,* 5:97-103.

Morgan, W. 1981. C.H. McCloy research lecture: Psychophysiology of self-awareness during vigorous physical activity. *Res. Q. Exerc. Sport* 52:385-427.

Noble, B., K. Metz, K. Pandolf, and E. Cafarelli. 1973. Perceptual responses to exercise: A multiple regression study. *Med. Sci. Sports* 5:104-9.

Ross, G. 1978. *Essentials of human physiology.* Chicago: Year Book Medical.

Sherrington, C.S. 1900. The muscular sense. In *Textbook of physiology,* ed. E. Schafer. Edinburgh and London: Pentland.

III

PART

Clinical Applications and Global Perspectives

Ratings of perceived exertion are used in the clinical setting to assess exercise tolerance and to prescribe and regulate therapeutic training intensity. Systematic quantification of perceived exertion increases the clinical sensitivity of disease diagnosis, exercise prescription, and work tolerance evaluation. Such clinical application assumes that perceptual responses have corollary physiological mediators that are specific to exercise performance.

The functional interdependence of perceptual and physiological responses during exercise performance provides an empirical rationale for the interpretation and subsequent clinical application of subjective estimates of physical exertion. This rationale is an extension of Borg's thesis that the response to an exercise stimulus involves three main effort continua: *perceptual, physiological,* and *performance*. The effort continua are theoretical constructs that depict the relation between physiological demands of an exercise performance and the perception of exertion associated with that exercise performance. The performance continuum involves exercise undertaken in therapeutic, sport, and pedagogical settings. The three continua operate as a complex psychophysiological feedback mechanism that contributes to homeostasis during exercise performance.

The interdependence of the perceptual, physiological, and performance continua is demonstrated by six overlapping intensity zones. These intensity zones are positioned consecutively along the functional length of each continuum. When examined sequentially, the zones depict the growth in perceptual responsiveness as the intensity of exercise performance increases, i.e., (1) minimal effort, (2) relative minimum, (3) preference level, (4) stress level, (5) relative maximum, and (6) maximum. These intensity zones have corollary positions on both the physiological and perceptual continua. As such, they can be defined in terms of metabolic units (i.e., heart rate, METs, absolute or relative oxygen uptake, lactate threshold) or physical units (i.e., speed, time, distance) that are typically used in clinical settings to prescribe exercise intensity.

However, the location of the intensity zones on the perceptual continuum are subjectively oriented. That is, their absolute beginning and ending points must have perceptual anchors. It follows that the physiological characteristics of each zone take on clincial significance only after their response limits have been psychologically quantified. Therefore, the functional link between the three effort continua indicates that perceptual responses provide much of the same information regarding exercise performance as do physiological responses. In the clinical setting, perceptual responses can then be used adjunctively with physiological measurements to evaluate exercise tolerance and to prescribe exercise intensity. As the upper and lower limits of the intensity zones reflect the influence of physical fitness, therapeutic training, and disease processes such adjunctive use of perceptual measurements enhances the clinical sensitivity of exercise evaluation and prescription.

The functional relation betwen the perceptual, physiological, and performance continua can be modified by such factors as clinical status, psychological mood states, exercise mode, and ability to use sensory scales. Quantification of the relation between the perceptual and physiological continua is dependent on systematic identification of a broad range of these modifying factors. Clinical application of scaled perceptions of exertion can then be undertaken, recognizing the limitations imposed by the interindividual variation in sensory responsiveness that is associated with such factors.

Once physiological and psychological inputs to the effort sense have been identified and clinical applications of RPE have been validated, it is important to place the entire field of study into a global perspective. Such a global outlook addresses the totality of the perceptual experience during physical exercise, attending to all factors that shape the intensity of the undifferentiated and differentiated exertional signal for a wide range of clinical states, activity modes, and performance milieus.

Part III contains three chapters. Chapter 10, "The Role of RPE in Graded Exercise Testing" initially reviews the methodological components of a graded exercise test. Perceptually based submaximal and maximal test protocols are then examined. Emphasis is placed on RPE as both an *independent* and *dependent* test variable when assessing functional aerobic power. Several perceptually based tests of anaerobic power are also described. The use of perceptual discriminate function analysis in determining the presence and severity of cardiopulmonary disease is explained.

Chapter 11, "The Role of RPE in Exercise Prescription" begins with an overview of the basic components of an exercise prescription. Specific attention is then directed to the use of RPE in both prescribing and regulating exercise intensity. Consideration is given to intra- and intermodal perceptually based exercise prescriptions. The prescriptive use of a "standard" RPE that is equivalent to the ventilatory and lactate thresholds is also explored.

Chaper 12 considers global perspectives and future directions in the study of perceived exertion. Initially, a distinction is made between *sensation* and *perception* from both a neurophysiological and functional point of view. A global explanatory model of the perceptual experience during dynamic exercise is then proposed. Each of the model's components is examined within the context of the "perceptual flow" from exercise stimulus to exertional response. Finally a list of experimental and clinical research questions that should be examined in future investigations is presented.

10

CHAPTER

The Role of RPE in Graded Exercise Testing

Graded exercise testing (GXT) involves the gradual, progressive, and systematic administration of an exercise stimulus to assess exertional tolerance in clinical, research, and sport settings. Ratings of perceived exertion are frequently used as an adjunct to standard physiological and clinical responses during a GXT. Combining objective physiological measures with subjective psychological measures during a GXT provides a robust assessment of the strain imposed by exercise and the capacity of the individual to tolerate that strain (Skinner, Borg, and Buskirk 1969). It has been established in chapters 4 through 7 that selected physiological responses mediate the intensity of exertional perceptions. Therefore, perceptual responses during a GXT provide much of the same information as do physiological responses when determining functional aerobic power, submaximal endurance performance, and tolerance for occupationally related physical activity. In addition, under certain conditions RPE can be used independently of physiological responses when testing exercise tolerance. The *adjunctive* and *independent* application of RPE during graded exercise testing provides dual themes upon which this chapter is organized.

Measurement of exertional perceptions during exercise testing is inexpensive, is noninvasive, and requires no bioelectrical instrumentation. Therefore, comparatively large numbers of individuals can be tested in a short time period. This is especially true when RPE is used as the principal dependent variable in low-risk, submaximal tests that are administered periodically during an exercise or therapeutic training program. Additional advantages are as follows:

1. The RPE scale is generalizable to a variety of populations and clinical subsets differing in gender, age, and athletic type.
2. RPE has wide application in home- and hospital-based rehabilitative programs.
3. Category scales to assess RPE are reliable and valid psychophysical tools.

4. Minimal scaling expertise is required on the part of the test administrator (i.e., exercise scientist, clinician, teacher, coach) or the individual being tested, i.e., experimental subject, patient, student, athlete (Noble 1982; Pollock, Jackson, and Foster 1986).

This chapter initially presents a brief overview of standard GXT procedures. Both the adjunctive and independent use of RPE during exercise testing is examined in the remaining sections. Specific attention will be given to (1) mode and protocol selection, (2) test applications, (3) special methodological considerations, and (4) clinical diagnosis.

Components of a Graded Exercise Test

Graded exercise tests are widely applied in clinical, research, and sport settings. Selected applications of the GXT within each of these settings are summarized in table 10.1. A graded exercise test has four components:

1. Format—continuous, intermittent, ramp
2. End point—submaximal, maximal, symptom limited
3. Mode—treadmill, cycle ergometer, arm ergometer, step bench, running track
4. Protocol—speed and grade (treadmill)
   brake resistance and pedal or crank rate (cycle and arm ergometer)
   step height and frequency (step bench)
   time and distance (running track)
   stage duration (all modes)

Table 10.1   Graded Exercise Testing: Settings and Applications

Settings	Applications
Clinical	• Diagnostic evaluation of clinical status • Assess therapeutic progress • Determine functional aerobic impairment • Develop exercise prescription • Determine ability to undertake daily tasks • Instill patient confidence
Research	• Determine maximal or peak oxygen uptake • Evaluate effect of experimental intervention/perturbation • Systematic assessment of perceptual and physiological responses to a standard exercise stimulus
Sport	• Preparticipation screening • Assess training progress • Predict performance capacity

Reprinted from American College of Sports Medicine 1991.

The remainder of this section describes each of the preceding GXT components. This description is a selected summary of a comprehensive chapter on graded exercise testing that can be found in the textbook by Pollock, Wilmore, and Fox (1984). The reader is referred to this text for more detailed information pertaining to the components, selection, application, and interpretation of a GXT.

Test Format

A GXT employs either a continuous, intermittent, or ramp format (fig. 10.1; deVries 1986). Selection of the test format often depends on the setting in which the evaluation takes place. Continuous, multistage GXTs are typically used in clinical settings where ease of administration, diagnostic sensitivity, and longitudinal monitoring of patient progress are desirable. This format uses progressive, uninterrupted increments in exercise intensity from one stage to the next until test termination criteria are achieved. The principal advantage of the continuous, multistage test is that the evaluation can be completed in a single session. Its disadvantage is that a plateau in physiological responses at peak exercise intensities is only seen in approximately 70% of tests. A plateau in test responses at peak exercise is considered the most important criterion for the identification of a true maximal end point. As a result, valid maximal data may not be obtained under some test conditions when a continuous, multistage format is employed.

An intermittent test format progressively increments exercise intensity from one stage to the next with rest periods of predetermined length interspersed between each test stage. The intermittent test continues until termination criteria are met (Taylor, Buskirk, and Henchel 1955; Mitchell, Sproule, and Chapman 1958). This format is most often used in the experimental setting, where attainment of true maximal responses is critical for test validity. That is, the intermittent format is terminated only when a plateau in oxygen uptake is observed between contiguous test stages at the highest exercise intensities. A disadvantage of the intermittent format is the length of time required to complete the evaluation. Because the intermittent stages are normally 5 to 8 min in length and are separated by a 30-min rest period, only two to three stages are presented in a single testing session. It is likely that several visits to the research laboratory will be necessary to ensure that maximal responses have been obtained.

The ramp format involves a constant, progressive increase in the exercise intensity until test termination criteria are obtained. This format is used almost exclusively in laboratory research to study oxygen kinetics during dynamic exercise or to assess anaerobic power.

Test End Points

Maximal Criteria

Two different criteria are used to establish the end point of a maximal GXT. The first involves volitional termination of the test by the individual being

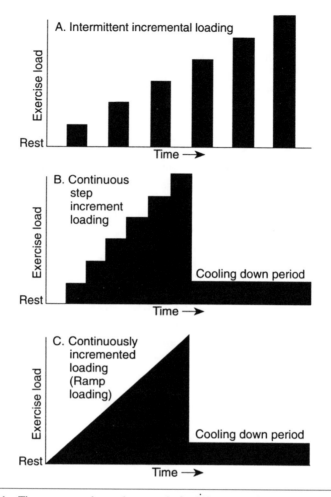

Figure 10.1   Three commonly used protocols for V̇O₂max testing.
Reprinted from deVries and Housh 1994.

evaluated owing to physiological or psychological fatigue. The second involves
the attainment of one or more of the following physiological criteria: (1) a plateau
in $\dot{V}O_2$ as exercise intensity continues to increase, (2) peak heart rate within ±5
b/min⁻¹ of age-adjusted maximum, (3) blood lactic acid concentration > 7 to 8
mmol/L, or (4) respiratory exchange ratio (RER) ≥ 1.2. The most frequent
variables measured at the termination of a maximal test are oxygen uptake,
ventilation, respiratory rate, heart rate, respiratory exchange ratio, blood pressure,
lactic acid concentration, and electrocardiographic wave forms. A GXT that
employs a maximal end point is considered the most accurate procedure to assess
peak physiological and/or clinical responses for purposes of medical diagnosis,
exercise prescription, and experimental research.

Submaximal Criteria

When the GXT is terminated prior to attaining maximal intensities, the evaluation is termed submaximal. The submaximal test is normally terminated when one of the following predetermined criterion responses is attained: (1) absolute $\dot{V}O_2$ [L/min or ml/kg^{-1}/min^{-1}] or heart rate (b/min^{-1}), (2) relative $\dot{V}O_2$ (%$\dot{V}O_2$max) or heart rate (%HR range), (3) RPE, or (4) absolute power output. Tests that employ a submaximal end point are particularly useful for physical fitness assessment when large numbers of individuals are to be evaluated. Functional exercise tolerance tests for those that are at low risk for coronary heart disease also employ submaximal end points. Under appropriately monitored conditions, a submaximal GXT can be administered periodically to monitor patient progress during cardiac exercise therapy. Provided that the end point of these periodic submaximal tests does not exceed the upper intensity of the patient's prescribed training zone, these evaluations can be very useful in promoting patient compliance. That is, feedback regarding beneficial changes in aerobic fitness and clinical status bolster the patient's confidence in the therapeutic intervention, reinforcing the necessity to maintain a regular exercise regime. Submaximal test results that are obtained in the cardiac rehabilitation setting also provide the clinician and exercise specialist with valuable information concerning the patient's response to therapeutic exercise, the accuracy of the exercise prescription, and the frequency of untoward clinical symptoms that appear during exercise therapy even when intensity is maintained within the training zone. Because the submaximal test is comparatively low risk and technically simple, it can be administered more frequently than a test that is terminated either at the point of physiological exhaustion or upon the appearance of clinical signs and symptoms contraindicating continued evaluation.

Symptom-Limited Functional Exercise Tolerance

When testing patients with cardiovascular or pulmonary disease, peak exercise is often defined by the onset of specific signs and symptoms of exertional intolerance. These symptoms are typically associated with untoward clinical manifestations of coronary or pulmonary insufficiency. Such clinical end points as anginal pain, ECG abnormalities (e.g., ST segment depression or excessive ectopic activity), inappropriate blood pressure responses, marked dyspnea, and arterial desaturation all serve as indicators that the GXT should be terminated. Sudden, profuse sweating, pallor, and unsteady gait are also indicative of insufficient myocardial oxygen supply or inadequate diffusion of oxygen from alveoli to the pulmonary capillary bed. The $\dot{V}O_2$ or MET level at the point of test termination is taken as the symptom-limited functional aerobic power. This value marks the upper limit of the functional metabolic range, providing the basis upon which a clinically appropriate exercise prescription is developed. The frequency and severity of clinical signs and symptoms noted at the point of GXT termination also provide valuable diagnostic information regarding disease status or its rate of progression. The reader is referred to the American College of Sports Medicine's authoritative publication *Guidelines for Exercise Testing and Prescription* (1991) for a comprehensive discussion of clinical factors that mark the end point of a symptom-limited GXT.

Mode and Protocol Selection

The most common modes used in graded exercise testing are the treadmill, cycle ergometer, arm ergometer, and step bench (Pollock, Wilmore, and Fox 1984). Selection of the test mode depends on the clinical and physiological characteristics of the individual to be evaluated, along with certain technical and practical factors associated with test administration. That is, for individuals who are not clinically or functionally restricted, a treadmill test is preferable. On the other hand, when testing a patient who is morbidly obese or who has an extremely low functional aerobic power, a stationary cycle ergometer may be the mode of choice. An arm ergometer is used when evaluating individuals with limited lower body mobility and is also preferred when testing pulmonary patients. A step test can be employed in physical education settings, where fitness assessment often involves a large number of young, healthy students who must be evaluated in a comparatively short period of time.

The GXT protocol determines the rate and manner by which exercise intensity is increased. Protocols increment exercise intensity according to a systematic, standardized pattern that is consistent from one testing session to the next. The individual's clinical status and aerobic fitness, as well as test objectives, exercise mode, and practical considerations, dictate the protocol choice. Quite often the protocol is identified by the name of the investigator who is credited with its development and validation. As an example, the Bruce treadmill protocol is named for Dr. Robert A. Bruce, a noted cardiologist who is widely credited with the earliest clinical application of exercise testing.

In general, the test protocol and test mode are functionally linked. Table 10.2 lists the major components of the GXT according to test mode and protocol. It should be noted that one or multiple protocol components can be manipulated at any given test stage in order to systematically increase exercise intensity.

A concept fundamental to the selection of a test protocol involves its *aggressiveness*. Protocol aggressiveness is defined as the magnitude of increase in $\dot{V}O_2$ [$ml/kg^{-1}/min^{-1}$; L/min; % of maximum] or METs with each successive test stage. The greater the $\dot{V}O_2$ or MET increment per stage, the more aggressive is the test protocol. In general, clinical status or functional aerobic power of the individual to be evaluated plays a major role in selecting the appropriate protocol aggressiveness. A lower level of aggressiveness should be used for individuals with clinical limitations (i.e., coronary or pulmonary patients) and poor aerobic fitness. High levels of protocol aggressiveness should be used when testing healthy, young, or middle-aged individuals who have good to excellent aerobic fitness. In actuality, peak physiological responses (i.e., $\dot{V}O_2$, HR, $\dot{V}_E$, RER, BP, [Hla]) do not markedly vary among protocols that differ widely in level of aggressiveness.

Table 10.2 Protocol Type and Level of Aggressiveness According to Test Mode, Clinical Status, and Aerobic Fitness

Mode	Clinical status[a]	Functional aerobic fitness	Level of aggressiveness			
			Initial stage	Increment	Stage duration	Suggested protocol
Treadmill (variable speed & grade)	CHD Pul.	Poor-low < 10 METs	2 METs	1 MET	3 min	Naughton
	Normal	Mod-high > 10 METs	2-3 METs	1-3 METs	1-3 min	Modified Bruce
	Athletic	> 14 METs	3+ METs	3+ METs	3+ METs	Åstrand
Cycle ergometer (50-80 rpm)	CHD Pul.	Poor-low < 10 METs	150 kgm/min	150 kgm/min	3 min	Sjostrand
	Normal	Mod-high > 10 METs	150-300 kgm/min	150-300 kgm/min	1-3 min	
Arm ergometer (50-60 rpm)	CHD Pul.	Poor-low < 10 METs	0 kgm/min	25-50 kgm/min	3 min	Sjostrand
	Normal	Mod-high > 10 METs	75-100 kgm/min	75-100 kgm/min		
Step platform (30 step/min)	Normal	Low to high	3 cm	2-4 cm	1-2 min	Nagle, Balke, Naughton

[a]CHD—Coronary heart disease
Pul.—Pulmonary disease

Therefore, the magnitude of increase in exercise intensity is of primary concern during the protocol stages immediately proceeding the attainment of the test end point. It is at these high submaximal stages that sufficient time must be provided to ensure accurate measurement of physiological responses and for clinical symptoms to develop. Physiological and clinical assessments at high intensities provide important information for exercise prescription and diagnostic assessment. If the test is too aggressive, termination may occur prematurely. Resultant physiological and clinical information may be distorted, negating the full value of the GXT. Table 10.2 can be used as a guideline in selecting the appropriate level of protocol aggressiveness.

Treadmill Protocols

Presented in figure 10.2 (Pollock, Wilmore, and Fox 1984) are the speeds, grade settings, and stage durations for some of the more commonly used treadmill test protocols (i.e., Bruce, Balke, Naughton, Ellestad, and Åstrand). In general, these protocols span a range of test intensities, beginning with the least (Balke) and progressing to the most (modified Åstrand) aggressive.

The Balke protocol is used when evaluating individuals who have low to moderate levels of aerobic fitness. When testing highly fit individuals, the Balke protocol may be excessively long, owing to its low level of aggressiveness. In such cases, localized leg fatigue may limit test performance prior to achieving an exercise intensity that maximally stresses the oxygen transport system. By contrast, the Åstrand protocol is best suited for young, healthy, athletic men and women because it employs an extremely high level of test aggressiveness. The Naughton protocol is usually preferred for predischarge testing of coronary heart disease patients and when evaluating older individuals who have very low functional aerobic power (i.e., < 6 METs). The Bruce and Ellestad protocols are the most flexible and are appropriate for men and women, athletes and nonathletes, and young to middle-aged individuals. Because the Bruce protocol is widely used in clinical settings, a large amount of normative data is available for comparative purposes. However, the speed settings for stages III (3.4 mph) and IV (4.2 mph) of the Bruce protocol are often judged awkward, with neither a walking nor running mode considered comfortable. Confusion regarding whether to change from a walking to running mode often results. In this context, Noble et al. (1973) found the locomotor speed at which an individual prefers to change from a walking to a running mode (i.e., mode change velocity; MCV) is approximately 4.0 mph (fig. 10.3). At speeds below the MCV, RPE is higher when running than when walking, whereas the reverse is true at speeds that are faster than the MCV. Therefore, irrespective of the treadmill protocol, the individual will normally elect to change from a walking to running mode when treadmill speed reaches approximately 4.0 mph, a decision consistent with his or her perception of exertion.

Distinctions are not normally made between submaximal and maximal treadmill protocols. The test end point as described earlier determines whether the

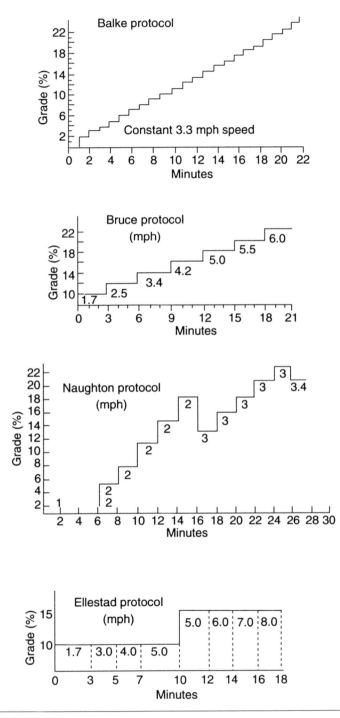

Figure 10.2 *(continued on next page)*

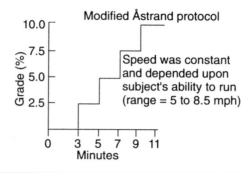

Figure 10.2 *(continued)* The Balke, Bruce, Naughton, Ellestad, and Åstrand treadmill protocols are the most commonly used. Ellestad has modified his testing protocol: The treadmill speed of 5 mph is maintained from minutes 10 to 12 and is increased to 6 mph from minutes 12 to 14, and so on.

Reprinted from Pollock, Wilmore, and Fox 1984.

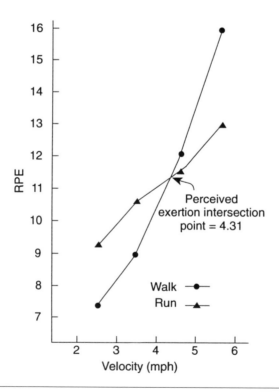

Figure 10.3 Perceived exertion response to walking and running at various velocities.
Reprinted from Noble 1973.

evaluation is terminated at maximal intensities or at a predetermined submaximal stage.

Cycle Protocols

A cycle ergometer has several advantages over other test modalities. Most stationary cycles are portable, can be easily stored, and emit comparatively little noise even at the highest power outputs. Thus, they are often preferred when testing is undertaken in a busy clinic where space may be at a premium. Of practical importance is that there is very little upper body movement during cycle ergometer testing, facilitating blood pressure measurement and reducing ECG baseline distortion. However, maximal values for $\dot{V}O_2$, $\dot{V}_E$, and heart rate may be as much as 10% lower during cycle than during treadmill testing. Comparisons of maximal physiological responses between cycle and treadmill modes should be made with these differential responses in mind. In contrast, clinical responses (e.g., ECG abnormalities, angina pectoris) at the point of symptom-limited test termination usually do not differ between cycle and treadmill tests. Accordingly, the cycle mode is often chosen when exercise tolerance is limited by peripheral vascular claudication, an ischemic response which is exacerbated to a comparatively greater extent by treadmill than by cycle exercise.

The two most commonly used cycle ergometer protocols are the Sjostrand multistage test and the Åstrand-Rhyming single stage test. The former protocol is terminated at either a submaximal or maximal intensity, whereas the latter employs a submaximal end point. The Sjostrand protocol holds pedal rate constant, usually within a range of 50 to 80 rpm. The initial power output is either 300 or 450 kgm/min. Pedal resistance is incremented by 150 or 300 kgm/min at the beginning of each 3-min test stage. When a submaximal test end point is employed, exercise is terminated at a predetermined heart rate such as 150 or 170 bpm. The power output achieved at this reference heart rate is taken as the physical work capacity at 150 or 170 bpm, that is, PWC_{150} or PWC_{170}. The maximal protocol is terminated when exercise can no longer be performed at the preestablished pedal rate owing to fatigue.

The Åstrand-Rhyming protocol employs a low-intensity warm-up followed immediately by the presentation of a single power output intended to elicit a heart rate response between 120 and 170 bpm. An age- and gender-based nomogram is then used to estimate $\dot{V}O_2$max from steady-state heart rate responses recorded during the final 2 min of the test. A detailed description of this test protocol can be found in Noble's (1986) textbook. The rationale underlying both the Sjostrand and Åstrand-Rhyming cycle protocols assumes a linear relation between heart rate and $\dot{V}O_2$ for a wide range of power outputs. Therefore, at a given power output, an individual with a higher functional aerobic power will have a lower heart rate than an individual with a lower level of aerobic fitness.

A third cycle protocol has been developed by the YMCA and is used for fitness testing in younger, healthy individuals. The protocol progressively increments power output, much as the Sjostrand protocol does. However, the amount by which the power output is incremented per test stage (i.e., aggressiveness) depends on the heart rate response to the previous stage. The lower the heart rate, the larger is the power output increment. The YMCA protocol is voluntarily terminated by the test subject when it is no longer possible to continue exercise due to fatigue. A detailed description of this protocol can be found elsewhere (Pollock, Wilmore, and Fox 1984).

Arm Ergometer Protocol

Exercise tests involving an arm ergometer are less common than treadmill or cycle evaluations. Upper body testing using arm ergometry is normally indicated when the more traditional leg modes cannot be used owing to clinical limitations (i.e., amputation, spinal cord injury, peripheral vascular claudication, spastic neuromuscular dysfunction, and obesity). Because upper body exercise produces a greater $\dot{V}_E$ than lower body exercise at a given power output, the arm ergometer is the mode of choice when evaluating pulmonary patients. In addition, arm ergometry is often employed when testing the functional aerobic power of athletes who engage in upper body competition.

There are several disadvantages associated with arm testing. Because of significant upper body movement, ECG tracings may be distorted by motion artifact, and blood pressure measures using auscultation are technically difficult to obtain. As a result, the arm mode may not be appropriate for patients who have recently experienced myocardial infarction or myocardial revascularization surgery. It should also be noted that, because of the smaller muscle mass involved in arm testing, peak values for $\dot{V}O_2$ and heart rate may be as much as 20% to 30% lower than would be obtained during leg exercise. Therefore, it is inappropriate to prescribe exercise intensity for leg exercise using results of an arm ergometer test. Similarly, the determination of $\dot{V}O_2$peak using data derived from arm testing cannot be generalized to peak responses for other modes of exercise, that is, leg or combined arm-and-leg activities.

The test protocol typically used with an arm ergometer is conceptually the same as the Sjostrand protocol previously described for cycle ergometer testing. However, the arm protocol employs comparatively lower initial power outputs and smaller step increments in power output per test stage. As in the leg protocol, crank rate is held constant throughout the test, usually ranging between 50 and 80 rpm. The arm test protocol can be terminated at either a submaximal or maximal end point, depending on test objectives. If a submaximal end point is selected, the test is terminated when a predetermined absolute or relative heart rate is attained. The maximal test is volitionally terminated by the subject when exercise can no longer be continued due to fatigue.

Step Test Protocol

The step test is typically employed when cycle or treadmill modes are not available or when large numbers of individuals are to be evaluated in a short time period. A step test is used to assess aerobic fitness and is rarely employed for clinical diagnosis of cardiovascular or pulmonary disease.

Ideally, the step apparatus should employ an adjustable step height. In this way the step height can be set according to leg length or body height, a notable advantage when testing heterogeneous population subsets.

The test protocol sets the step frequency and duration of each stage. Step cadence follows a left-up, right-up, left-down, right-down pattern, normally executed at 30 cycles per min. The four-count step pattern can be regulated by a metronome. The step protocol is terminated after a predetermined period of exercise, usually 3 to 5 min. Heart rate is measured during the final minute of the test using ECG telemetry. If such an electronic monitoring system is not available, heart rate can be measured during the initial 10 s of a standing or sitting recovery period using a stethoscope or radial artery palpation. The physiological rationale underlying the step test is that the lower the heart rate for a given step frequency and test duration, the higher is the level of functional aerobic power. Therefore, $\dot{V}O_2$peak can be predicted using submaximal heart rate responses to a step test.

Run Test

The run test is performed on a level track that has a measured circumference and preferably a synthetic surface. The test is used to classify aerobic fitness of healthy young men and women. Well-trained, middle-aged individuals can also be evaluated with the run test, although this application is comparatively limited. The test is particularly advantageous when large numbers of individuals are to be evaluated in a single session. A field test of this type should not be used for diagnostic purposes. The test protocol requires that the individual run the greatest distance possible in a given time period (e.g., 9 min) or to run a given distance (e.g., 1 mi) as fast as possible. Both dependent variables (i.e., distance and time) have a high correlation ($r = .75$ to $.85$) with actual laboratory measurement of $\dot{V}O_2$max (Pollock, Wilmore, and Fox 1984).

Test Applications Using RPE

Ratings of perceived exertion can be used during graded exercise testing as either an independent or adjunctive measure of functional exercise tolerance. As discussed in previous chapters, exertional perceptions are related to respiratory-metabolic and peripheral physiological mediators. Therefore, RPE provides much of the same information regarding functional exercise tolerance as do physiological responses. The independent application of RPE is seen in simple field tests of aerobic fitness, where a single criterion measure is all that is required to assess training status. More typically, however, RPE is employed as an adjunct to standard physiological measures during exercise testing, especially in the clinical setting. In this context, RPE provides a subjective measure of exercise tolerance that complements objective physiological measures. By example, both RPE and heart rate are measured every minute of a graded treadmill test as a means of approximating the relative exercise intensity and to determine the patient's capacity to continue the evaluation.

A GXT is constructed around two types of variables: independent and dependent. The independent variable provides a criterion from which the dependent variable is measured during testing. However, depending on the test protocol, the same measure can be either an independent or dependent variable. As an example, the Sjostrand cycle ergometer test identifies the power output (i.e., the dependent variable) that is equivalent to a criterion heart rate (i.e., the independent variable). The higher the power output at the criterion heart rate, the higher is the level of aerobic fitness. In contrast, the heart rate response (dependent variable) to a fixed power output (independent variable) can also be determined during a submaximal cycle ergometer test. A lower heart rate at a fixed power output indicates a higher level of aerobic fitness.

In an analogous manner, RPE is used as either an independent or dependent variable during a GXT. That is, a predetermined RPE can serve as a criterion measure to determine changes in power output subsequent to exercise training. Conversely, RPE can be measured at a fixed power output prior to and following training. Under the former test protocol, RPE is the independent variable, while under the latter protocol, the perceptual response serves as the dependent variable. A number of cycle and field tests that variously employ RPE as either an independent or dependent variable are explored more fully later in this section.

An assumption basic to the application of RPE in clinical testing is that perceptual and physiological responses are linearly related across a variety of exercise modes and intensities (Gutmann et al. 1981; Stamford 1976; Skinner et al. 1973; Gamberale 1972). Interpretation of GXT responses that employ RPE as either an independent or dependent variable must satisfy this assumption if the test is to be judged valid using physiological or clinical criteria. The linear relation between RPE and such variables as heart rate, oxygen uptake, and power output is particularly important when measures are to be obtained during a submaximal test and used to predict maximal aerobic power. Such a linear relation allows extrapolation from a single criterion measure to a fixed end point that determines maximal responses.

The following section examines the application of RPE in a number of clinical and performance-based exercise evaluations. Specific attention is given to the following:

- Control of test progression
- Perceptually modified Sjostrand cycle test
- Perceptually based run test
- Anaerobic power tests
- Selected testing applications

Perceptually Guided GXT

One of the most common and perhaps earliest applications of RPE in a clinical setting involves the use of perceptual responses to guide the progression of a GXT. In this context RPE serves two very important methodological functions. First, when the terminal RPE (i.e., the highest scale category) is reported, it provides subjective confirmation that clinical or physiological end points of the GXT have been achieved. Peak physiological and clinical responses are not always sufficiently sensitive criteria to terminate a GXT. At peak intensity, both HR and $\dot{V}O_2$ are subject to marked interindividual variability (Squires, Rod, and Pollock 1982; Morgan and Borg 1980), especially when evaluating coronary and pulmonary patients. Therefore, age-adjusted normative values for these physiological responses may not accurately identify the test end point. In contrast, RPE reaches its terminal value at the test end point regardless of the population or clinical subset being evaluated. It follows that the test end point will coincide in a temporal manner with the terminal perceptual rating. Therefore, if functional aerobic power or performance time change in response to an exercise or therapeutic intervention while the terminal RPE remains at its highest scale value, the test results represent a true alteration in cardiorespiratory fitness or clinical status (Pollock, Wilmore, and Fox 1984). The results are not biased by the patient's unwillingness to undertake the test or lack of motivation to pursue the test to peak physiological or clinical end points, a circumstance not unusual when evaluating nonathletic groups.

Second, the intensity of exertional perception at a given time during testing indicates the point within the functional metabolic range to which the evaluation has progressed. That is, RPE is a valuable adjunct to such physiological measures as HR, $\dot{V}O_2$, RER, and blood [Hla] in guiding the progression of a GXT. The increment in RPE from one test stage to the next can be used to estimate the rate of progress toward the test end point. Under some testing conditions, RPE is a better indicator of the relative metabolic stress than heart rate (Borg 1971). As an example, beta-blocking medications such as propranolol attenuate the HR response during a GXT. RPE, on the other hand, is unaffected by pharmacological beta-blockade (fig. 10.4). In this instance, RPE provides a more sensitive measure of test progression relative to physiological or clinical end points than does heart rate. As the RPE approaches 15 to 17 on the Borg scale, preliminary procedures to safely terminate the test should be initiated, even though the HR response may indicate that the evaluation is not nearing its end point.

RPE may also provide a more accurate marker of the relative metabolic stress than does HR when individuals of various ages are evaluated using the same test protocol. The HR response at a given submaximal power output or $\dot{V}O_2$ is largely unaffected by age. In contrast, RPE at a given power output or $\dot{V}O_2$ increases with age, owing to chronological decrement in functional aerobic power (Borg 1970). If only HR is used to guide the GXT, both younger and older individuals would appear to be at the same point in the test progression. However, the higher RPE in the older individual than in the younger individual indicates

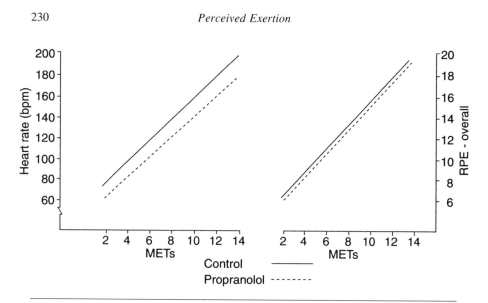

Figure 10.4   Effect of beta-blocking medication on heart rate and RPE during graded exercise testing.

a comparatively greater level of metabolic stress and more rapid progression toward the test end point.

Several practical rules of thumb apply when test progression is guided by RPE. Noble (1982) observed that coronary heart disease patients generally will not complete more than one additional stage of the Bruce treadmill protocol after responding with an RPE of 15 to 17 on the Borg scale. In this situation, RPE responses to progressive test stages indicate the time when test administrators should prepare to terminate the evaluation. It should also be noted that test progression can be monitored more effectively by anticipating the rate of increase in RPE as a function of both exercise intensity and mode. When walking on a horizontal treadmill, a 1.7-km/h increment in speed produces a two-category increase on the Borg RPE scale (Smutok, Skrinar, and Pandolf 1980). A 1.7-km/h increment in treadmill running speed results in a one-category increase on the Borg RPE scale. Speed increments that are less than 0.6 km/h are below the difference threshold necessary to alter RPE. When performing on an outdoor running track, RPE will increase by approximately three categories on the Borg scale for every 1-m/s increase in running speed (Van Den Burg and Ceci, 1986). In a similar manner, the difference threshold for a one-category increment on the Borg RPE scale during cycle ergometer testing is 300 kgm/min (Kamon, Pandolf, and Cafarelli 1974). Finally, RPE at the lactate or ventilatory threshold ranges from 12 to 14 and remains relatively stable over fitness level, training state, and gender (Hill et al. 1987). It therefore marks the lower intensity of the training window (i.e., target training range) for aerobic fitness. When appropriate instrumentation is available during a GXT, accurate assessment of the RPE that corresponds to the lactate or ventilatory threshold proves useful in developing an exercise prescription. This exercise prescription procedure is examined in more detail in chapter 11.

The foregoing guidelines are intended only as general rules to estimate test progression using RPE responses. Their utility may vary between individuals and test protocols. This precautionary point is particularly important, because the subjects used to develop these guidelines were primarily young, healthy, and at least moderately active. Therefore, the absolute increase in exercise intensity required to produce a change in RPE for a given test mode may vary as a function of clinical condition, aerobic fitness, and training status. The use of RPE to guide the progress of a GXT should not be undertaken within a clinical or physiological vacuum (Pollock, Wilmore, and Fox 1984). Rather, perceptual signals should be used in conjunction with pertinent clinical, physiological, and psychological information to guide test progress and evaluate functional exercise tolerance. Table 10.3 lists a number of intensity thresholds that are useful in tracking the progression of a GXT according to the projected increment in RPE.

Submaximal Cycle Ergometer Tests

Exercise evaluations involving a cycle ergometer normally employ a protocol that either systematically increases power output until a predetermined end point is reached or uses a fixed power output that is performed for a predetermined period of time. RPE can be employed to estimate functional aerobic power using both of these protocols. When power output is systematically increased until test termination, perceptual responses serve as the independent variable. By contrast, when power output is held constant, perceptual responses become a dependent variable. In both cases, RPE is used to estimate aerobic power in a manner analogous to the way that heart rate is employed in submaximal cycle testing. The validity of a perceptually based cycle ergometer test is based on the linear relation between power output and both RPE and heart rate across a wide range of exercise intensities (Borg 1962, 1978).

Table 10.3   Intensity Thresholds for Increments in RPE: Suggested Guidelines

Mode	Intensity	Increment RPE (15-pt scale)	Reference
Treadmill			
(walking)	1.7 km/h	2	Smutok, Skrinar, and Pandolf 1980
(running)	1.7 km/h	1	
Track	1 m/s	2.7	Van Den Burg and Ceci 1986
Cycle	300 kgm/min	1	Kamon, Pandolf, and Cafarelli 1974

The perceptually modified Sjostrand physical work capacity (PWC) test systematically increases power output until the test termination criterion is attained (Sjostrand 1947). In this protocol, pedal rate is set at 50 rpm, while power output is incremented by 150 or 300 kgm/min every 3 min. RPE is measured at the end of each 3-min stage (Borg 1971, 1978). The test is terminated when a predetermined RPE is attained. Normally, terminal measures, called criterion values, are set at an RPE of 15 on the Borg scale. As shown in figure 10.5, PWC is determined by plotting RPE responses as a function of power output (PO; Robertson et al. 1993). A horizontal line is drawn from the criterion value on the y axis (i.e., RPE of 15) to the reference line. A vertical line is then drawn downward from the point of intersection on the reference line to the x axis, where PO at an RPE of 15 (PO_{R15}) is determined. The same procedure can be applied for any criterion RPE (e.g., 13, 15, 17). The perceptually modified Sjostrand protocol can be used for both intra- and interindividual comparisons. Intraindividual comparisons are typically employed to determine the effect of a training program on cardiorespiratory fitness. Upon completion of an aerobic training program, the reference line depicting the relation between RPE and power output will be adjusted rightward. The same criterion RPE that was used during the pretraining evaluation is again employed to determine the posttraining PO_R. As demonstrated in figure 10.5, a horizontal line is drawn from a criterion RPE of 15 to the posttraining reference line. A vertical line is then drawn downward from the point of intersection on the reference line to the x axis, identifying PO_{R15}. The pretraining-to-posttraining change in PO at an RPE of 15 indicates the magnitude of improvement in cardiorespiratory fitness following aerobic training. The physiological rationale underlying the perceptually modified Sjostrand protocol holds that as functional aerobic power increases, a higher power output can be performed at a given criterion RPE.

Interindividual comparisons of functional aerobic power based on the perceptually modified Sjostrand protocol can be used to stratify population subsets according to their level of cardiorespiratory fitness. In this context RPE may be a better criterion variable than heart rate. There is large interindividual variability in maximal heart rate for a given age. As such, a submaximal criterion heart rate can represent widely different relative exercise intensities among individuals. Interindividual comparison of functional aerobic power derived using a criterion heart rate may be inappropriate. In contrast, the terminal (i.e., highest) RPE on a category scale is the same for all individuals, regardless of age, gender, clinical status, or aerobic fitness. Therefore, a given criterion RPE represents the same level of perceptual stress for all individuals, facilitating interindividual comparison of PO_R.

The perceptually modified Sjostrand protocol has been validated by correlating PO measures that were separately derived using a criterion RPE and a criterion HR. The validity coefficients range from $r = .60$ to $r = .75$ (Borg 1962; Borg and Ohlsson 1975). In addition, PO at an RPE of 17 (PO_{R17}) correlated reasonably well ($r = .50$) with performance on such field criteria as running, skiing, lumber work, and military activities (Borg 1962).

An alternative perceptually based submaximal cycle ergometer protocol employs a constant power output intended to produce a heart rate response between 120 and

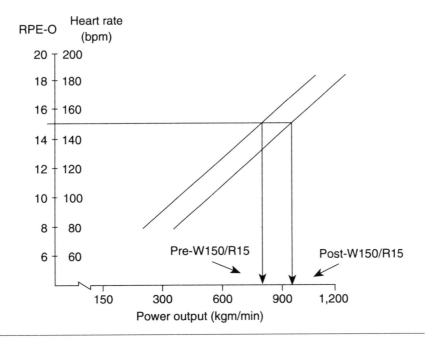

Figure 10.5 Perceptually modified submaximal Sjostrand cycle ergometer test of aerobic fitness. RPE-O = RPE-Overall; Pre= pretraining; Post = posttraining; W_{150}/R_{15} = power output at a heart rate of 150 b · min^{-1} and RPE of 15.
Reprinted from Robertson, Goss, and Metz.

170 bpm. The absolute power output used is dependent on the level of aerobic fitness and gender. Normally, a higher power output is required for more fit individuals than for less fit individuals and for men than for women. However, highly fit women may require higher power outputs than less fit men. As a rule of thumb, power outputs ranging from 300 to 900 kgm/min usually fall within the desired heart rate range. The protocol employs an 8-min exercise period, allowing sufficient time to achieve physiological and perceptual steady state. Pedaling rate is set at 50 rpm and is usually regulated by a metronome or calibrated tachometer. The first 3 min of exercise are used as a warm-up. If the heart rate response has not reached the lower level of the desired range (i.e., 120 bpm) at the conclusion of the warm-up, the power output should be incremented by 150 or 300 kgm/min. RPE is measured at the end of each exercise minute. The rationale underlying this test protocol is that at a fixed power output, the dependent measure (i.e., RPE) will be lower for the more aerobically fit individual.

Run Test

The perceptually based run test is a low-risk, submaximal evaluation that can be easily administered as part of a daily training program to assess progress or to classify aerobic fitness (Borg 1970). Periodic assessment of aerobic fitness is an important adjunct to a training program. Unfortunately, many tests of aerobic fitness require expensive, time-consuming, and electronically complex procedures that allow only one individual to be evaluated at a time. Such technically involved testing procedures may not be practical in certain clinical, sport, and physical education settings where assessment must be undertaken on a gymnasium floor or running track. The run test is ideally suited for these settings because it

- employs moderate exercise intensities (i.e., is low risk),
- requires minimal instrumentation,
- evaluates a number of individuals at the same time,
- is easy to administer,
- uses a common mode of exercise that stimulates interest and reduces variability, and
- requires exercise periods that are short enough to motivate subjects to continue but long enough to optimally stress the cardiorespiratory system (Borg and Ohlsson 1975).

The run test reverses the normal independent-dependent variable system that is customarily employed in treadmill testing (Borg 1970; Robertson et al. 1993). Running speed is self-selected according to perceptual preference, thereby becoming a dependent variable (Borg 1970; Robertson et al. 1993). This is in contrast to treadmill testing, in which speed is a precisely controlled independent variable. At a criterion RPE, the higher the level of aerobic fitness, the faster will be the self-selected running speed. The use of a criterion RPE in this manner is analogous to the perceptually modified Sjostrand cycle ergometer test described earlier.

The run test requires that three separate self-selected speeds be performed. These speeds vary according to the individual's interpretation of test instructions (Borg 1970) and the level of running experience (i.e., a faster pace will be selected by trained runners; Michael and Eckard 1972). During the first test trial, subjects are instructed to run very slowly at a constant speed. In the second trial, the instructions require the individuals to run somewhat faster but at a moderate pace. During the third trial the individual is instructed to run a little faster than the previous trial (Borg 1984). The instructions provide for the subjective identification of test speeds that are linearly related to RPE. Very slow and very fast speeds are not used because they violate the assumption of linearity between RPE and running velocity, invalidating the test (Borg and Ohlsson 1975). The distance for each test trial can range from 600 to 1,200 m (Edgren and Borg 1975; Borg and Ohlsson 1975). The test distance should be selected so that the trial is 3 to 5 min in duration, allowing sufficient time to achieve a physiological steady state. A 1- to 5-min recovery period is provided between test trials. In general, the lower the individual's aerobic fitness, the shorter is the test distance. A measured running track or gymnasium perimeter provides the best setting to ensure that the requisite distance has been traversed. Shorter lap distances allow more frequent measurement of RPE, reducing test variability.

RPEs are determined at the end of each lap. Normally, the RPEs for the last two laps are averaged and used to compute test responses. Total time to perform the test distance is also recorded and converted to running speed. RPEs from the three test trials are then plotted as a function of their respective running speeds. This procedure can be facilitated by using linear regression analysis (fig. 10.6; Robertson, Goss, and Metz 1993). The plotting procedure assumes that RPE is a linear function of the subjectively selected test speeds. A criterion RPE is then selected, usually 13, 15, or 17 on the Borg scale. Using the plot, a horizontal line is drawn from the criterion RPE on the y axis to the reference line depicting the relation between independent and dependent variables. A vertical line is then drawn downward from the point of intersection on the reference line to the x axis, identifying the running speed (V_R) that is equivalent to the criterion RPE. The faster the V_R, the higher is the individual's level of aerobic fitness. The run test can be administered prior to and following an aerobic training program. An increase in V_R after completion of training indicates that functional aerobic power has improved.

The run test has been validated for distances between 600 and 1,200 m using runners, general sport participants, and nonexercisers. Correlations between V_R and cycle ergometer physical work capacity and between V_R and 1,500 m run time and predicted $\dot{V}O_2$max range from $r = .57$ to .74 (Borg 1984; Borg and Ohlsson 1975), indicating acceptable validity for the test procedure. Test-retest reliability is high ($r = .93$; Borg 1984).

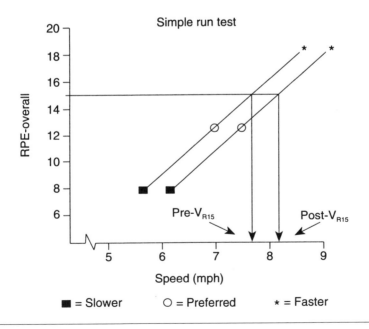

Figure 10.6   Perceptually based run test of aerobic fitness.
Reprinted from Robertson, Goss, and Metz.

Anaerobic Power

Perceptually based tests of anaerobic power are less common than tests of aerobic power. This is probably because anaerobic power tests are typically of short duration and very high intensity. Therefore, RPE responses reach the high terminal scale category for all individuals, reducing the interindividual discriminative power of the evaluation. However, Borg (1982) has developed a test of anaerobic power that employs submaximal RPE responses. Called the maximum work (Wmax) test, the evaluation predicts the highest power output that can be maintained on a cycle ergometer for 30 s.

The maximum work test employs a modified ramp protocol. The initial power output is set at 50 W. Power output is then incremented by 50 W every 30 s until test termination. Pedal rate is held constant at 60 rpm throughout the test. RPE (Borg 15-category scale) is determined at the end of each 30-s test stage. The test is terminated at an RPE of 17. As shown in figure 10.7 (Borg 1982), RPE is then plotted as a function of power output. Using the slope of the plot, a line is extrapolated to an RPE of 20. From the point of intersection, a vertical line is drawn downward to intersect the x axis, identifying the Wmax power output. This is taken as the highest power output that can be maintained for 30 s, that is, a perceptually based prediction of anaerobic power.

When the perceptually extrapolated value for Wmax was compared to the measured value, a correlation coefficient of $r = .96$ was found for a mixed sample of men and women (Borg 1982). In addition, when the extrapolated Wmax was actually performed, the test duration was 30.4 s, a performance time very close to the test criterion. It can be concluded that RPE determined during a very short exercise period (i.e., 30 s) at submaximal intensities provides a valid prediction of anaerobic power.

A particular advantage of the maximum work test protocol is that pedal rate is held constant throughout the evaluation. This procedure is subjectively preferable and provides precise control of the exercise intensity. In contrast, some tests of anaerobic power—most notably the Wingate protocol—hold resistance constant and increment pedal rate; this procedure may be biomechanically awkward for some individuals.

The cycling strength and endurance test (CSET) assesses anaerobic power by determining 10 intermittent maximal exercise thresholds (Edgren et al. 1976). The CSET does not use RPE responses to calculate anaerobic power. Its principal variable is the peak power output attained at each maximal threshold. The test is described in this chapter mainly because it was developed by Gunnar Borg as part of his early studies of human exercise performance. As such, CSET responses were often used to validate other tests, many of which use RPE as a variable. For example, anaerobic power determined by the perceptually based maximum work test described earlier correlates very highly ($r = .90$) with anaerobic power derived from the CSET (Borg 1982).

The CSET protocol employs 10 intermittent trials, each of approximately 45 s duration. A 15-s rest period separates each trial. The initial power output for each

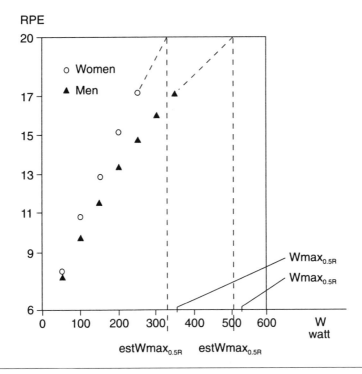

Figure 10.7   Means of RPE values plotted against work loads for men and women. Estimates of maximal performances from ratings, estWmax$_{0.5R}$ (= W$_{0.5R}$), are also given together with the actual maximal performances measured, Wmax$_{0.5}$, for men and women. Reprinted from Borg 1982.

trial is set at 1,500 kgm/min and is incremented by 40 kgm/(min · s) using a ramplike format. The maximal threshold (kgm/min) for each trial is determined as the point where a 60 rpm pedaling rate cannot be maintained. The mean of the first three thresholds is a measure of anaerobic power, while the mean of the last three thresholds measures cycle-specific muscular endurance.

Flexible Work Test

An important methodological component of the GXT is the pattern by which exercise intensity is progressively incremented. Most GXTs employ equal power output increments from one protocol stage to the next. This causes interindividual variation in physiological strain and perceived exertion at a given submaximal power output. Total test time also varies between individuals. Under some circumstances, these test conditions may not be satisfactory. Borg proposes an alternative protocol that employs a perceptual feedback mechanism as part of a standard

Sjostrand physical work capacity test (Borg, Edgren, Marklund 1970). Exercise stages are subjectively the same, while power output at each test stage varies between individuals. The increase in power output is guided by a feedback system that uses RPE and heart rate responses from the preceding test stages. Using this feedback system, peak power output is attained in the last 4 min of the test. Termed the Flexible Work Test, the evaluation provides a perceptual measure of physical work capacity expressed as the highest power output that can be sustained for 4 min (i.e., W^4max; Borg, Edstrom, and Marklund 1970). Total test time is 10 min for all individuals. The power output is incremented in steps that represent a similar point in each subject's perceived range of exertion. The reader is referred to Borg, Edstrom, and Marklund (1970) for a detailed explanation of the procedures to administer the flexible work test.

Training Progress

Throughout this chapter it has been noted that RPE can be used to monitor training outcomes. This is accomplished by measuring RPE at a fixed metabolic (i.e., $\dot{V}O_2$) reference point during a GXT. Serial administration of the GXT during an aerobic training program provides a perceptual check on training progress. As functional aerobic power increases over the course of training, the reference submaximal $\dot{V}O_2$ represents a progressively lower relative metabolic rate. Because the intensity of the perceptual signal is linked to the relative metabolic rate (i.e., $\%\dot{V}O_2max$), RPE is also lower at the fixed reference point. When submaximal GXTs are administered periodically during the course of a training program, RPE responses provide convenient, technically simple measures of training progress. As an example, Ekelund et al. (1986) measured RPE at a fixed $\dot{V}O_2$ (2.5 L/min) during graded exercise testing prior to and following a therapeutic training program for hypertensive patients. Following training, RPE at the metabolic reference point was lower than at pretraining, irrespective of whether patients were or were not receiving beta-blocking therapy. A number of other investigations also report attenuation of exertional perceptions following therapeutic and competitive aerobic training regimes when comparisons were made at a constant metabolic rate (Ekblom and Goldbarg 1971; Gutmann et al. 1981; Pandolf, Burse, and Goldman 1975; Lewis et al. 1980; Knuttgen et al. 1973).

Special Considerations

Perceptual Preference

Patient compliance with evaluation procedures can be enhanced by selecting test modes that are perceptually preferable. Perceptual preference is expressed as those exercise conditions that are associated with the lowest RPE. Attention to perceptual preference when selecting the GXT protocol helps to eliminate the influence of patient motivation on end-point criteria. That is, clinical and physiological measures can be interpreted knowing that they represent true peak responses and are not biased by end points that reflect poor motivation to continue the evaluation. A few examples may serve to underline this point. Cycle ergometer test protocols typically increment exercise intensity by increasing brake resistance while holding pedal rate constant. A less frequently employed protocol holds resistance constant while pedal rate is increased. Maximal aerobic power does not differ between the two protocols (Moffatt and Stamford 1978). Therefore, both are physiologically acceptable procedures to assess functional exercise tolerance. However, as Moffatt and Stamford (1978) noted, perceptual preference of both men and women favored the protocol that incremented pedal rate. When perceptual preference is of concern in selecting a cycle ergometer protocol, comparatively greater increments in pedal rate than brake resistance appear desirable.

Under test conditions where cycle ergometer brake resistance is progressively incremented, it is often practical to select a pedal rate that is both metabolically and perceptually optimal. For most individuals, pedal rates that fall within a range of 60 to 80 rpm have the highest metabolic efficiency, while rates approximating 40 and 120 rpm have the lowest efficiency (Coast, Cox, and Welch 1986). In general, RPE is lowest at the midrange pedal rates and highest at the extremes of the range (Stamford and Noble 1974; Pandolf and Noble 1973; Robertson et al. 1979). The 60- to 80-rpm pedal rates are therefore both perceptually and metabolically optimal for most individuals, with the possible exception of highly trained cyclists, who usually prefer somewhat higher rates.

Selection of a treadmill protocol can also be based on subjective preference. McConnell and Clark (1988) examined four maximal test protocols wherein treadmill speeds were incremented in 1-min stages, in 2-min stages, according to the average daily training speed, and by a self-selected pace that reflected perceptual preference. Maximal values for $\dot{V}O_2$, HR, and RER did not differ among protocols, underlining the subjective utility of self-selected treadmill speeds when evaluating maximal aerobic power of trained runners.

Accommodating perceptual preference is comparatively less important when choosing between treadmill and cycle testing modes. This is especially the case when the GXT reaches higher intensities. Sidney and Shephard (1972) noted that RPE did not differ between treadmill and cycle exercise when comparisons were made at heart rates above 150 bpm. Therefore, both exercise modes are perceptually acceptable when the test end point is defined as maximal aerobic power.

An important consideration when incorporating a self-selected training pace into an exercise prescription is to ensure that the perceptually preferred intensity elicits a physiological response that falls within the stimulus zone for improvement of cardiorespiratory fitness (Dishman 1994). Investigations by Farrell et al. (1982) and Dishman, Farquhar, and Cureton (1994) involving self-selected training pace suggest that this is a reasonable expectation. In the Farrell et al. (1982) experiment, trained male runners were allowed to freely select a pace that they deemed appropriate for a 30-min exercise bout. Dishman, Farquhar, and Cureton (1994) instructed middle-aged men to select a training speed that they considered to be "comfortable." In both of these investigations, preferred training intensities elicited relative metabolic rates that ranged from 65% to 75% $\dot{V}O_2$peak. These relative exercise intensities fall within the training zone for improvement of cardiorespiratory fitness. A finding common to both investigations was that the RPE corresponding to the preferred training intensities ranged from 9 to 14 on the Borg scale. These numerical categories were generally associated with verbal scale descriptors of "very light" to "somewhat hard" and seemed compatible with the notion of a preferred exercise intensity that is subjectively tolerable over prolonged training periods.

Perceived exertion responses at preferred exercise intensities are largely independent of aerobic fitness level. Dishman, Farquhar, and Cureton (1994) instructed a group of physically active and a group of physically inactive young men to select a cycle ergometer intensity that they preferred during a 20-min training bout. RPE was similar between groups, with responses ranging from 11 to 14 (Borg scale) over the 20-min training bout. This occurred despite a 25- to 50-W greater absolute power output in the trained than in the untrained subjects. It is of note that exertional symptoms (i.e., task aversion, general fatigue, local fatigue) did not differ between groups, suggesting a contributory role of these subjective responses in the selection of preferred training intensities for prolonged, steady-state exercise. There was also a significant reduction in state anxiety traits immediately following termination of exercise in the trained group. Such mood state shifts may reinforce the subjective preference for a specific training intensity during subsequent exercise sessions. Dishman, Farquhar, and Cureton (1994) concluded that the RPE associated with preferred exercise intensities can dissociate from selected physiological mediators that typically define the relative exercise intensity during grade- or load-incremented tests or intensity-production tasks.

A final note with regard to perceptual preference during a GXT involves the type of muscular contraction required by the protocol. In general, RPE for equivalent metabolic rates is lower when the test mode involves concentric rather than eccentric muscular contractions (Henriksson, Knuttgen, and Bonde-Peterson 1972). When a choice is available, selection of a test mode that minimizes eccentric contractions appears preferable.

Medications

Symptom-limited functional aerobic power is an important and frequently used assessment in cardiac and pulmonary rehabilitation programs. In many cases, tests of functional aerobic power are administered to patients who are taking cardioactive medications. The pharmacological action of these medications can alter hemodynamic responses to graded exercise tests. When this occurs, measures such as heart rate and rate-pressure product may not be useful indices of exertional tolerance. A well-documented affect of beta-adrenergic blocking medications such as propranolol is to attenuate heart rate at a given oxygen uptake or power output (Davies and Sargeant 1979). Conversely, atropine accelerates the heart rate response during graded exercise testing (Davies and Sargeant 1979). Therefore, reliance on heart rate alone to determine test progression may result in overestimation of exercise tolerance when propranolol is used and in underestimation when atropine is used. In both cases, test progress is not accurately assessed, making it difficult to measure clinical and physiological responses at or near peak exercise, where sensitive diagnostic information is needed. On the other hand, RPE is largely independent of cardioactive medications, making it ideal to monitor test progression (Ekblom and Goldbarg 1971; Davies and Sargeant 1979; Pollock, Jackson, and Foster 1986; Squires, Rod, and Pollock 1982; Van Herwaarden et al. 1979). For example, Davies and Sargeant (1979) alternately administered practolol and atropine to healthy subjects prior to graded exercise testing. At a reference oxygen uptake of 2.0 L/min, heart rate was reduced with practolol and increased with atropine in comparison to a placebo condition. On the other hand, exertional perceptions were unaffected by either medication (fig. 10.8). Findings indicated that exertional perceptions can be used to accurately assess test progress relative to predetermined clinical or physiological end points, facilitating the timing of critical measurements.

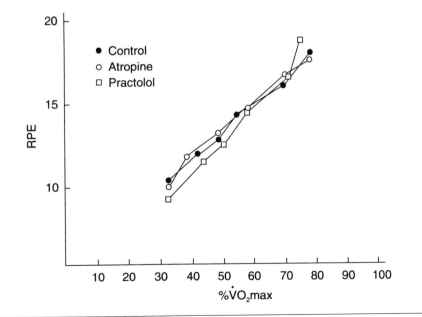

Figure 10.8   RPE in progressive exercise, plotted against %$\dot{V}O_2$max.
Reprinted from Davies and Sargeant 1979.

Methodological Factors

A number of factors involving test methods, individual characteristics, and environmental conditions can influence perceptual responses during an exercise evaluation. If these factors are not controlled, both intra- and interindividual comparisons of test responses may be difficult.

Muscle Mass

Selection of a test mode is often influenced by clinical characteristics of the individual to be evaluated or by the type of ergometer available. The volume of active muscle mass varies with the test mode, generally being lowest for arm exercise and highest for combined arm and leg exercise. At a given submaximal oxygen uptake or power output, RPE is higher for those test modes requiring smaller rather than larger muscle mass (Sargeant and Davies 1977; Sargeant and Davies 1973; Skinner et al. 1973). This occurs because the smaller the muscle mass required during testing, the lower is the $\dot{V}O_2max$ for that particular mode. Therefore, the reference oxygen uptake (i.e., L/min) represents a higher relative metabolic rate (%$\dot{V}O_2max$) for the test mode requiring the smaller muscle mass than for that requiring the larger muscle mass. The intensity of the perceptual signal is linked to the relative metabolic rate. It follows that the perceptual signal will be most intense for test modes that require the highest relative metabolic stress per area of active muscle tissue.

Comparisons of submaximal perceptual responses between modes requiring different levels of muscle mass may not be appropriate when the absolute oxygen uptake (L/min) is used as a physiological reference. An alternative procedure to compare perceptual responses among different test modes is to employ the relative oxygen uptake (i.e., %$\dot{V}O_2max$) as the physiological reference. Under these conditions, RPE does not vary between modes that require different amounts of active muscle mass. This concept is demonstrated in figure 10.9. RPE at a fixed oxygen uptake was highest during single-arm testing and lowest during two-leg testing. However, when comparisons were made at a given %$\dot{V}O_2max$, RPE was the same among all four tests. The effect of the volume of active muscle mass on the relative metabolic rate accounted for these perceptual responses.

Age, Gender, Menstrual Cycle

A number of individual characteristics can affect perceptual responses during exercise testing. The following are a few examples. When men and women of a similar age are evaluated using either a treadmill or cycle ergometer protocol, RPE does not differ between genders (Borg and Linderholm 1970; Noble et al. 1981). This occurs when comparisons are made at a relative (%$\dot{V}O_2max$) as opposed to an absolute physiological reference point. In contrast, Henriksson, Knuttgen, and Bonde-Peterson (1972) noted that females rated the intensity of

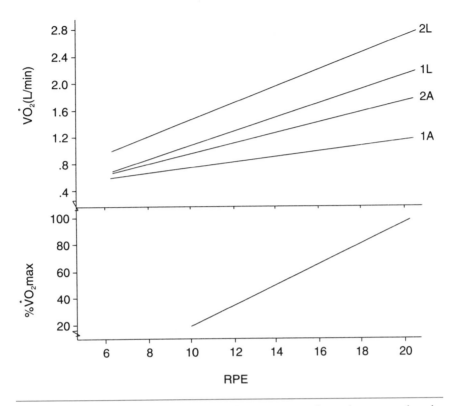

Figure 10.9   Effect of exercise involving different amounts of muscle mass on the relationship between ratings of perceived exertion (RPE) and oxygen uptake ($\dot{V}O_2$). 1L = one leg; 2L = two legs; 1A = one arm; 2A = two arms.

perceived exertion greater than males during both concentric and eccentric exercise when comparisons were made at a fixed $\dot{V}O_2$. This gender difference in perceptual response may reflect a higher maximal aerobic power for the male than for the female subjects. The absolute physiological reference therefore represented a comparatively higher relative metabolic rate for the females, causing RPE to be higher.

The chronological age of the individual appears to have varying effects on perceptual responsiveness. Bar-Or (1977) observed that when comparisons are made at a given exercise heart rate, RPE is generally lower for younger (10-12 yr) than for older (31-68 yr) individuals. However, when factors such as level of aerobic fitness and daily physical activity are controlled, age differences in perceptual responsiveness during testing may not be present (Hughes et al. 1984). One additional note regarding the possible differential influence of age on test responses involves the RPE–HR ratio. The original notion that exercise heart rate could be determined by multiplying RPE by 10 may be valid for middle-aged and older individuals. The ratio is not accurate for children, adolescents, or young adults, being somewhat higher than $10 \times$ RPE in these age groups (Bar-Or 1977).

Finally, normal menstrual function has no differential effect on RPE during cycle ergometer exercise testing (Stephenson, Kolka, and Wilderson 1982).

Testing Conditions

Sleep deprivation can affect perceptual responses to a GXT. In general, as sleep loss progresses, the intensity of exertional perceptions increases commensurately (Faria and Drummond 1982; Martin and Gaddis 1981). The effect of sleep loss on GXT performance and RPE appears to follow a diurnal pattern. Faria and Drummond (1982) found that while oxygen uptake remained constant during intermittent exercise testing over a 24-h period, RPE was highest between 2:00 A.M. and 4:00 A.M. It is speculated that sleep loss lowers alertness and contributes to poor cognitive adaptation. The resulting low level of neuronal excitation causes a communicative dissociation between active skeletal muscle and cognitive function.

Control of ambient temperature in the testing area is essential if physiological, clinical, and perceptual measures are to be compared to normative data. At a given submaximal power output or test stage, RPE will increase as ambient temperature increases relative to thermoneutral conditions (Pollock, Wilmore, and Fox 1984). In this regard, it is particularly important that serial testing to determine clinical or training progress be undertaken at the same ambient temperature throughout the period of assessment, preferably under thermoneutral conditions (i.e., 24°-27° C).

Protocol Type–Exercise Mode Differential Effect

When RPE is used as a dependent variable during an exercise evaluation, the interaction between test protocol and exercise mode may have a differential effect on responses. During treadmill exercise, RPE as well as $\dot{V}O_2$, $\dot{V}_E$, HR, and lactic acid are higher for intermittent than for continuous protocols when the same total work is performed under both conditions (Edwards et al. 1972). In contrast, when a test is performed on a combined arm and leg ergometer, RPE does not differ between intermittent and continuous exercise. This result holds when 25% or less of the total power output is distributed to the arms (Gutin, Ang, and Torrey 1988). Recognizing the potential for differential perceptual responsiveness is important when comparing test results that employ varying exercise modes and protocols.

Ventilatory Threshold

Identification of the ventilatory threshold and its corresponding RPE value during a GXT provides useful information for the prescription of exercise intensity. In fact, many computerized respiratory-metabolic systems can be programmed to automatically identify the ventilatory threshold. Normally, the ventilatory threshold varies between 40% and 80% $\dot{V}O_2$max, depending on training status, limb involvement, aerobic fitness, and exercise mode. However, RPE at the ventilatory threshold is relatively constant (12-14 Borg scale) for both trained and untrained men and women (DeMello et al. 1987). The comparatively stable perceptual response at the ventilatory threshold provides a reference point upon which to prescribe exercise intensity. The reader is referred to chapter 11 on exercise prescription for a more detailed explanation of this procedure.

Clinical Diagnosis

Perceptual Discriminate Function Analysis

Clinical diagnosis can often be facilitated by determining both physiological and psychological responses to an exercise challenge. The objective of the diagnosis is to *discriminate* between normal and pathological responses during the exercise test. Diagnostic discriminate function analysis uses normal responses to an exercise challenge as a clinical reference. Perceptual responsiveness during a graded exercise test has proven to be a useful diagnostic criterion for discriminate function analysis of coronary artery disease (Gutmann et al. 1981; Borg and Linderholm 1970; Pollock, Jackson, and Foster 1986), chronic obstructive pulmonary disease (Linderholm 1986; Silverman et al. 1988), psychiatric disorders (Borg and Linderholm 1970), neuromuscular dysfunction (Bar-Or and Reed 1986), and selected atherogenic risk factors (Hughes et al. 1984). The use of exertional perceptions in clinical discriminate function analysis was first undertaken by Borg and Linderholm (1970), who collaboratively developed a diagnostic classification of disease severity for coronary and pulmonary patients. They reasoned that when there is a clinical or physiological discrimination between pathological and normal responses to a GXT, there is a corresponding perceptual discrimination. Therefore, perceptual responses during exercise testing differentially classify the severity of disease for such clinical subsets as coronary and pulmonary patients.

Several examples may elucidate the power of perceptual responsiveness for diagnostic discrimination during a graded exercise test. Clinical diagnosis of coronary atherosclerosis and subsequent classification of disease severity can be facilitated by comparing RPE at a fixed submaximal power output or oxygen uptake between normal individuals and patients with various degrees of pathology (Gutmann et al. 1981; Borg and Linderholm 1970; Pollock, Jackson, and Foster 1986; Hughes et al. 1984; Tukulin, Zamlic, and Pegan 1972). The more severe the disease, the higher the RPE will be at the test reference point when comparisons are made to clinically normal individuals. This occurs because functional aerobic power typically declines as disease severity progresses. The reference $\dot{V}O_2$ or power output therefore represents a comparatively higher relative metabolic rate for the patient with advanced disease. Because the exertional signal is linked to the relative metabolic rate, RPE increases commensurately with the progression of disease severity. Therefore, RPE during a GXT reflects patient status and can be used in conjunction with physiological and clinical responses to discriminate between various degrees of disease severity.

A similar diagnostic procedure can be used to classify the comparative severity of pulmonary disease, particularly when the perceptual rating is differentially linked to respiratory function (Linderholm 1986; Silverman et al. 1988). In this example, RPE is used as the independent test variable, while selected measures of respiratory function serve as the dependent variables. As shown in figure 10.10, at a given reference RPE, respiratory rate was approximately 5 breaths/min higher in pulmonary patients than in clinically normal individuals (Linderholm 1986). The foregoing example employed the undifferentiated RPE for the overall body. However, the sensitivity of pulmonary exercise testing can be further enhanced if perceptual signals are specifically differentiated to the chest. Such differentiated RPEs are directly linked to respiratory-metabolic function during dynamic exercise (Robertson 1982) and are diagnostically reproducible during repeated exercise tests (Silverman et al. 1988).

Mahler and Horowitz (1994) described the use of the Borg CR-10 scale to develop a severity index of chronic obstructive pulmonary disease (COPD) based

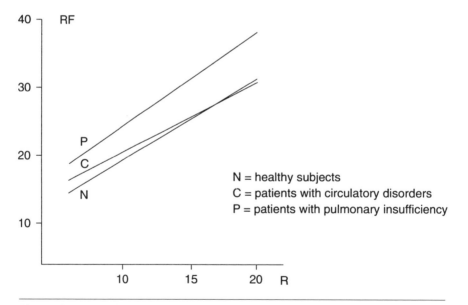

Figure 10.10 Respiratory frequency (RF) in relation to rating of perceived exertion (R) in the normal (N), circulatory disorder (C), and pulmonary insufficiency (P) groups, represented by linear regression lines.
Reprinted from Linderholm 1986.

on the ratio of power output to ratings of dyspnea. Patients with severe COPD (FEV_1 < 50% predicted) estimated dyspnea to be more intense than patients with mild or moderate COPD (FEV_1 > 50% predicted) when comparisons were made for a given submaximal power output during a load-incremented cycle ergometer protocol. It was concluded that the power output–dyspnea ratio determined during a cycle ergometer test is a sensitive measure to discriminate between patients presenting COPD of varying severity.

Perceptual discriminate function analysis is also an effective diagnostic procedure when evaluating the severity of psychiatric disorders and progressive neuromuscular spasticity (Borg 1978; Bar-Or and Reed 1986). The more severe the pathology, the more intense is the perceptual signal when comparisons are made between patient and normal groups at a fixed physiological reference point. The comparatively more intense perceptual signals in these patient groups may be due in part to a lower functional aerobic power secondary to chronic disability. The underlying psychophysical mechanisms for this response are the same as those previously described for coronary and pulmonary patients. However, while a low functional aerobic power may characterize many individuals in these clinical subsets, other factors having both psychological and biomechanical origins are likely also important determinants of the comparatively more intense perceptual responsiveness observed in psychiatric and neuromuscular patients during testing.

Differentiated Anginal Scaling

Category scaling of the pain and discomfort symptomatic of angina pectoris yields ratings that increase as a positively accelerating function of exercise intensity for most test modalities (Karlsson et al. 1984; Borg, Holmgren, and Lindblad 1981; Aström 1986). The intensity of anginal pain can be quantified using the same category scale format as employed in measuring the intensity of exertional perceptions (Borg, Holmgren, and Lindblad 1981). The advantage of this procedure is that the patient uses a single scale format during testing to estimate the intensity of two different perceptual domains, that is, anginal pain and physical effort. Measurement is then simplified, making it possible to scale both anginal symptoms and perceptions of exertion at the same time points throughout the GXT. Provided clear and unequivocal scaling instructions are presented prior to the GXT, patients are able to reliably distinguish between and differentially rate the intensity of anginal pain and perceived exertion (Borg, Holmgren, and Lindblad 1981; Maresh and Noble 1984; Aström 1986).

The use of a standardized category scale to measure the intensity of anginal pain during a GXT serves two interrelated diagnostic functions. First, ratings of anginal pain at a fixed submaximal power output discriminate between individuals who differ in symptom-limited functional aerobic power. As an example, Borg, Holmgren, and Lindblad (1981) used a specially modified, nine-category RPE scale to measure the intensity of anginal pain. Three groups of angina pectoris patients varying in severity of coronary atherosclerosis were evaluated during

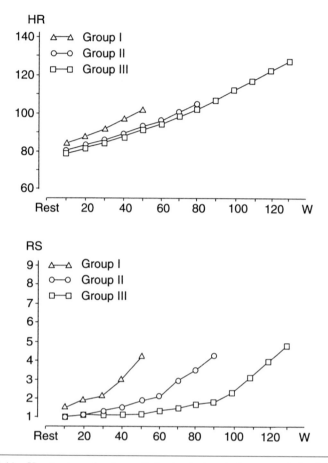

Figure 10.11   Heart rate and ratings of chest pain in relation to work load. Groups: I—low, II—moderate, III—high functional aerobic power.
Reprinted from Borg, Holmgren, and Lindblad 1980.

a cycle ergometer GXT. Figure 10.11 (Borg, Holmgren, and Lindblad 1980) demonstrates that at a given power output, anginal pain was greatest for patients with the lowest as compared to the highest symptom-limited functional aerobic power. Ratings of chest pain discriminated between patients who varied in symptom-limited functional aerobic power. These variations likely reflected differences in the severity of underlying coronary atherosclerosis.

Second, when a predetermined anginal rating is employed as a test termination criterion, it is possible to discriminate between patients of varying disease severity and symptom-limited exercise tolerance. Normally, it is recommended that a test of functional exercise tolerance be terminated at an anginal rating of six on a nine-point scale. Using this termination criterion, patients with the least advanced disease will have the highest symptom-limited functional aerobic power, with

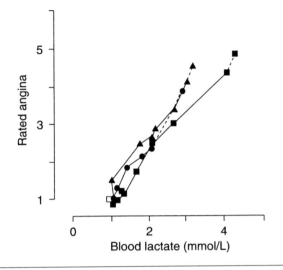

Figure 10.12   Mean rated anginal pain versus blood lactate concentration at rest and during exercise: ❑ = supine rest; ● = low functional aerobic power; ▲ = moderate functional aerobic power; ■ = high functional aerobic power.
Reprinted from Karlsson et al. 1984.

the reciprocal holding for patients with the most advanced disease (Borg, Holmgren, and Lindblad 1981). A uniform test termination criterion based on a standardized rating of anginal pain facilitates both intra- and interindividual comparison of symptom-limited functional exercise tolerance.

A methodological note regarding the use of category scales to measure the intensity of exercise-induced angina pectoris is offered at this juncture. Karlsson et al. (1984) propose that blood lactic acid concentration provides a better physiological reference point than the absolute level of oxygen uptake when making interindividual comparisons of anginal pain. The principal assumption underlying this procedure is that lactic acid concentration is a generalized marker of the relative metabolic rate during most modes of dynamic exercise. When anginal ratings are plotted against lactic acid concentration, responses do not differ between clinical subsets in spite of large variations in symptom-limited functional aerobic power (fig. 10.12) This facilitates comparisons between the intensity of anginal pain and the intensity of exertional perceptions at a given time point in an exercise test.

Summary

This chapter considered the role of RPE in exercise testing for functionally normal and clinically impaired children and adults. The exercise test has four components: format, end point, mode, and protocol. Each of these components is selected with respect to the clinical, research, or sport setting within which the test is used to assess exercise tolerance.

Exercise tests involving RPE are used to assess both aerobic and anaerobic metabolic function. During exercise testing, RPE is used either as an independent or dependent variable. That is, a predetermined RPE can serve as a criterion measure to determine changes in power output subsequent to exercise training. In this case, RPE is an independent variable. For example, the perceptually modified Sjostrand submaximal cycle ergometer protocol identifies the power output equivalent to a criterion RPE of 15 on the Borg scale. An increase in the power output equivalent to RPE-15 from pre- to postexercise training indicates an improvement in functional aerobic power. Similar conclusions can be drawn from the run test when locomotor speed at a criterion RPE-15 is determined pre- and posttraining. Conversely, when RPE is measured at a fixed power output during exercise testing, it becomes a dependent variable. In this case, a lower RPE at a criterion power output following a training program indicates that aerobic fitness has improved.

Other types of exercise tests that use RPE as a criterion measure include the maximum work test and the flexible work test. In the former, the maximum power output that can be sustained for 30 s at an RPE of 20 is taken as a measure of anaerobic power. In the latter test, the power output at each exercise stage is subjectively determined according to a perceptual feedback system. The measure of exercise tolerance is taken as the highest power output that can be sustained for 4 min.

Also discussed were a number of special methodological factors that should be considered when perceptually based tests are used to assess exertional tolerance in both normal and clinical populations. As an example, test intensity (e.g., walking speed or pedal frequency), format, and mode should be selected in accordance with the subject's perceptual preference. The presence of cardioactive medications should also be considered during a GXT. These medications have comparatively little effect on perceptual responses to a GXT but can have a marked effect on physiological responses. In this context RPE is often a better indicator of the point within the metabolic range to which the test has progressed and of the time remaining until test termination than are more traditional measures such as heart rate and oxygen uptake. Muscle mass, age, gender, exercise mode, and the ventilatory threshold all exert a systematic influence on RPE during exercise testing. An attempt should be made to standardize test conditions in order to control for the possible influence of these factors on perceptual responses.

Finally, consideration was given to the use of RPE as a diagnostic tool in discriminating between clinically normal and pathological responses to a GXT. Diagnostic discriminate function analysis uses normal perceptual responses to an exercise challenge as a clinical reference in determining disease severity. Category scaling of the pain and discomfort symptomatic of exercise-induced angina pectoris is an extension of this diagnostic procedure.

References

American College of Sports Medicine. 1991. *Guidelines for exercise testing and prescription.* 4th ed. Philadelphia: Lea and Febiger.

Åström, H. 1986. Rating perceived symptoms during exercise in heart disease. In *The perception of exertion in physical work,* ed. G. Borg and D. Ottoson, 199-206. London: Macmillan.

Bar-Or, O. 1977. Age related changes in exercise perception. In *Physical work and effort,* ed. G. Borg, 255-66. New York: Pergamon Press.

Bar-Or, O., and S.L. Reed. 1986. Ratings of perceived exertion in adolescents with neuromuscular disease. In *The perception of exertion in physical work,* ed. G. Borg and D. Ottoson, 137-48. London: Macmillan.

Borg, G. 1962. Physical performance and perceived exertion. In *Studia psychologia et paedagogica,* vol. 11, 1-35. Lund, Sweden: Gleerup.

———. 1970. Perceived exertion as an indicator of somatic stress. *Scand. J. Rehab. Med.* 2:92-98.

———. 1971. The perception of physical performance. In *Frontiers of fitness,* ed. R.J. Shepard, 280-94. Springfield, IL: Charles C Thomas.

———. 1978. Subjective effort in relation to physical performance and working capacity. In *Psychology: From research to practice,* ed. H.L. Pick, 333-61. New York: Plenum Press.

———. 1982. Ratings of perceived exertion and heart rates during short-term cycle exercise and their use in a cycling strength test. *Int. J. Sports Med.* 3:153-58.

———. 1984. *Some characteristics of a simple run test and its correlation with a bicycle ergometer test of physical work capacity.* Reports from the Institute of Applied Psychology, no. 625. Stockholm: Univ. of Stockholm.

Borg, G., B. Edgren, and G. Marklund. 1970. *A flexible work test with a feedback system guiding the test course.* Reports from the Institute of Applied Psychology, no. 8. Stockholm: Univ. of Stockholm.

Borg, G., C. Edstrom, and G. Marklund. 1970. *A new method to determine the exponent for perceived force in physical work.* Reports from the Institute of Applied Psychology, no. 4. Stockholm: Univ. of Stockholm.

Borg, G., A. Holmgren, and I. Lindblad. 1980. *Perception of chest pain during physical work in a group of patients with angina pectoris.* Reports from the Institute of Applied Psychology, no. 81. Stockholm: Univ. of Stockholm.

Borg, G., A. Holmgren, and I. Lindblad. 1981. Quantitative evaluation of chest pain. *Acta Med. Scand.* 644 (Suppl.): 43-45.

Borg, G., and H. Linderholm. 1970. Exercise performance and perceived exertion in patients with coronary insufficiency, arterial hypertension and vasoregulatory asthenia. *Acta Med. Scand.* 187:17-26.

Borg, G., and M. Ohlsson. 1975. *A study of two variants of a simple run-test for determining physical working capacity.* Reports from the Institute of Applied Psychology, no. 61. Stockholm: Univ. of Stockholm.

Coast, J.R., R.H. Cox, and H.G. Welch. 1986. Optimal pedalling rate in prolonged bouts of cycle ergometry. *Med. Sci. Sports Exerc.* 18:225-30.

Davies, C.T., and A.J. Sargeant. 1979. The effects of atropine and practolol on the perception of exertion during treadmill exercise. *Ergonomics* 22:1141-46.

DeMello, J.J., K.J. Cureton, R.E. Boineau, and M.M. Singh. 1987. Ratings of perceived exertion at the lactate threshold in trained and untrained men and women. *Med. Sci. Sports Exerc.* 19:354-62.

deVries, H.A. 1986. *Physiology of exercise.* Dubuque, IA: Brown.

Dishman, R.K. 1994. Prescribing exercise intensity for healthy adults using perceived exertion. *Med. Sci. Sports Exerc.* 26:9; 1087-94.

Dishman, R.K., R.P. Farquhar, and K.J. Cureton. 1994. Responses to preferred intensities of exertion in men differing in activity levels. *Med. Sci. Sports Exerc.* 26:783-90.

Edgren, B., and G. Borg. 1975. *The reliability and stability of the indicators in a simple run test.* Reports from the Institute of Applied Psychology, no. 57. Stockholm: Univ. of Stockholm.

Edgren, B., G. Marklund, O. Norderjo, and G. Borg. 1976. The validity of four bicycle ergometer tests. *Med. Sci. Sports Exerc.* 8:179-85.

Edwards, R.H.T., A. Melcher, C.M. Hesser, O. Wigebtz, and L.G. Ekelund. 1972. Physiological correlates of perceived exertion in continuous and intermittent exercise with the same average power output. *Eur. J. Clin. Invest.* 2:108-14.

Ekblom, B., and A.N. Goldbarg. 1971. The influence of physical training and other factors on the subjective rating of perceived exertion. *Acta Physiol. Scand.* 83:399-406.

Ekelund, L.G., J.A. Blumenthal, M.C. Morey, and C.C. Ekelund. 1986. The effect of nonselective and selective betablockade on perceived exertion during treadmill exercise in mild hypertensive type A and B males and the interaction with aerobic training. In *The perception of exertion in physical work,* ed. G. Borg and D. Ottoson, 191-98. London: Macmillan.

Faria, I.E., and B.J. Drummond. 1982. Circadian changes in resting heart rate and body temperature, maximal oxygen consumption and perceived exertion. *Ergonomics* 25:381-86.

Farrell, P.A., W.K. Gates, M.G. Maksud, and W.P. Morgan. 1982. Increases in plasma β-endorphin/β-lipotropin immunoreactivity after treadmill running in humans. *J. Appl. Physiol. Respir. Environ. Exerc. Physiol.* 52:1245-49.

Gamberale, F. 1972. Perception of exertion, heart rate, oxygen uptake and blood lactate in different work operations. *Ergonomics* 15:545-54.

Gutin, B., K.E. Ang, and K. Torrey. 1988. Cardiorespiratory and subjective responses to incremental and constant load ergometry with arms and legs. *Arch. Phys. Med. Rehab.* 69:510-13.

Gutmann, M.C., R.W. Squires, M.L. Pollock, C. Foster, and J. Anholm. 1981. Perceived exertion–heart rate relationship during exercise testing and training in cardiac patients. *J. Cardiac Rehab.* 1:52-59.

Henriksson, J., H.G. Knuttgen, and F. Bonde-Peterson. 1972. Perceived exertion during exercise with concentric and eccentric muscle contractions. *Ergonomics* 15:537-44.

Hill, D.W., K.J. Cureton, S.C. Grisham, and M.A. Collins. 1987. Effect of training on the rating of perceived exertion at the ventilatory threshold. *Eur. J. Appl. Physiol.* 56:206-11.

Hughes, J.R., R.S. Crow, D.R. Jacobs, Jr., M.B. Mittelmark, and A.S. Leon. 1984. Physical activity, smoking, and exercise-induced fatigue. *J. Behav. Med.* 7:217-30.

Kamon, E., K. Pandolf, and E. Cafarelli. 1974. The relationship between perceptual information and physiological responses to exercise in the heat. *J. Human Ergol.* 3:45-54.

Karlsson, J., H. Aström, A. Holmgren, C. Kaijer, and E. Orinius. 1984. Angina pectoris and blood lactate concentration during graded exercise. *Int. J. Sports Med.* 5:348-51.

Knuttgen, H.G., L.D. Nordesjo, B. Ollander, and B. Saltin. 1973. Physical conditioning through interval training with young male adults. *Med. Sci. Sports* 5:220-26.

Lewis, S., P. Thompson, N.H. Areskog, P. Vodak, M. Marconyak, R. DeBusk, S. Mellen, and W. Haskell. 1980. Transfer effects of endurance training to exercise with untrained limbs. *Eur. J. Appl. Physiol.* 44:25-34.

Linderholm, H. 1986. Perceived exertion during exercise in the discrimination between circulatory and pulmonary disorders. In *Perception of exertion in physical work,* ed. G. Borg and D. Ottoson, 199-206. London: Macmillan.

Mahler, D.A., and M.B. Horowitz. 1994. Perception of breathlessness during exercise in patients with respiratory disease. *Med. Sci. Sports Exerc.* 26:9; 1078-81.

Maresh, C.M., and B.J. Noble. 1984. Utilization of perceived exertion ratings during exercise testing and training. In *Cardiac rehabilitation: Exercise testing and prescription,* ed. L.K. Hall, 155-73. New York: Spectrum Books.

Martin, B.J., and G.M. Gaddis. 1981. Exercise after sleep deprivation. *Med. Sci. Sports Exerc.* 13:220-23.

McConnell, T.R., and B.A. Clark. 1988. Treadmill protocols for determination of maximum oxygen uptake in runners. *Br. J. Sports Med.* 22:3-5.

Michael, E.D., and L. Eckard. 1972. The selection of hard work by trained and non-trained subjects. *Med. Sci. Sports* 4:107-10.

Mitchell, J.H., B.J. Sproule, and C.B. Chapman. 1958. The physiological meaning of the maximal oxygen intake test. *J. Clin. Invest.* 37:538-47.

Moffatt, R.J., and B.A. Stamford. 1978. Effects of pedalling rate changes on maximal oxygen uptake and perceived effort during bicycle ergometer work. *Med. Sci. Sports* 10:27-31.

Morgan, W.P., and G.A. Borg. 1980. Perception of effort in the prescription of physical activity. In *Mental health and emotional aspects of sports,* ed. T. Craig. Chicago: American Medical Association.

Noble, B.J. 1973. Perceived exertion during walking and running—II. *Med. Sci. Sports* 5 (2): 116-20.

———. 1982. Clinical applications of perceived exertion. *Med. Sci. Sports Exerc.* 14:406-11.

———. 1986. *Physiology of exercise and sport.* St. Louis: Times Mirror/ Mosby College.

Noble, B.J., C.M. Maresh, and M. Ritchey. 1981. Comparison of exercise sensations between males and females. In: *Women and Sport,* J. Borms, M. Hebbelinck, and A. Venerando (Eds). Basel: S. Karger. 175-179.

Noble, B.J., K.F. Metz, K.B. Pandolf, and E. Cafarelli. 1973. Perceptual responses to exercise: A multiple regression study. *Med. Sci. Sports* 5:104-9.

Pandolf, K.B., R.L. Burse, and R.F. Goldman. 1975. Differentiated ratings of perceived exertion during physical conditioning of older individuals using leg-weight loading. *Percept. Motor Skills* 40:563-74.

Pandolf, K.B., and B.J. Noble. 1973. The effect of pedalling speed and resistance changes on perceived exertion for equivalent power outputs on the bicycle ergometer. *Med. Sci. Sports* 5:132-36.

Pollock, M.L., A.S. Jackson, and C. Foster. 1986. The use of the perception scale for exercise prescription. In *The perception of exertion in physical work,* ed. G. Borg and D. Ottoson, 161-78. London: Macmillan.

Pollock, M.L., J.H. Wilmore, and S.M. Fox. 1984. *Exercise in health and disease: Evaluation and prescription for prevention and rehabilitation.* Philadelphia: Saunders.

Robertson, R.J. 1982. Central signals of perceived exertion during dynamic exercise. *Med. Sci. Sports Exerc.* 14:390-96.

Robertson, R.J., F.L. Goss, and K.F. Metz. Ratings of perceived exertion (RPE) in cardiac rehabilitation: application and validation. In: Proceedings of the Vth World Congress on Cardiac Rehabilitation. J.P. Broustet (ed.) Intercept Limited, Andover, Hampshire, England. p151-159.

Robertson, R.J., R.L. Gillespie, J. McCarthy, and K.D. Rose. 1979. Differentiated perceptions of exertion: Part II. Relationship to local and central physiological responses. *Percept. Motor Skills* 49:691-97.

Sargeant, A.J., and C.T. Davies. 1973. Perceived exertion during rhythmic exercise involving different muscle masses. *J. Human Ergol.* 2:3-11.

———. 1977. Perceived exertion of dynamic exercise in normal subjects and patients following leg injury. In *Physical work and effort,* ed. G. Borg, 345-56. New York: Pergamon Press.

Sidney, K.H., and R.J. Shephard. 1972. Perception of exercise in the elderly, effects of aging, mode of exercise, and physical training. *Percept. Motor Skills* 44:999-1000.

Silverman, M., J. Barry, H. Hellerstein, J. Janos, and S. Kelsen. 1988. Variability of the perceived sense of effort in breathing during exercise in patients with chronic obstructive pulmonary disease. *Am. Rev. Respir. Dis.* 137:206-9.

Sjostrand, T. 1947. Changes in the respiratory organs of workmen at an ore smelting works. *Acta Med. Scand.* 196 (Suppl.): 687-99.

Skinner, J.S., G. Borg, and E.R. Buskirk. 1969. Physiological and perceptual reactions to exertion of young men differing in activity and body size. In *Exercise and fitness,* ed. B.D. Franks, 53-66. Chicago: Athletic Institute.

Skinner, J.S., R. Hustler, V. Bersteinova, and E.R. Buskirk. 1973. Perception of effort during different types of exercise and under different environmental conditions. *Med. Sci. Sports* 5:110-55.

Smutok, M.A., G.S. Skrinar, and K.B. Pandolf. 1980. Exercise intensity: Subjective regulation by perceived exertion. *Arch. Phys. Med. Rehab.* 61:569-74.

Squires, R.W., J.L. Rod, and M.L. Pollock. 1982. Effects of propranolol on perceived exertion soon after myocardial revascularization surgery. *Med. Sci. Sports Exerc.* 14:276-80.

Stamford, B.A. 1976. Validity and reliability of subjective ratings of perceived exertion during work. *Ergonomics* 19:53-60.

Stamford, B.A., and B.J. Noble. 1974. Metabolic cost and perception of effort during bicycle ergometer work performance. *Med. Sci. Sports* 6:226-31.

Stephenson, L.A., M.A. Kolka, and J.E. Wilderson. 1982. Perceived exertion and anaerobic threshold during the menstrual cycle. *Med. Sci. Sports Exerc.* 14:218-22.

Taylor, H., E. Buskirk, and A. Henchel. 1955. Maximal oxygen intake as an objective measure of cardiorespiratory performance. *J. Appl. Physiol.* 8:73-80.

Tukulin, K., B. Zamlic, and U. Pegan. 1972. Exercise performance and perceived exertion in patients after myocardial infarction. In *Physical work and effort,* ed. G. Borg, 357-66. New York: Pergamon Press.

Van Den Burg, M., and R. Ceci. 1986. A comparison of a psychophysical estimation and a production method in a laboratory and a field condition. In *Perception of exertion in physical work,* ed. G. Borg and D. Ottoson, 35-46. London: Macmillan.

Van Herwaarden, C.L., R.A. Binkhorst, J.F. Fennis, and A. Van 'T Laar. 1979. Effects of propranolol and metroprolol on haemodynamic and respiratory indices and on perceived exertion during exercise in hypertensive patients. *Br. Heart J.* 41:99-105.

11

CHAPTER

The Role of RPE in Exercise Prescription

Exercise training in athletic, recreational, and therapeutic settings should follow a carefully developed and individualized prescription if optimal performance benefits are to be realized. An individually prescribed exercise program provides a training stimulus that is physiologically effective and clinically safe (Fardy, Yanowitz, and Wilson 1988). The principal components of an exercise prescription are

1. intensity,
2. duration,
3. frequency,
4. progression, and
5. activity mode (American College of Sports Medicine 1991).

Of these five components, the prescription of exercise intensity requires the most precision, relying heavily on periodic monitoring of perceptual, physiological, and clinical responses to ensure that the target training zone is attained and maintained. Therefore, this chapter focuses on those factors that are fundamental to the prescription and regulation of exercise *intensity* for the healthy individual as well as for the coronary heart disease (CHD) patient. The reader is referred to the American College of Sports Medicine's *Guidelines for Exercise Testing and Prescription* (1991) for a more thorough discussion of the remaining four components of the prescription process.

The prescription of exercise intensity is based on physiological [i.e., oxygen uptake ($\dot{V}O_2$), heart rate (HR), ventilation ($\dot{V}_E$)], clinical (e.g., ECG abnormalities, anginal pain, and blood pressure abnormalities), and perceptual (i.e., RPE) responses to a graded exercise test (GXT). Because these responses are functionally related, RPE can be used for both the *prescription* and *regulation* of exercise intensity. A perceptually regulated exercise prescription assumes that a predetermined aerobic metabolic rate can be attained and maintained by using a target

RPE in a manner analogous to a target HR (Robertson et al. 1990). This prescriptive process is attractive for sport, clinical, and recreational applications because it (1) uses simple and inexpensive instrumentation, (2) requires comparatively little perceptual scaling expertise so that a minimum of instruction is needed, and (3) may be generalized over a wide range of activity modes.

As an example, runners and swimmers often prescribe and regulate the pace (i.e., intensity) of their training or competitive performances using perceptions of physical exertion (Ulmer 1986). At the outset of a race, the athlete and coach jointly develop a tactical arrangement that sets the pace for a winning performance. During the race, perceptions of fatigue and discomfort arising from peripheral skeletal muscle and respiratory-metabolic processes necessitate that tactics and hence pace be modified. This perceptual feedback system allows the competitor to adjust the race pace around a physiological set point whose associated limits are consistent with an optimal performance.

Perceptual regulation of exercise intensity is also applicable in settings other than highly structured athletic training programs. In fact, we use perceptual feedback to regulate the pace of many daily physical activities, often doing so without conscious awareness. The intensity of home, recreational, and even some occupational activities is often self-regulated using exertional perceptions that reflect local and general fatigue, thermal stress, and dyspnea. In most cases, the pace with which these activities is undertaken allows their successful completion without undue physiological strain. This happens even though many of the perceptual signals used to regulate the intensity of the activity occur on a subconscious level of sensory processing and as such are not cognitively evaluated.

The prescription of exercise intensity using exertional perceptions may also have a favorable impact on adherence to training and rehabilitation programs (Dishman 1982). An exercise prescription that exceeds the subjective tolerance for physiological stress may contribute to poor program adherence, especially among new exercise participants or those undergoing cardiovascular rehabilitation. Because a perceptually regulated prescription reflects a "behavioral training dosage," program adherence is optimized (Dishman 1982). The objective of a behaviorally derived exercise prescription is to establish a balance between the ideal physiological dosage and a manageable perceptual dosage. The outcome is to match perceived stress with actual physiological stress so that the exercise task is judged manageable, making the training or rehabilitation process more enjoyable. From a behavioral standpoint, the more enjoyable the exercise experience, the better is the adherence to the prescribed training or therapeutic regime.

Components of the Exercise Prescription

An important prerequisite to undertaking an aerobic exercise program is the development of an individualized exercise prescription. As noted earlier, the exercise prescription has five components: intensity, duration, frequency, progression, and mode. Following is a summary of how these components are organized to form the training dosage (Pollock, Wilmore, and Fox 1984). The *intensity* of an aerobic exercise program is initially set at 50% to 70% of either the heart rate range (HRR) or maximal oxygen uptake ($\dot{V}O_2$max). As physiological adaptation takes place, the intensity progresses between 70% and 85% of the HRR or $\dot{V}O_2$max. This progression usually takes place over the first 6 to 10 weeks of training. The *duration* of a single exercise session should be 10 to 12 min during the initial phase of training and should progress to 20 to 60 min as cardiovascular fitness improves. During the initial phase of training, the *frequency* of exercise should be three times per week, preferably with sessions separated from 24 to 48 h. Over time, training frequency can progress to five or even seven days per week. However, it should be remembered that the incidence of exercise-related injuries increases substantially when the frequency of training moves from three to seven days per week (Pollock et al. 1977). Exercise *modes* that promote cardiovascular fitness involve dynamic, rhythmical contractions of large muscle groups and are often called aerobic activities. Walking, running, cycling, swimming, and rowing are examples of aerobic activities that promote cardiovascular fitness. Aerobic games and aerobic dancing can be included in the exercise prescription after an initial orientation period. Ideally, the mode of exercise training should not only improve cardiovascular fitness but should also be an enjoyable activity. In addition, cardiac rehabilitation programs should only employ exercise modes that allow accurate quantification of intensity and are easily supervised. The *progression* of exercise dosage for aerobic training was previously presented within the context of each prescription component.

Prescription of Exercise Intensity

Prescribing exercise intensity is a complex and precise process. Two separate approaches are commonly used. In the first, the exercise stimulus (i.e., training pace) is varied to attain a prescribed physiological response. The second approach prescribes a fixed exercise stimulus, which elicits a variable physiological response. This latter approach is not effective under exercise conditions where the terrain is uneven or where climatic conditions markedly alter weather and ambient temperature. In addition, prescribing exercise according to a fixed pace may be unsafe for cardiac rehabilitation in which a desired clinical outcome (e.g., ST depression < 0.5 mm) is linked to a predetermined physiological response. Therefore, each of the prescription methods described allows the training pace to vary in order to produce a predetermined physiological or clinical response.

The prescription of exercise intensity assumes that a predetermined level of oxygen uptake ($\dot{V}O_2$) is achieved during the stimulus portion of each training session. This $\dot{V}O_2$ should fall within the target training zone for cardiorespiratory fitness. There are three prescriptive methods that are consistent with this assumption. These methods are termed metabolic, heart rate, and RPE (Pollock, Wilmore, and Fox 1984).

Metabolic Method

The metabolic method of prescribing exercise intensity identifies a training pace that is equivalent to 50% to 85% of $\dot{V}O_2$max or peak METs (METSpeak). In this method, maximal levels of $\dot{V}O_2$ or METs are determined during a GXT. The prescribed percentage of $\dot{V}O_2$max or METSpeak that is to be achieved during training is then calculated using these test responses. However, in order to regulate exercise intensity, the prescribed %$\dot{V}O_2$max or %METSpeak must be linked to a target physiological response that can be easily monitored during training. Typically, this target response is the exercise heart rate. The target heart rate is determined by plotting heart rate responses during a GXT as a function of corresponding $\dot{V}O_2$ responses. The heart rate that is equivalent to the prescribed %$\dot{V}O_2$max or %METSpeak is then identified from this plot. During training, exercise intensity is adjusted until the target heart rate is achieved, ensuring that the prescribed relative metabolic rate (i.e., %$\dot{V}O_2$max or %METSpeak) is maintained.

A variant of the metabolic method uses normative tables that list the energy cost (i.e., kcal, $\dot{V}O_2$, METs[1]) of a wide range of aerobic activities. When the target metabolic rate has been calculated as previously described, the normative tables are used to choose an activity whose energy cost is equivalent to the prescribed level. In this method, the intensity of the activity is not usually regulated by a target heart rate, and often the exerciser must perform at a fixed pace. While convenient, the method has several drawbacks (Fardy, Yanowitz, and Wilson 1988). A prescription based on the average energy cost of an activity does not consider variations in caloric expenditure owing to individual differences in body size, aerobic fitness, and motor skill.

Also, energy cost tables often do not present the full range of caloric expenditure that may be required for a given activity. Some aerobic activities are performed at varying intensities within a given exercise session. If the full range of energy costs for such activities is not known, the target metabolic intensity may be under- or overestimated. Examples of such activities are aerobic dancing and racquet sports. While the average value presented in an energy cost table for these activities may be equal to the prescribed metabolic rate, a substantial part of an exercise session could actually be spent at intensities above or below the target training zone. Such a response invalidates the metabolic assumptions underlying the prescription process.

---

[1]One MET equals the resting VO_2 and is approximately 3.5 ml/(kg · min).

Heart Rate Method

Practical considerations frequently make it difficult to measure $\dot{V}O_2$ during graded exercise testing. However, heart rate can be determined easily and accurately during an exercise evaluation. Therefore, exercise intensity is often prescribed using only heart rate responses to a GXT. The physiological rationale underlying this prescriptive procedure is based on the comparatively linear relation between heart rate and $\dot{V}O_2$ for most dynamic exercise modes. Two HR methods are commonly employed. The first of these determines exercise intensity as a percentage of the heart rate range (HRR). The HRR is calculated by subtracting the resting heart rate from the maximal heart rate. The maximal heart rate is most accurately determined by measuring the highest value attained during a GXT terminated at the point of exhaustion (Noble et al. 1986). Alternatively, maximal heart rate can be estimated by using age-adjusted normative tables or by subtracting the individual's age from 220 for a male and 226 for a female. A predetermined percentage (70%-85%) of the HRR is calculated and then added to the resting heart rate. The resulting value is the target training heart rate. A given percentage of the HRR is equivalent to the same percentage of $\dot{V}O_2$max. That is, an exercise intensity that requires 85% of the HRR also requires 85% $\dot{V}O_2$max. As a result, prescription of exercise intensity by the HRR method is physiologically consonant with the metabolic method described previously.

Alternatively, exercise intensity can be prescribed by calculating a predetermined percentage of the maximal exercise heart rate (HRmax). The resulting value serves as the target training heart rate. A target heart rate that is derived as a percentage of HRmax is approximately 10% lower than that calculated by either the metabolic or the HRR method. Therefore, the $\dot{V}O_2$ attained during a training session is underestimated, partially invalidating the metabolic assumptions that are basic to the exercise prescription. This prescriptive procedure has further limitations when applied to the coronary patient. Often patients with cardiovascular disease have a high resting heart rate or a low HRmax. In either case, a target training heart rate that is calculated as a percentage of HRmax may be only marginally greater than the resting heart rate, minimizing the physiological stimulus and negating a training response. A similar limitation exists when HRmax is attenuated by beta-blocking medications (Fardy, Yanowitz, and Wilson 1988).

While the heart rate method of prescribing exercise intensity is easy to calculate, it has a number of drawbacks (Pollock, Wilmore, and Fox 1984; Pollock, Jackson, and Foster 1986; Fardy, Yanowitz, and Wilson 1988; Gutmann et al. 1981). First, both of the foregoing heart rate methods require knowledge of the age-adjusted maximal heart rate. Actual measurement of the mode-specific maximal heart rate requires that exercise tests be carried out to the point of physiological exhaustion, thereby presenting a level of risk to the participant. Alternatively, the estimation of HRmax using normative tables is associated with considerable intraindividual error ($\pm10\%$). Second, the comparatively linear relation between HR and $\dot{V}O_2$ during dynamic exercise can be distorted by such factors as high ambient temperature, psychological stress, caffeine, and medications. The resulting change in heart rate response at a prescribed $\dot{V}O_2$ invalidates the exercise prescription. Third, because electronic heart rate monitoring is expensive and impractical in most nonclinical settings, exercise heart rate is often recorded by palpation. Unfortunately, many participants find it difficult to accurately monitor their own heart rate, owing to inexperience, pulse counting errors, and variations in the palpation site. In some extreme cases, exercisers become incessant "pulse counters," losing sight of the pleasurable aspects of the exercise program (Borg 1970).

RPE Method

The intensity of aerobic exercise can be prescribed using RPE either independently or as an adjunct to the heart rate method. RPE is not influenced by many of the perturbations described above for heart rate, thereby providing a method of exercise prescription that is applicable over a wide range of clinical, recreational, and athletic settings. As demonstrated earlier for heart rate, RPE is linearly related to $\dot{V}O_2$ during most dynamic exercise modes. This relationship is strongest when $\dot{V}O_2$ is expressed as a percentage of the mode-specific maximal value. The perceptually based exercise prescription is derived by first plotting the RPE that has been estimated during a GXT against corresponding $\dot{V}O_2$ responses (fig. 11.1). The RPE that is equivalent to the prescribed percentage of $\dot{V}O_2$max is then determined from this plot. During training, exercise intensity is adjusted until the prescribed (target) RPE is produced.

The prescription of exercise intensity using RPE is consistent with the physiological assumption underlying both the metabolic and HRR methods described earlier. In fact, when expressed as a function of the percentage of the HRR, RPE does not differ between groups ranging in age from 31 to 68 yr (Bar-Or 1977). As an example, figure 11.2 illustrates RPE plotted against exercise heart rate responses for young, healthy adults and coronary heart disease patients (Pollock, Wilmore, and Fox 1984). Heart rate responses are expressed as percentages of the HRR. The relation between RPE and the percentage of the HRR demonstrates a consistent pattern for all subject groups. Normally, the intensity of ambulatory training for an inpatient cardiac rehabilitation program is rated between 11 and 12 on the Borg RPE scale (Pollock, Wilmore, and Fox 1984). Activities undertaken in a second-phase outpatient program are rated between 12 and 13. As shown in figure 11.2, when the heart rates corresponding to these RPEs are calculated as a percentage of the HRR, the target training stimulus is reasonably consistent across groups that are divergent in both clinical status and functional aerobic power.

RPE can also be used as an adjunct to a target heart rate in regulating exercise intensity (Pollock, Jackson, and Foster 1986). During the initial phase of training, exercise intensity should be regulated by both heart rate and RPE. Adjunctive use of perceptual monitoring helps to refine the exercise prescription by subjectively matching the performance intensity with the training zone. As the training program progresses, heart rate monitoring by palpation can be reduced or eliminated,

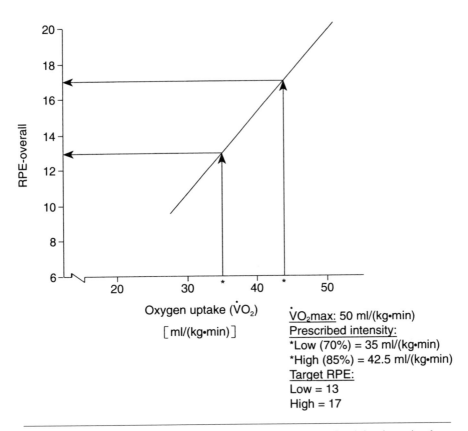

Figure 11.1   Determination of target RPEs for the regulation of training intensity during aerobic exercise.

especially when clinically normal individuals are involved. Regulation of the prescribed exercise intensity can then be accomplished by producing a target RPE. An advantage of this procedure is that exercise need not be interrupted for periodic heart rate measurements.

Development of the Perceptually Regulated Exercise Prescription

A perceptually based exercise prescription assumes that a target RPE that has been *estimated* during a GXT can be used to regulate exercise intensity by *producing* a similar level of exertion during training or rehabilitative therapy. Perceptual regulation of exercise intensity is considered physiologically and

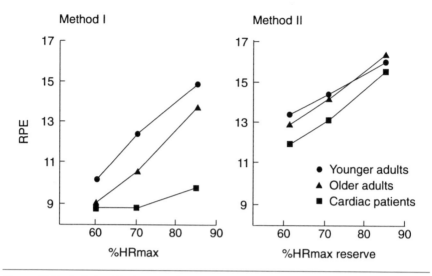

Figure 11.2   Relationship between heart rate (HR) and perceived exertion (RPE) with two methods of calculating training heart rate. %HRmax (method I) was calculated on the basis of the percentage of the difference between zero and peak HR attained. %HRmax reserve (method II) was calculated according to Karvonen et al. (1957) and represents the percentage difference between the resting and maximal HR added to the resting HR.
Reprinted from Pollock, Wilmore, and Fox 1984.

clinically valid if HR, $\dot{V}O_2$, rate-pressure product, or ECG criteria do not differ when comparisons are made at similar levels of exertion between a GXT (i.e., estimation trial) and an individual training session (i.e., production trial). A number of laboratory and field-based experiments have examined the physiological and clinical validity of the perceptual estimation-production paradigm in prescribing and regulating exercise intensity. While some inconsistencies exist, these experiments generally agree that a target RPE estimated during a GXT can be produced during a training session in order to regulate exercise intensity. The following sections describe experiments that used both perceptual estimation paradigms and perceptual estimation-production paradigms to regulate exercise intensity.

Estimation Prescriptions

Experimental paradigms employing only a perceptual estimation procedure require that perceived exertion be rated during both a GXT and an individual training session. Comparisons of selected criterion responses such as heart rate, $\dot{V}O_2$, or power output at a given RPE are made between the GXT and training session. When the criterion responses are the same between the GXT and training sessions,

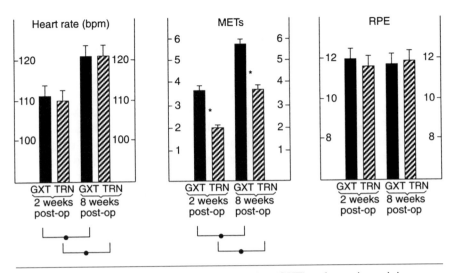

Figure 11.3   Comparison of graded exercise testing (GXT) and exercise training (TRN) for heart rate, exercise intensity (METs), and rating of perceived exertion (RPE) at two and eight weeks after surgery. Means $\pm$ *SE; *$*p < .01$.
Reprinted from Gutmann et al. 1981.

perceptually regulated exercise intensity is considered physiologically valid. The first of these investigations was undertaken by Borg and Linderholm (1970) using a mixed sample of healthy and hypertensive men and women. Power output was the same when determined at a heart rate of 130 bpm or at an RPE of 13, suggesting that exercise intensity could be subjectively regulated. However, in the absence of a training condition in which subjects are actually required to produce a prescribed target RPE, the foregoing conclusion must be interpreted conservatively.

Using a somewhat different experimental paradigm, Gutmann et al. (1981) examined the perceptual responses of coronary artery revascularization patients during testing and therapeutic exercise training. Heart rate was matched between a GXT and a daily training session involving prolonged treadmill and cycle exercise. When compared at heart rates of 110 bpm and 120 bpm, RPE-Overall did not differ between testing and training conditions (fig. 11.3). These responses support the conjunctive use of RPE and heart rate in regulating exercise intensity, especially for cardiac rehabilitation.

Estimation-Production Prescriptions

In actual practice, a perceptually regulated exercise prescription requires the use of an estimation-production procedure. Physiological validation of this prescriptive procedure has been established in both laboratory and field settings (Van Den Burg and Ceci 1986; Ceci and Hassmen 1991; Burke and Collins 1983; Myles

1985; Eston, Davies, and Williams 1987; Bayles et al. 1990). As an example, Van Den Burg and Ceci (1986) compared heart rate responses between a multistage treadmill test and a treadmill training session. RPE was estimated for each stage of the treadmill test. During training, subjects were instructed to select a treadmill speed that produced an RPE of 13. The heart rate responses equivalent to an RPE of 13 did not differ between the treadmill test (145 bpm) and the training session (149 bpm; fig. 11.4). These findings provide physiological evidence that a target RPE estimated during a GXT can be used to regulate the intensity of a treadmill training session. Van Den Burg and Ceci (1986) also found that the self-selected training speed was faster than that attained during testing when comparisons were made at the prescribed perceptual reference point. This was likely due to the cumulative effect of progressive increments in exercise intensity during the GXT, resulting in a comparatively higher RPE and heart rate for a given speed. A faster speed is then required during training to produce the target RPE and corresponding heart rate. However, a discrepancy in speed between a GXT and an individual training session does not invalidate the assumptions underlying the perceptual estimation-production method of exercise prescription. It should be remembered that the objective of the exercise prescription is to achieve a target RPE or heart rate, not a predetermined physical stimulus such as running speed.

A number of other laboratory experiments have used an estimation-production paradigm to examine the physiological validity of a perceptually regulated exercise prescription (Eston, Davies, and Williams 1987; Burke and Collins 1983; Glass, Knowlton, and Becque 1992; Smutok, Skrinar, and Pandolf 1980; Bayles et al. 1990, Dunbar et al. 1992). In general, these investigations support the prescriptive application of RPE for a wide range of exercise intensities and for individuals of

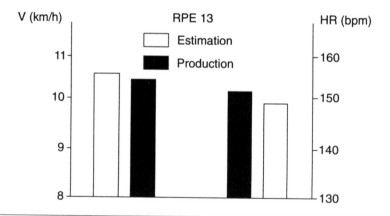

Figure 11.4   Comparison of velocity of running (V) and heart rate (HR) at RPE 13 during an estimation and a production method in a laboratory situation.
Reprinted from Van Den Burg and Ceci 1986.

varying age, fitness, clinical status, and level of fatigue. Self-regulation of exercise intensity using RPE has also been found to be physiologically valid when production trials were administered in random order and when perceptual scaling instructions were periodically reinforced by a special feedback procedure.

It is of particular importance that a perceptually based exercise prescription be physiologically valid over a wide range of exercise intensities if the procedure is to be used with individuals who vary in functional aerobic power. A majority of laboratory investigations indicate that perceptual regulation of exercise intensity is effective for aerobic activities requiring relative metabolic rates that span the training zone for cardiorespiratory fitness (i.e., 50%-85% $\dot{V}O_2$max). A good example is the perceptual estimation-production experiment undertaken by Dunbar et al. (1992). Estimation trials were conducted on a treadmill and cycle ergometer at 50% and 70% $\dot{V}O_2$peak. RPEs for the overall body were estimated and heart rate measured at the two relative exercise intensities for both test modes. Subjects were subsequently instructed to produce the previously estimated target RPE during simulated training sessions using both treadmill and cycle ergometer modes. Four estimation-production paradigms were examined: (1) treadmill-treadmill, (2) treadmill-cycle, (3) cycle-cycle, and (4) cycle-treadmill, respectively. Each of the estimation-production paradigms was undertaken at n intensity equivalent to 50% and 70% $\dot{V}O_2$peak. Physiological validation of the perceptual prescription procedure was taken as the difference in heart rate response between the estimation and production trials. Figure 11.5 demonstrates that the heart rate across the four intra- and intermodal conditions ranged from 0.26 to 26.85 bpm. These data provide physiological validation of perceptually regulated exercise intensity using an estimation-production paradigm.

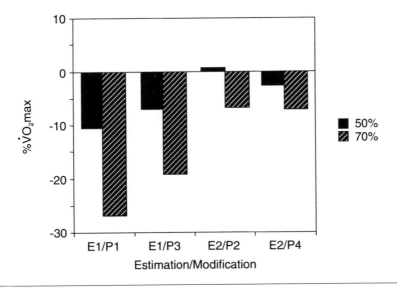

Figure 11.5   Differences (δ) in heart rate between estimation and production trials.

Caution is necessary regarding the amount of time that separates identification of a target RPE during exercise testing and actual implementation of the exercise prescription during training. In the experiment by Van Den Burg and Ceci (1986) previously described, subjects were asked to select a running speed on an outdoor track that produced an RPE of 13. Heart rate during the outdoor training session (164 bpm) was significantly higher than that achieved during graded exercise testing (145 bpm) when comparisons were made at a reference RPE of 13. However, a period of two months separated the GXT and the outdoor training session. Quite possibly "perceptual memory" had faded over the interim period, necessitating that the exercise conditions associated with the target RPE be reestablished through a follow-up GXT.

In summary, laboratory experiments where exercise intensity is regulated by producing a previously estimated RPE support the physiological validity of a perceptually based exercise prescription. This prescriptive procedure must next be validated in actual field settings involving athletic, clinical, and recreational training programs.

Problems and Solutions

The perceptual regulation of exercise intensity using an estimation-production prescriptive procedure has a number of methodological problems. It is not unusual to find that for a given RPE or HR, both power output and MET level are higher during a training session than during graded exercise testing (Gutmann et al. 1981; Van Den Burg and Ceci 1986). During a training session, the slope of the relation between RPE and power output is greater than the slope of the same relation during a GXT. As a result, a comparatively higher power output is required to produce the target RPE during training. This distortion of the relation between RPE and power output is in part due to the longer time typically required for an individual training session (30 min) than is needed to administer a GXT (i.e., 12 min; Maresh and Noble 1984; Gutmann et al. 1981). However, it should be remembered that the intent of an exercise prescription is to produce a target RPE or HR, not a fixed power output or locomotor speed. The somewhat higher power output or speed that is required to produce a given RPE during training as compared to testing does not invalidate a perceptually regulated exercise prescription.

Under most conditions, the regulation of exercise intensity according to a target RPE yields heart rate responses that fall within the prescribed training zone as defined during a GXT. Occasionally, however, the training heart rate that is equivalent to the target RPE is not the same as that prescribed from the GXT (Davies and Sargeant 1979). Such inconsistencies in heart rate response may be attributable to multistage testing protocols wherein power output is systematically increased until termination criteria are attained. The cumulative physiological effect of the preceding stages results in a higher heart rate during exercise testing than during training when comparisons are made at the prescribed RPE. Prescription errors of this type can be eliminated if both the estimation and production trials are administered within training sessions only. As an example, Chow and Wilmore (1984) instructed subjects to estimate the RPE that was equivalent to a prescribed exercise intensity during an orientation session that duplicated the salient features of an actual training session. This target RPE was then used to regulate exercise intensity during actual training sessions. Perceptual regulation of exercise intensity using this modified estimation-production procedure was found to be 48.5% accurate. That is, 48.5% of the heart rate responses were within the prescribed training zone. This compared favorably with the 55.3% accuracy of the traditional heart rate palpation method to regulate exercise intensity.

Noble's Titration Test

Noble developed a titration test to correct perceptual estimation-production errors when prescribing exercise intensity according to a target RPE (Maresh and Noble 1984). The titration test identifies the target RPE corresponding to a prescribed heart rate that has been previously determined during a GXT. This test is administered during the first several days of a training program using the following procedures:

1. Instruct the participant to walk at a natural but constant pace over a measured distance so that the total time exceeds 3 min. This provides sufficient time to establish a physiological steady state.
2. At the end of step 1, record the exact time required for the walk. This will be used to calculate speed in feet per second. Heart rate and RPE should be recorded during the first 10 s of the postexercise period.
3. If the recorded heart rate is below that prescribed from the GXT, repeat step 1 at a slightly accelerated pace. Then repeat step 2.
4. Repeat steps 1 and 2 until one heart rate falls above and one below the prescribed target heart rate.
5. Figure 11.6 presents an example of how the target RPE and training speed are determined. In this plot, a horizontal line (A) is drawn from the target heart rate to line B, which expresses heart rate as a function of speed. From the point of intersection, a vertical line (C) is dropped to the speed axis to determine training speed. Again, starting from the intersection point a vertical line (D) is drawn upward to the line E, which expresses the estimated RPE as a function of speed, and then horizontally over to the RPE axis. The point of intersection with the RPE axis identifies the target RPE that will be produced during training.
6. Convert speed to lap time so that training intensity can be controlled by a large pace clock.
7. Finally, the training pace is produced at the calculated lap time for a 3-min period during which RPE and heart rate are checked. After two or three trials during which the participant learns to correlate RPE with heart rate and pace, exercise intensity can be effectively controlled by producing a target RPE alone.

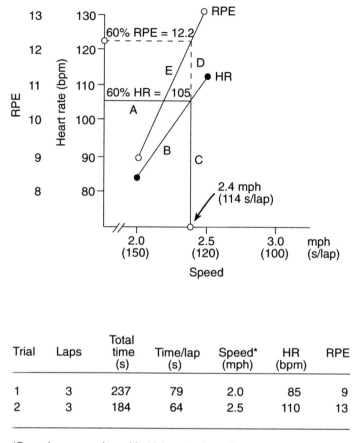

Figure 11.6   Illustration of a method to determine training movement speed and RPE from a single titration test.
Reprinted from Maresh and Noble 1984.

Trial	Laps	Total time (s)	Time/lap (s)	Speed* (mph)	HR (bpm)	RPE
1	3	237	79	2.0	85	9
2	3	184	64	2.5	110	13

*Based on gym size with 12 laps to the mile

Perceptual Feedback Protocol

Bayles et al. (1990) developed a *practice protocol* that enhances the precision of a perceptually regulated exercise prescription. The perceptual protocol uses a modification of the standard Borg RPE scale to provide cognitive feedback regarding the type and strength of various signals that influence RPE. The scale modification includes the addition of verbal descriptors that define the intensity of exertional perceptions at various points in the response continuum. Written instructions that elucidate these verbal descriptors are presented in conjunction with the modified scale during both exercise testing and training sessions (fig. 11.7). The error in replicating training speed decreased from 18% when the

6. . . .	6. . . .
	very, very light
	cool
7. very, very light	7. no breathing difficulties
	no discomfort
	high motivation
8. . . .	8. . . .
9. very light	9. very light
10. . . .	10. . . .
11. fairly light	11. fairly light
12. . . .	12. . . .
	somewhat hard
	warm
13. somewhat hard	13. minor breathing difficulties
	minor discomfort
	moderate motivation
14. . . .	14. . . .
15. hard	15. hard
16. . . .	16. . . .
17. very hard	17. very hard
18. . . .	18. . . .
	very, very hard
	hot
19. very, very hard	19. major breathing difficulties
	major discomfort
	low motivation
20. . . .	20. . . .

Figure 11.7 Modified Borg 6-20 category-rating scale with additional verbal descriptors.
Reprinted from Borg 1985.

standard Borg scale was employed to 7.5% when the perceptual feedback protocol was used (fig. 11.8). The feedback protocol was found to be physiologically valid during both treadmill and track running at exercise intensities equivalent to 60% and 80% of the heart rate range.

Lactate and Ventilatory Inflection Points: Prescriptive Anchors

The lactate and ventilatory inflection points serve as physiological markers upon which a perceptually regulated exercise prescription can be developed (Haskvitz et al. 1992; Seip et al. 1991; Hetzler et al. 1991). The lactate inflection point is defined as the $\%\dot{V}O_2$max or power output just below which blood lactate begins to exponentially increase above resting levels (1.0 mmol/L) during dynamic

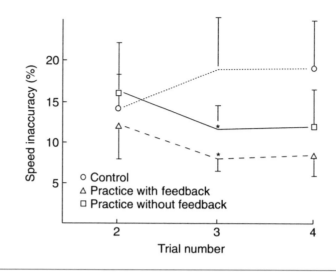

Figure 11.8   Mean percentage inaccuracy scores for speed at trials 2, 3, and 4 for each experimental group. *Trials 3 and 4 significantly less than trial 2, $p < .05$. Reprinted from Bayles et al. 1990.

exercise (Brooks and Fahey 1985). In an analogous manner, the ventilatory inflection point is the $\%\dot{V}O_2max$ or power output just below which pulmonary ventilation evinces a nonlinear increase in relation to $\dot{V}O_2$ (Wasserman et al. 1973). The lactate and ventilatory inflection points generally occur at exercise intensities that range from 50% to 80% $\dot{V}O_2max$ during arm, leg, and combined arm and leg exercise. It is assumed that the two inflection points are physiologically linked in that a nonlinear increase in the ventilatory equivalent for oxygen indicates buffering of metabolic acidosis secondary to blood lactate accumulation. However, it is also important to note that considerable disagreement exists as to whether or not the appearance of either the lactate or ventilatory inflection point signals the onset of anaerobic metabolism in muscle.

Despite such disagreement, the lactate and ventilatory inflection points are measurable with an acceptable degree of precision, are indicative of peripheral training adaptation, and, most important, fall within the training zone for cardiorespiratory fitness. Therefore, exercise intensity can be regulated by exertional perceptions using these points as physiological references (Purvis and Cureton 1981; DeMello et al. 1987). RPE at the lactate and ventilatory inflection points ranges from 12 to 14 on the Borg scale for arm, leg, and combined arm and leg exercise. The comparative stability of RPE at the lactate and ventilatory inflection points holds for men and women of varying age and training experience and also persists from one training session to the next (DeMello et al. 1987; Hill et al. 1987; Gutin, Ang, and Torrey 1988; Purvis and Cureton 1981;

Burke 1986). All of these factors contribute to the precision and utility of an exercise prescription that uses the RPE at the lactate or ventilatory inflection point as the reference upon which to regulate training intensity. The relative metabolic rates (i.e., 50%-80% $\dot{V}O_2$max) that define the lactate and ventilatory inflection points fall within the training zone for cardiorespiratory conditioning. Therefore, the regulation of exercise intensity by producing an RPE that corresponds to these points provides an appropriate overload stimulus to improve functional aerobic power and can be considered a physiologically valid prescriptive procedure. Of importance to training progression is the consistency of RPE at the lactate and ventilatory inflection points even though the $\dot{V}O_2$ and power output that mark these points increase as a function of training adaptation (Hill et al. 1987). As training progresses, a higher absolute intensity will be required to produce the target RPE (i.e., 12-14) equivalent to the lactate and ventilatory inflection points. Perceptually regulated exercise intensity will then remain equal to the lactate or ventilatory inflection points throughout the training program.

The prescription of exercise intensity according to the RPE that corresponds to the lactate or ventilatory inflection point employs an estimation-production procedure. First, lactate or ventilatory responses to the GXT are used to identify their respective inflection points. RPEs that have been estimated during a GXT are plotted as a function of either $\dot{V}O_2$ or power output. A target RPE corresponding to either the $\dot{V}O_2$ or power output that marks the inflection point is then determined from the plot. During training, the intensity of exercise is adjusted to produce this target RPE. Therefore, the relative metabolic rate that is attained during training is equivalent to the inflection point. This procedure also allows the adjustment of exercise intensity to levels that fall within the normal training zone but are somewhat higher or lower than the lactate or ventilatory inflection points. As an example, competitive runners often train at an intensity equivalent to 115% of their lactate or ventilatory inflection point (Gutin, Ang, and Torrey 1988). Once the $\dot{V}O_2$ that corresponds to 115% of the inflection point is identified, the corresponding target RPE is derived from the RPE-$\dot{V}O_2$ plot as described earlier.

The link between RPE and the lactate and ventilatory inflection points likely reflects the influence of both peripheral and respiratory-metabolic mediators (DeMello et al. 1987). The lactate and ventilatory inflection points serve as metabolic markers for the exercise intensity at which pH begins to decrease and lactate concentration begins to increase in blood and muscle. These peripheral physiological events signal the onset of metabolic acidosis during moderate to heavy exercise. Ventilatory buffering of metabolic acidosis is in turn initiated. As noted in previous chapters, both metabolic acidosis and ventilatory drive serve as physiological mediators for, respectively, peripheral and respiratory-metabolic exertional signals. The intensity of exertional perceptions at the lactate and ventilatory inflection points at least in part reflects the mediating influence of these underlying physiological events.

Perceptually Based Cross-Modal Exercise Prescription

Exercise programs in both clinical and competitive settings often use a number of different aerobic activities in a single training session. As an example, programs often employ a circuit training format, wherein a different activity is undertaken at each exercise station. When the stations are performed sequentially and without interruption, circuit training is a very effective procedure to enhance cardiorespiratory fitness. Normally, an exercise prescription for circuit training is based on graded exercise tests that are specific to each mode used in the program (Robertson et al. 1990). However, mode-specific exercise testing is often impractical and expensive, especially when a comparatively large number of activities are involved. An alternative approach is to develop a cross-modal prescription of exercise intensity using RPE (Robertson et al. 1990). Perceptually based cross-modal prescriptions do not have to be derived from a graded exercise test that involves the same muscle groups as used in training. Providing a variety of activity modes is a more practical approach to the regulation of exercise intensity.

Robertson et al. (1990) examined the validity of a perceptually based cross-modal exercise prescription using treadmill, stationary cycle, and hand-weighted bench-stepping exercise. The latter activity was chosen because it combines arm and leg movements in a unique form of total body exercise that has low impact on joints, requires comparatively little equipment, and can be easily included in group or home exercise programs (Goss et al. 1987; Auble, Schwartz, and Robertson 1987). In this experiment, RPE-Overall (RPE-O) that was estimated during treadmill exercise was compared with RPE-O responses during cycling and hand-weighted bench stepping. The latter two modes were performed at an intensity equivalent to both an absolute $\dot{V}O_2$ of 39.8 ml/(kg · min) and a relative value equivalent to 70% $\dot{V}O_2$peak. The treadmill test that served as the reference mode was performed at an intensity equivalent to 70% of peak oxygen uptake for treadmill exercise. RPE-O was the same for the treadmill reference test and the relative tests for cycling and hand-weighted bench stepping. In contrast, RPE-O was significantly higher during the two absolute tests than during the treadmill reference test (fig. 11.9). These responses are a function of differences in $\dot{V}O_2$peak among the three exercise modes. Peak oxygen uptake was lower in cycling and hand-weighted bench stepping than in treadmill exercise, owing to the smaller total muscle mass required in the first two modes. Consequently, the absolute submaximal $\dot{V}O_2$ represented a higher relative aerobic demand for cycling and hand-weighted bench stepping than for treadmill exercise (fig. 11.10). The higher RPE-O for the two absolute tests reflects a comparatively greater relative aerobic stress. As expected, when exercise intensity was set equal to 70% of mode specific $\dot{V}O_2$peak, perceptual responses did not differ between experimental tests. Therefore, a perceptually based cross-modal exercise prescription is physiologically valid when intensity is set equal to the relative rather than the absolute $\dot{V}O_2$. These findings indicate a close relation between exertional perceptions for the overall body and the relative $\dot{V}O_2$, a relation that has been observed for a wide range of exercise modalities (Robertson 1982; see chapter 5).

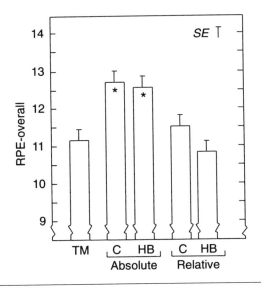

Figure 11.9 Ratings of perceived exertion (RPE) for the overall body during treadmill (TM), cycle (C), and hand-weighted bench-stepping (HB) exercise at absolute and relative intensities. An * indicates that the mean for that mode and intensity is higher ($p <$ .05) than the treadmill mean.
Reprinted from Robertson et al. 1990.

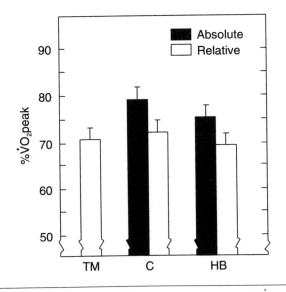

Figure 11.10 Percentage of mode-specific peak oxygen uptake (%$\dot{V}O_2$peak) attained during the absolute and relative experimental tests. Values are means $\pm$ SE for treadmill (TM), cycle (C), and hand-weighted bench-stepping (HB) exercise.
Reprinted from Robertson et al. 1990.

In practice, this laboratory experiment suggests that the intensity of cycle and hand-weighted bench-stepping exercise can be subjectively regulated to achieve a target metabolic rate (%$\dot{V}O_2$peak) that has been prescribed from treadmill testing. Of importance is that the $\dot{V}O_2$ and associated RPE-O that are achieved during cycling and hand-weighted bench stepping are the same as those which would be obtained from their respective mode-specific tests, had they been used to prescribe exercise intensity. Therefore, a target RPE-O that is equivalent to the prescribed %$\dot{V}O_2$peak can be derived during graded treadmill exercise and generalized to a variety of modes ranging from leg-only exercise (e.g., cycling) to combined arm and leg exercise (e.g., hand-weighted bench stepping).

A similar conclusion was drawn by Pollock, Jackson, and Foster (1986) using a modified perceptual production procedure. Exercise intensity was adjusted on a treadmill and arm ergometer to produce RPEs ranging from 11 to 15 on the Borg scale. Oxygen uptake and heart rate were lower for arm than for leg exercise. However, %$\dot{V}O_2$max did not differ between modes, validating the cross-modal regulation of exercise intensity using a target RPE.

RPE-Overall Versus Heart Rate

The use of a target RPE in cross-modal prescription of exercise intensity may be more advantageous than a target heart rate. In the cross-modal experiment previously described, heart rate was lower during the relative tests for cycling and hand-weighted bench stepping than during the treadmill test. This occurred despite the similarity in RPE-O among the three modes when exercise was performed at 70% $\dot{V}O_2$peak. The lower heart rate responses during the relative cycle and hand-weighted bench-stepping tests were consistent with the lower absolute $\dot{V}O_2$ for the same modes. Under cross-modal conditions, the adjustment of exercise intensity to achieve a target heart rate based on a predetermined percentage of treadmill $\dot{V}O_2$max would result in a higher than prescribed $\dot{V}O_2$ for cycling and hand-weighted bench stepping. This would erroneously elevate the target training zone. In contrast, when exercise is prescribed according to a target RPE-O, the appropriate training intensity is achieved over a range of modes.

In addition, heart rate for a given $\dot{V}O_2$ is generally higher for arm than for leg exercise. This further complicates cross-modal prescription when the reference mode involves treadmill exercise but the training mode involves arm exercise (e.g., hand-weighted bench stepping). However, RPE is not linked in a causal way to heart rate (Robertson 1982). Rather, RPE is mediated by the relative metabolic rate (%$\dot{V}O_2$peak). Therefore, the relation between RPE and %$\dot{V}O_2$peak remains constant across exercise modes, facilitating cross-modal prescription.

Differentiated RPE and Cross-Modal Prescription

Ratings of perceived exertion that are differentiated to the limbs and chest are somewhat less useful than RPE-Overall in cross-modal prescription of exercise intensity (Robertson et al. 1990). The strength of the peripheral (i.e., RPE-Legs

[RPE-L] and RPE-Arms [RPE-A]) and respiratory-metabolic (i.e., RPE-Chest [RPE-C]) perceptual signals varies respectively with the number of limbs involved during exercise and the pulmonary ventilation necessary to meet a given aerobic requirement. Limb involvement is determined by the exercise mode. Therefore, RPE-A and RPE-L are not effective in cross-modal prescription of exercise intensity when either lower- or upper-body muscular involvement varies substantially between modes. The respiratory-metabolic signal is closely linked to the pulmonary ventilation necessary to sustain a given $\dot{V}O_2$ (Robertson 1982). In the cross-modal experiment described earlier in this section, $\dot{V}O_2$, $\dot{V}_E$, and RPE-C were the same for the treadmill test and for the absolute tests for cycling and hand-weighted bench stepping (Robertson et al. 1990). In contrast, $\dot{V}O_2$ and $\dot{V}_E$ during cycling and hand-weighted bench stepping were lower than during treadmill exercise when each was performed at 70% of mode-specific $\dot{V}O_2$peak. RPE-C was correspondingly lower under the relative conditions for the cycle and hand-weighted bench-stepping modes. Therefore, cross-modal prescription of exercise intensity using the differentiated rating for the chest is not physiologically valid when the absolute $\dot{V}O_2$ that is equivalent to a prescribed %$\dot{V}O_2$peak varies among exercise modes. In general, the rating of perceived exertion for the overall body is more useful than the differentiated peripheral and respiratory-metabolic perceptual signals when prescribing exercise intensity over a range of activity modes (Robertson et al. 1990).

Implementation of a perceptually regulated exercise prescription assumes that the generalization of a target RPE from a graded exercise test to a constant-intensity submaximal training bout is a physiologically valid procedure. Central to this prescription process is the expectation that a target RPE estimated during a load- or grade-incremented test protocol transfers in a numerically invariant form to prolonged steady-state exercise. In general, the assumption of invariant transfer properties of target training RPEs appears valid. As an example, Dishman (1994) used heart rate response as a physiological criterion to validate a field-based walk-jog training program that was regulated by target RPEs. The perceptually regulated training intensity was intended to elicit heart rate responses that were equivalent to 60% of the heart rate range. When the target RPE was produced during training, the actual heart rate attained was within +3 bpm of the expected value. In contrast, when exercise intensity was regulated by a target heart rate, the actual training response was 18 to 23 bpm greater than the prescribed value, an error margin that is unacceptable in the presence of certain clinical conditions.

Experimental evidence suggests that the transfer properties of a target RPE are largely invariant and therefore are independent of systematic differences in test and training protocols. This conclusion appears to hold for estimation-production paradigms involving intra- and intermodal perceptually regulated exercise prescriptions (Ceci and Hassmen 1991; Dunbar et al. 1992; Dishman 1994). Nevertheless, it is suggested that three learning trials under actual, field-based conditions be incorporated at the beginning of an aerobic training program to ensure that even small perceptual production errors are within clinically acceptable levels for asymptomatic adult males (Dishman 1994). An alternative approach is to reduce the target RPE range as determined from the incremental exercise test by two Borg scale units. Ceci and Hassmen (1991) reported that when such a ''perceptual adjustment'' was applied during production trials under actual field conditions, heart rate and locomotor velocity at the target RPE were equivalent between treadmill testing and a jog-run training bout. In general, when either heart rate or oxygen uptake are used as the validation criterion, RPE production errors during actual training approximate only 5%. This is a readily acceptable error margin, minimizing the risk of untoward clinical events during exercise therapy.

Walk-Run Trading Functions

An exercise prescription can be made more flexible by alternating walking and running modes in the same training session. Perceptual regulation of an exercise prescription that involves both walking and running requires identification of the perceived exertion intersection point (PEIP) (Noble et al. 1973). This intersection point is operationally identified by plotting walking and running RPE responses as a function of locomotor speed (fig 11.11). On average, RPE

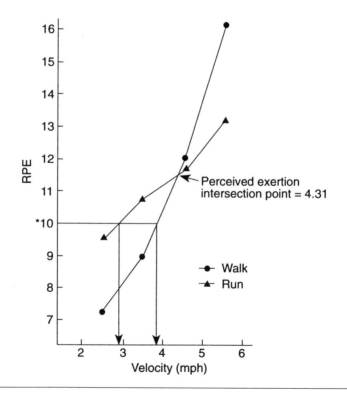

Figure 11.11   Perceived exertional response to walking and running at various velocities. * = target RPE.

will increase by two scale units for each 1.7-km/h increase in walk speed and one scale unit for each 1.7-km/h increase in run speed (Smutok, Skrinar, and Pandolf 1980). The PEIP is defined as the locomotor speed at which the walk and run RPE curves intersect. For young, healthy individuals, the PEIP is approximately 4.3 mph and is associated with an RPE of 11.5 (Noble et al. 1973; Smutok, Skrinar, and Pandolf 1980). At speeds below the PEIP, walking is perceived to be less effortful than running. The reciprocal is true for speeds above the PEIP; that is, walking is perceptually more effortful than running. Therefore, the training speed required to produce a target RPE will be slower for running than for walking if the exercise intensity is below the PEIP. When the exercise intensity is above the PEIP, the training speed will be faster for running than walking. The PEIP then becomes a reference point upon which walking and running exercise intensity is prescribed. For example, figure 11.11 presents a typical exercise prescription that employs walking and running perceptual trading functions. A horizontal line is drawn from the target RPE on the y axis so that it intersects both the walking and running curves. Vertical lines are then drawn downward to the x axis from the points of intersection on the walk and run curves. The target RPE is attained by selecting either a comparatively faster walking speed or a slower running speed.

A perceptually regulated exercise prescription that interchanges (i.e., trades) walking and running modes at speeds above and below the PEIP adds flexibility to a training program. The mode that is perceptually acceptable for a particular exercise session can be selected without compromising the physiological validity of the prescription. The participant's activity interests can then be more easily accommodated within the exercise prescription, promoting long-term program adherence (Dishman 1982).

Perceptual and Physiological Adaptation to Training

Ratings of perceived exertion can be used independently or in conjunction with heart rate responses to indicate (1) when it is necessary to adjust the intensity of a training stimulus (Pollock, Wilmore, and Fox 1984) and (2) the magnitude of physiological adaptation to an aerobic training program. Both RPE and heart rate at a given training intensity will decrease as functional aerobic power increases. This response reflects a positive training adaptation. The exercise intensity should then be increased until the target RPE is again produced during the stimulus portion of each training session. The prescribed physiological stimulus is maintained through perceptual regulation of exercise intensity that takes into account training adaptation.

Ratings of perceived exertion are an accurate indicator of training adaptation in exercise programs that involve cardiac and hypertensive patients as well as clinically normal participants (Hill et al. 1987; Gutmann et al. 1981; Ekelund et al. 1986). For example, Gutmann et al. (1981) found that for a given submaximal $\dot{V}O_2$, both RPE and heart rate decreased during an aerobic training program

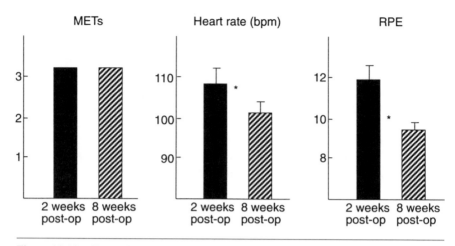

Figure 11.12   Comparison of heart rate and rating of perceived exertion (RPE) during graded exercise testing for the 3.2 MET level at two and eight weeks after myocardial revascularization surgery (means ± *SE*; * = $p < .01$).
Reprinted from Gutmann et al. 1981.

involving myocardial revascularization patients (fig. 11.12). The reciprocal of these responses also occurred; that is, both the heart rate and MET equivalent of a given RPE increased following six weeks of cardiac exercise therapy. Such changes in perceptual and physiological responses to exercise therapy indicate that functional aerobic power has improved and that the exercise intensity should be increased in order to maintain the training stimulus within the target zone.

The use of RPE to assess training adaptation is most effective when perceptual signals are assessed during graded exercise tests that involve the same muscle mass as used during training. Lewis et al. (1980) observed that RPE and submaximal heart rate decreased following an 11-week aerobic training program. The posttraining change in heart rate was apparent when testing involved untrained as well as trained limbs. In contrast, the posttraining attenuation of RPE at a given submaximal oxygen uptake or power output was specific to trained limbs only. Therefore, when using RPE to monitor physiological adaptation, it may be advantageous to measure peripheral signals that are differentiated to trained limbs.

Clinical Aspects

Exercise therapy for cardiovascular rehabilitation is typically presented in three sequential phases. Phase 1 provides in-hospital ambulatory activities that are performed during the first 10 to 14 days following myocardial infarction or revascularization surgery. Phase 2 is administered on a hospital outpatient basis and requires constant electronic monitoring of physiological and clinical responses to exercise therapy. Phase 3 exercise rehabilitation takes place in a community setting where therapeutic sessions are supervised by specialists but constant electronic monitoring is not indicated. Exertional perceptions can be used to regulate the intensity of exercise therapy in all three phases of rehabilitation. However, they are primarily employed during phases 2 and 3, often in conjunction with a target training heart rate. Gutmann et al. (1981) observed that myocardial revascularization patients effectively used RPE to regulate the intensity of therapeutic exercise during a six-week, phase 2 rehabilitation program. Perceptual regulation of exercise intensity was found to be a physiologically valid and clinically safe prescriptive procedure for phase 2 coronary rehabilitation. Once the patient progresses to a phase 3 community-based rehabilitation program, there is comparatively greater reliance on perceptual regulation of exercise intensity with a concomitant reduction in clinical and physiological monitoring. Self-regulation of exercise intensity using exertional perceptions makes phase 3 therapy similar in format to a traditional recreational fitness program. Therefore, one of the behavioral advantages of a perceptually based phase 3 format is to build the patients' confidence that their therapy is progressing satisfactorily and their functional capacities are approaching normal or near normal levels. Such confidence contributes to higher levels of program adherence.

The physiological and clinical assumptions underlying the prescription of exercise for the coronary patient are—with one notable exception—the same as those previously described for the clinically normal individual. The exception to normal prescriptive procedures involves the need to set exercise intensity within the functional or clinical constraints imposed by the ischemic threshold. From a physiological standpoint, the ischemic threshold is reached when myocardial oxygen demand exceeds supply. Clinical signs and symptoms of exercise-induced ischemia include ECG abnormalities, anginal pain, and inappropriate blood pressure responses. (See Pollock, Wilmore, and Fox [1984] for a more detailed explanation of these ischemic signs and symptoms.) As with the normal individual, the objective of an exercise prescription for the coronary patient is to achieve a total body oxygen uptake that falls within a predetermined training zone for cardiorespiratory fitness. However, for the coronary patient, the cardiac output needed to meet a prescribed total body oxygen uptake must not require a level of left ventricular work that compromises myocardial oxygen supply. When oxygen supply is inadequate for myocardial work, the ischemic threshold is exceeded, producing symptoms of coronary insufficiency and exertional intolerance. The physiological and clinical characteristics of the ischemic threshold are identified through graded exercise testing. Once identified, the ischemic threshold provides a prescriptive reference upon which the intensity of exercise is established. This is normally accomplished by selecting a therapeutic training zone that is equal to or approximately one MET below the ischemic threshold (Pollock, Jackson, and Foster 1986). The RPE that corresponds to the therapeutic training zone is then identified from a plot that expresses exertional perceptions as a function of METs. These data are obtained during the graded exercise test. Both perceptual and physiological responses can then be used to maintain exercise intensity within a clinically safe training zone that does not exceed the ischemic threshold.

Perceptions of exertion can be used in conjunction with heart rate to regulate exercise intensity during phase 1 therapy. It is recommended that the upper training heart rate for an inpatient ambulatory program be 20 bpm above the value for standing rest. The corresponding RPEs for this training intensity are 11 to 12 on the Borg category scale (Pollock, Jackson, and Foster 1986). This intensity is equal to the physiological demands of most inpatient ambulatory activities. However, neither a target heart rate nor RPE should be chosen that requires an exercise intensity that produces ischemic symptoms.

Anginal Pain and Exercise Intensity

Patients with exertional angina pectoris present a clinical reference point upon which to develop a therapeutic exercise prescription. It is often necessary to define the target training zone according to the perceived intensity of anginal pain (Borg, Holmgren, and Lindblad 1980). Exercise-induced anginal pain is an ischemic symptom secondary to coronary atherosclerosis. It appears as pain, tightness, or discomfort in the chest, back, jaw, or arms. The sensation of angina is often characterized as radiating from a focal point. Angina pectoris is a complex perceptual experience that includes frank sensation of pain as well as emotional and cognitive factors (Borg, Holmgren, and Lindblad 1980). As such, ratings of anginal pain during exercise must take into account individual differences in both sensory experience and personality. Borg, Holmgren, and Lindblad (1980) have developed a nine-category perceived anginal scale for use during dynamic exercise (fig. 11.13). The scale allows the patient to describe and communicate the perceived intensity of anginal pain during exercise testing and training. Instructions to the patient emphasize the association between the scale's verbal descriptors and the various numerical scale categories as follows: 1—freedom from pain, 5 to 6—pain that forces the patient to stop walking in everyday life, and 8 to 9—severest anginal pain ever felt. As shown in figure 11.14, the anginal threshold is highest for those with the least severe coronary disease. Therefore, the scale is a useful clinical tool when quantifying symptom-limited functional aerobic power in the angina patient.

The prescription of a target training intensity for the angina patient should be based on the appearance of pain. Owing to a built-in sensory alarm system that is triggered by the onset of angina pain, it is possible to maintain the intensity of exercise therapy within a clinically safe and physiologically effective training zone for these patients. The appearance of anginal pain usually coincides with the exercise intensities that span the ischemic threshold. Therefore, exercise is undertaken at an intensity that elicits a perceived anginal rating equivalent to the ischemic threshold. Rarely does this target anginal rating exceed a scale response of 6 (on the 9-point scale).

1. None at all

2. Extremely light

3. Very light

4. Rather light

5. Not so light, rather strong

6. Strong

7. Very strong

8. Extremely strong

9. Maximum, unbearable

Figure 11.13   Rating scale for anginal pain.
Reprinted from Borg, Holmgren, and Lindblad 1980.

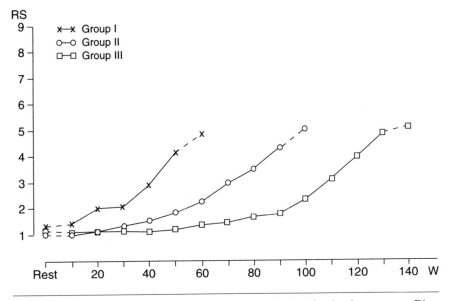

Figure 11.14   Mean pain ratings as a function of work load for the three groups. Disease severity: I=most; II=moderate; III=least.

Medication Effects

Medications such as beta-blocking agents and cardiac stimulants are routinely used by patients who are undergoing cardiovascular exercise rehabilitation. Many of these cardioactive medications alter the normal heart rate response to exercise. As an example, beta-blocking agents such as propranolol and atenolol attenuate exercise heart rate, whereas cardiac stimulants such as atropine accelerate the exercise heart rate. The regulation of exercise intensity according to a target heart rate is complicated when the dosage of these medications is periodically titrated to achieve optimal therapeutic benefit. In such cases, it may be advantageous to regulate the intensity of exercise therapy according to a target RPE. Exertional perceptions are generally stable in the presence of cardioactive medications (Davies and Sargeant 1979; Ekblom and Goldbarg 1971; Squires et al. 1982; Grimby and Smith 1978; Van Herwaarden et al. 1979; Sjoberg, Frankenhaeuser, and Bjurstedt 1979). Therefore, despite alterations in exercise heart rate that occur when medication dosage is changed, the prescribed exercise intensity can be maintained according to a target RPE.

The only exercise condition under which RPE can be affected by beta-blockade occurs when the medication reduces $\dot{V}O_2max$ (Ekelund et al. 1986). The mechanism that accounts for this reduction in the maximal level of oxygen transport involves an attenuation of cardiac output at peak exercise intensity. This response is most often observed when comparatively high doses of beta-blocking agents are used. Ekelund et al. (1986) compared RPE between exercise trials in which beta-blocking medications or a placebo were used. At a fixed submaximal $\dot{V}O_2$ (2.5 L/min), RPE was two to three units higher with beta-blockade than under the placebo condition. However, it should be noted that the submaximal reference $\dot{V}O_2$ represented a higher relative metabolic rate under beta-blockade than under placebo conditions owing to the attenuating effect of the medication on maximal aerobic power. If comparisons are made at a constant $\%\dot{V}O_2max$, RPE is normally not affected by beta-blocking therapy (Robertson 1982; Sargeant and Davies 1973). This observation has a direct implication for the regulation of exercise intensity using RPE. As noted earlier in this chapter, the intensity of an exercise prescription is set equal to a predetermined $\%\dot{V}O_2max$ that falls within the physiological training zone. The target RPE for the regulation of exercise intensity is also equivalent to this predetermined $\%\dot{V}O_2max$. Therefore, the intensity of a perceptually regulated exercise prescription is self-adjusted to offset changes in $\dot{V}O_2max$ that may occur when beta-blocking therapy is used. As long as the target RPE is produced during the training session, the prescribed relative metabolic rate will be attained irrespective of an attenuation in $\dot{V}O_2max$ secondary to medications.

In conclusion, it is recommended that during the initial phases of cardiac rehabilitation, RPE should be used in conjunction with heart rate to regulate the intensity of exercise (Monahan 1988). The conjunctive use of RPE and heart rate allows the coronary patient to regulate the intensity of therapeutic exercise within the context of clinical symptoms and physiological responses. After the patient learns to regulate exercise intensity using RPE in the therapeutic setting, the same technique can be transferred to everyday activities (Monahan 1988).

General Prescription Guidelines

The exercise intensities that define the perceptual and physiological training zone for cardiorespiratory fitness are summarized in table 11.1. These intensities are presented as general guidelines for the development of perceptually regulated exercise prescriptions. The target training zone is defined by RPEs that range from 12 to 16 on the Borg scale. This perceptual range parallels a physiological range that is equivalent to 50% to 85% $\dot{V}O_2$max. The perceptual training zone is generally constant and is not influenced by gender, level of aerobic fitness, or competitive experience. These prescription guidelines can also be applied to game activities in which movement is sustained over an extended period and the intensity of exercise varies with the competitive situation (Pollock, Wilmore, and Fox 1984). As an example, the following holds when exertional perceptions are used to regulate the intensity of a racquetball game:

RPE	Intensity	Energy cost (kcal/min)
12-13	Moderate	10
14-15	Moderate to hard	12.5
16-17	Very hard	15

Partitioning the levels of perceptual control to achieve low, medium, and high energy costs may be necessary when recreational games are used as part of a therapeutic conditioning program and where the functional aerobic power of participants varies markedly.

Table 11.1   Perceptual and Physiological Training Zones for Cardiorespiratory Conditioning Programs

	RPE (Borg 6-20 scale)				
	12	13	14	15	16
%HRR	60	70	"Preferred"	85	90
%$\dot{V}O_2$max	50			85	

Values are for the percentage of heart rate range (%HRR) and percentage of maximal oxygen uptake (%$\dot{V}O_2$max). Data from Gutmann et al. 1981; Maresh and Noble 1984; Eston, Davies, and Williams 1987; Burke and Collins 1983; Pollock, Jackson, and Foster 1986; Pollock, Wilmore, and Fox 1984.

Preferred Training Zone

The preferred training zone for cardiorespiratory fitness corresponds to RPEs of 13-15 (table 11.1). An exercise pace that falls within the preferred zone is considered perceptually acceptable. Where possible, it is advantageous to develop an exercise prescription that uses the preferred level of exertion to set the training pace. Provided that the target physiological response for cardiorespiratory fitness is attained, an exercise prescription that is also perceptually acceptable promotes program compliance and helps to establish a positive attitude toward physical activity (Dishman 1982).

A slightly different approach to the identification of a perceptually acceptable training pace is required during cycle ergometer exercise. When power output is held constant, exertional perceptions are normally lowest for pedal frequencies between 60 and 80 rpm and highest when pedaling at 40 or 120 rpm (Coast, Cox, and Welch 1986). Therefore, when participants other than competitive cyclists select a pedal frequency for purposes of exercise training, it normally falls between 60 and 80 rpm, a pace that is not only metabolically efficient but perceptually acceptable for prolonged activity.

The selection of a physiologically appropriate training pace that is perceptually acceptable may reflect a link between the preferred level of exertion and the metabolic rates that delineate the target conditioning zone. For example, Michael and Eckard (1972) asked subjects to select a treadmill running speed that corresponded to a "hard exercise workout" that would cause fatigue in 15 min. Both trained runners and untrained students selected treadmill speeds that were slower for incline than for horizontal running. Nevertheless, aerobic metabolic cost ($\dot{V}O_2$) did not differ between the two treadmill runs for both the trained and untrained groups.

Continuous Versus Intermittent Exercise

Perceptual regulation of exercise intensity can be used during intermittent as well as continuous training (Fardy, Yanowitz, and Wilson 1988). Intermittent exercise training has application in both competitive and clinical settings. An intermittent format allows a greater amount of physiological work to be done in a given period of time than is possible when using continuous training. The intensity of intermittent exercise is regulated by producing target RPEs that correspond to metabolic rates (%$\dot{V}O_2$max) set alternately at the low and high end of the physiological training zone. As an example, exercise can be performed 5 min at an intensity that produces an RPE of 17 and for 2 min at an intensity that produces an RPE of 13 (fig. 11.15). These oscillating intensities are repeated for a prescribed time period.

However, Edwards et al. (1972) observed that RPE was higher during intermittent than during continuous exercise when the same total amount of work was performed during both training formats. Oxygen uptake, heart rate, and blood lactic acid concentration were also higher for the intermittent than for the continuous format.

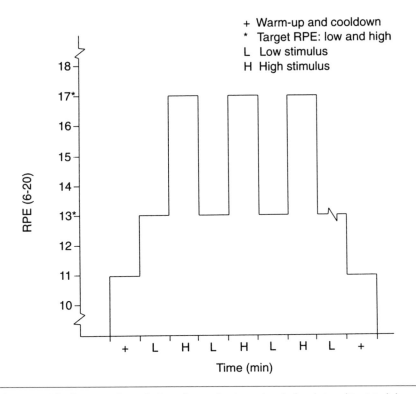

Figure 11.15   Perceptual regulation of exercise intensity during intermittent training.

These perceptual and physiological responses indicate a greater relative metabolic demand when performing intermittent exercise than when performing continuous exercise at the same average power output. Careful monitoring of exercise intensity is necessary if a perceptually based exercise prescription involves continuous and intermittent training formats that are employed conjunctively within a single session or that are presented according to a predetermined alternating sequence. Under these conditions, the precision of the prescription can be increased if target RPEs are established separately for continuous and intermittent training. Noble's titration test, described earlier in this chapter, which establishes target exercise intensities using RPE and heart rate responses to an actual training session, may be particularly helpful in this regard.

The perceptual and physiological differences between intermittent and continuous training notwithstanding, an intermittent format has important benefits when prescribing exercise for individuals with low functional aerobic power or for patients with cardiopulmonary disease. Certain physical activities require a higher relative metabolic rate than can be tolerated by individuals who have limited aerobic power. Performance of these activities may be possible only when an intermittent exercise format is used. In addition, because functional aerobic power is often limited by clinical symptoms, cardiac and pulmonary patients may not be able to sustain a prescribed exercise intensity for a period of time sufficient to produce a training stimulus. An intermittent format allows the patient to achieve the prescribed training stimulus, while the brief rest periods that are interspersed between exercise periods help to minimize clinical symptoms of exertional intolerance. The shortest rest period that is practicable should be used, and the exercise time should be less than that required to produce symptoms (Edwards et al. 1972). The full therapeutic impact of the exercise stimulus can then be realized.

Concentric Versus Eccentric Muscular Contractions

Caution is necessary when developing a perceptually based cross-modal exercise prescription involving activities that require both concentric and eccentric muscle contractions. Henriksson, Knuttgen, and Bonde-Peterson (1972) noted that for a given $\dot{V}O_2$ or heart rate, RPE is higher for concentric than for eccentric muscular activity. This differential perceptual response presents methodological problems in cross-modal exercise prescriptions where the target RPE is derived from a graded treadmill test that employs concentric muscle contractions but is applied to an exercise mode that uses eccentric contractions. Under these conditions, the precision of a perceptually regulated exercise prescription can be increased if the target RPE is derived from a graded exercise test that involves eccentric muscular contractions.

Effect of Fatigue

A unique advantage of a perceptually controlled exercise prescription is the ability to self-regulate training intensity to account for fatigue associated with sleep loss (Soule and Goldman 1973; Costa and Gaffuri 1977; Faria and Drummond 1982). Occasionally, the time of daily exercise must be adjusted to accommodate shift work or occupationally related travel. In such cases, exercise training is often undertaken following a period of sleep disruption, causing a higher level of exertional fatigue than is normally experienced. As fatigue increases, self-regulated exercise intensity is reduced to a lower energy requirement in order to produce the target RPE (Soule and Goldman 1973).

Summary

An exercise prescription for the improvement of cardiorespiratory fitness has five components: intensity, frequency, duration, mode, and progression. Of these components, the prescription of exercise intensity is the most complex, requiring the greatest precision. The prescription of exercise intensity assumes that a predetermined level of oxygen uptake is achieved during the stimulus portion of each training session. Three prescriptive methods are consistent with these assumptions: metabolic, heart rate, and RPE. Using these three methods, exercise intensity is set equal to 50% to 85% $\dot{V}O_2$max. The RPE method can be used independently or as an adjunct to the heart rate method. A perceptually based exercise prescription is derived by plotting RPEs that have been estimated during a GXT against corresponding $\dot{V}O_2$ responses. The RPE that corresponds to the prescribed percentage of $\dot{V}O_2$max is then determined from the plot. During training, exercise intensity is adjusted until the prescribed target RPE is produced. This perceptual estimation-production paradigm has been shown to be both physiologically and clinically valid for a wide range of exercise modes and intensities.

The lactate and ventilatory inflection points serve as physiological anchors upon which to develop a perceptually regulated exercise prescription. These points generally occur at exercise intensities ranging from 50% to 85% $\dot{V}O_2$max and therefore fall within the training zone to improve cardiorespiratory fitness. The RPE that corresponds to either point is identified from GXT responses. Training intensity is then adjusted to achieve the target RPE equivalent to the lactate or ventilatory inflection points.

A perceptually based cross-modal exercise prescription can be used to regulate the intensity of a circuit training program. The cross-modal prescription normally uses RPE-Overall responses that are obtained during treadmill testing. These perceptual responses are then used to regulate the intensity of such diverse activities as stationary cycling and hand-weighted bench stepping. The physiological validity of this procedure is based on the strong relation between RPE-Overall and %$\dot{V}O_2$max for a wide range of activity modes.

Ratings of perceived exertion can be used independently or in conjunction with heart rate to indicate when it is necessary to adjust the intensity of a training stimulus and to determine the magnitude of physiological adaptation to an aerobic training program. Such application is effective for the clinically normal individual as well as the coronary patient. However, for the purposes of a cardiac rehabilitation program, exercise intensity must be established within the functional or clinical constraints imposed by the ischemic threshold. In many cases the ischemic threshold is defined by anginal pain, the intensity of which can be measured by a category rating scale. Exercise therapy is undertaken at an intensity that elicits an anginal rating equivalent to the ischemic threshold (i.e., 6 on a 9-point scale).

In general, the target training zone for cardiorespiratory fitness is defined by RPEs that range from 12 to 16 on the Borg scale. This perceptual range parallels a physiological range that is equivalent to 50% to 85% $\dot{V}O_2$max. The preferred training zone for cardiorespiratory fitness corresponds to RPEs of 13 to 15. An exercise intensity that falls within the preferred zone is considered perceptually acceptable.

References

American College of Sports Medicine. 1991. *Guidelines for exercise testing and prescription.* 4th ed. Philadelphia: Lea and Febiger.

Auble, T.E., L. Schwartz, and R.J. Robertson. 1987. Aerobic requirements for moving handweights through various ranges of motion while walking. *Physician Sportsmed.* 15:133-40.

Bar-Or, O. 1977. Age related changes in exercise perception. In *Physical work and effort,* ed. G. Borg, 255-66. New York: Pergamon Press.

Bayles, C.M., K.F. Metz, R.J. Robertson, F.L. Goss, J. Cosgrove, and D. McBurney. 1990. Perceptual regulation of prescribed exercise. *J. Cardiopul. Rehab.* 10:25-31.

Borg, G. 1970. Perceived exertion as an indicator of somatic stress. *Scand. J. Rehab. Med.* 2:92-98.

Borg, G., A. Holmgren, and I. Lindblad. 1980. *Perception of chest pain during physical work in a group of patients with angina pectoris.* Reports from the Institute of Applied Psychology, no. 81. Stockholm: Univ. of Stockholm.

Borg, G., and H. Linderholm. 1970. Exercise performance and perceived exertion in patients with coronary insufficiency, arterial hypertension and vasoregulatory asthenia. *Acta Med. Scand.* 187:17-26.

Brooks, G.A., and T.D. Fahey. 1985. *Exercise physiology: Human bioenergetics and its applications.* New York: Macmillan.

Burke, E.J. 1986. Perceived exertion: Subjectivity and objectivity in work assessment. In *The perception of exertion in physical work,* ed. G. Borg and D. Ottoson, 149-59. London: Macmillan.

Burke, E.J., and M.L. Collins. 1983. Using perceived exertion for the prescription of exercise in healthy adults. In *Clinical sports medicine,* ed. R.C. Cantu, 93-105. Toronto: Collamore Press, D.C. Health.

Ceci, R., and P. Hassmen. 1991. Self-monitored exercise at three different RPE intensities in treadmill vs. field running. *Med. Sci. Sports Exerc.* 23:732-38.

Chow, R.J., and J.H. Wilmore. 1984. The regulation of exercise intensity by ratings of perceived exertion. *J. Cardiac Rehab.* 4:382-87.

Coast, J.R., R.H. Cox, and H.G. Welch. 1986. Optimal pedalling rate in prolonged bouts of cycle ergometry. *Med. Sci. Sports Exerc.* 18:225-30.

Costa, G., and E. Gaffuri. 1977. Studies of perceived exertion rate on bicycle ergometer in conditions reproducing some aspect of industrial work (shift work; noise). In *Physical work and effort,* ed. G. Borg, 297-306. New York: Pergamon Press.

Davies, C.T., and A.J. Sargeant. 1979. The effects of atropine and practolol on the perception of exertion during treadmill exercise. *Ergonomics* 22:1141-46.

DeMello, J.J., K.J. Cureton, R.E. Boineau, and M.M. Singh. 1987. Ratings of perceived exertion at the lactate threshold in trained and untrained men and women. *Med. Sci. Sports Exerc.* 19:354-62.

Dishman, R.K. 1982. Contemporary sport psychology. *Exerc. Sport Sci. Rev.* 10:120-59.

———. 1994. Prescribing exercise intensity for healthy adults using perceived exertion. *Med. Sci. Sports Exerc.* 26:9; 1087-94.

Dunbar, C.C., R.J. Robertson, R. Baun, M.F. Blandin, K. Metz, R. Burdett, and F.L. Goss. 1992. The validity of regulating exercise intensity by ratings of perceived exertion. *Med. Sci. Sports Exerc.* 24:94-99.

Edwards, R.H.T., A. Melcher, C.M. Hesser, O. Wigebtz, and L.G. Ekelund. 1972. Physiological correlates of perceived exertion in continuous and intermittent exercise with the same average power output. *Eur. J. Clin. Invest.* 2:108-14.

Ekblom, B., and A.N. Goldbarg. 1971. The influence of physical training and other factors on the subjective rating of perceived exertion. *Acta Physiol. Scand.* 83:399-406.

Ekelund, L.G., J.A. Blumenthal, M.C. Morey, and C.C. Ekelund. 1986. The effect of nonselective and selective betablockade on perceived exertion during treadmill exercise in mild hypertensive type A and B males and the interaction with aerobic training. In *The perception of exertion in physical work,* ed. G. Borg and D. Ottoson, 191-98. London: Macmillan.

Eston, R.G., B.L. Davies, and J.G. Williams. 1987. Use of perceived effort ratings to control exercise intensity in young healthy adults. *Eur. J. Appl. Physiol.* 56:222-24.

Fardy, P.S., F.G. Yanowitz, and P.K. Wilson. 1988. *Cardiac rehabilitation, adult fitness, and exercise testing.* 2d ed. Philadelphia: Lea and Febiger.

Faria, I.E., and B.J. Drummond. 1982. Circadian changes in resting heart rate and body temperature, maximal oxygen consumption and perceived exertion. *Ergonomics* 25:381-86.

Glass, S.C., R.G. Knowlton, and M.D. Becque. 1992. Accuracy of RPE from graded exercise to established exercise training intensity. *Med. Sci. Sports Exerc.* 24:1303-7.

Goss, F.L., R.J. Robertson, T.E. Auble, D.A. Cassinelli, R.J. Spina, E.E. Glickman, R.W. Galbreath, R.M. Silberman, and K.F. Metz. 1987. Are treadmill-based exercise prescriptions generalizable to combined arm and leg exercise? *J. Cardiopul. Rehab.* 7:551-55.

Grimby, G., and U. Smith. 1978. Beta-blockade and muscle function. *Lancet* 2 (8103): 1318-19.

Gutin, B., K.E. Ang, and K. Torrey. 1988. Cardiorespiratory and subjective responses to incremental and constant load ergometry with arms and legs. *Arch. Phys. Med. Rehab.* 69:510-13.

Gutmann, M.C., R.W. Squires, M.L. Pollock, C. Foster, and J. Anholm. 1981. Perceived exertion–heart rate relationship during exercise testing and training in cardiac patients. *J. Cardiac Rehab.* 1:52-59.

Haskvitz, E.M., R.L. Seip, J.Y. Weltman, A.D. Rogol, and A. Weltman. 1992. The effect of training intensity on ratings of perceived exertion. *Int. J. Sports Med.* 13-5:377-83.

Henriksson, J., H.G. Knuttgen, and F. Bonde-Peterson. 1972. Perceived exertion during exercise with concentric and eccentric muscle contractions. *Ergonomics* 15:537-44.

Hetzler, R.K., R.L. Seip, S.H. Boutcher, E. Pierce, D. Snead, and A. Weltman. 1991. Effect of exercise modality on ratings of perceived exertion at various lactate concentrations. *Med. Sci. Sports Exerc.* 23-1:88-92.

Hill, D.W., K.J. Cureton, S.C. Grisham, and M.A. Collins. 1987. Effect of training on the rating of perceived exertion at the ventilatory threshold. *Eur. J. Appl. Physiol.* 56:206-11.

Karvonen, M.J., E. Kentala, and O. Mustala. 1957. The effects of training heart rate: A longitudinal study. *Annales Medicinae Experimentalis et Biologiae Fenniae,* 35:307-15.

Lewis, S., P. Thompson, N.H. Areskog, P. Vodak, M. Marconyak, R. DeBusk, S. Mellen, and W. Haskell. 1980. Transfer effects of endurance training to exercise with untrained limbs. *Eur. J. Appl. Physiol.* 44:25-34.

Maresh, C.M., and B.J. Noble. 1984. Utilization of perceived exertion ratings during exercise testing and training. In *Cardiac rehabilitation: Exercise testing and prescription,* ed. L. K. Hall, 155-73. New York: Spectrum.

Michael, E.D., and L. Eckard. 1972. The selection of hard work by trained and non-trained subjects. *Med. Sci. Sports* 4:107-10.

Monahan, T. 1988. Perceived exertion: An old exercise tool finds new applications. *Physician Sportsmed.* 16:174-79.

Myles, W.S. 1985. Sleep deprivation, physical fatigue, and the perception of exercise intensity. *Med. Sci. Sports Exerc.* 17:580-84.

Noble, B.J., W.J. Kraemer, J.G. Allen, J.S. Plank, and L.A. Woodard. 1986. The integration of physiological cues in effort perception: Stimulus strength vs. relative contribution. In *Perception of exertion in physical work,* ed. G. Borg and D. Ottoson, 83-96. London: Macmillan.

Noble, B.J., K.F. Metz, K.B. Pandolf, C.W. Bell, E. Cafarelli, and W.E. Sime. 1973. Perceived exertion during walking and running—II. *Med. Sci. Sports* 5:116-20.

Pollock, M.L., L.R. Gettman, C.A. Mileses, M.D. Bah, J.L. Durstine, and R.B. Johnson. 1977. Effects of frequency and duration of training on attrition and incidence of injury. *Med. Sci. Sports* 9:31-36.

Pollock, M.L., A.S. Jackson, and C. Foster. 1986. The use of the perception scale for exercise prescription. In *Perception of exertion in physical work,* ed. G. Borg and D. Ottoson, 161-78. London: Macmillan.

Pollock, M.L., J.H. Wilmore, and S.M. Fox. 1984. *Exercise in health and disease: Evaluation and prescription for prevention and rehabilitation.* Philadelphia: Saunders.

Purvis, J.W., and K.J. Cureton. 1981. Ratings of perceived exertion at the anaerobic threshold. *Ergonomics* 24:295-300.

Robertson, R.J. 1982. Central signals of perceived exertion during dynamic exercise. *Med. Sci. Sports Exerc.* 14:390-96.

Robertson, R.J., F.L. Goss, T.E. Auble, R. Spina, D. Cassinelli, E. Glickman, R. Galbreath, and K. Metz. 1990. Cross-modal exercise prescription at absolute and relative oxygen uptake using perceived exertion. *Med. Sci. Sports Exerc.* 22:653-59.

Sargeant, A.J., and C.T. Davies. 1973. Perceived exertion during rhythmic exercise involving different muscle masses. *J. Human Ergol.* 2:3-11.

Seip, R.L., D. Snead, E.F. Pierce, P. Stein, and A. Weltman. 1991. Perceptual responses and blood lactate concentration: Effect of training state. *Med. Sci. Sports Exerc.* 23-1:80-87.

Sjoberg, H., M. Frankenhaeuser, and H. Bjurstedt. 1979. Interactions between heart rate, psychomotor performance and perceived effort during physical work as influenced by beta-adrenergic blockade. *Biol. Psychol.* 8:31-43.

Smutok, M.A., G.S. Skrinar, and K.B. Pandolf. 1980. Exercise intensity: Subjective regulation by perceived exertion. *Arch. Phys. Med. Rehab.* 61:569-74.

Soule, R.G., and R.F. Goldman. 1973. Pacing of intermittent work during 31 hours. *Med. Sci. Sports* 5:128-31.

Squires, R.W., J.L. Rod, M.L. Pollock, and C. Foster. 1982. Effects of propranolol on perceived exertion after myocardial revascularization surgery. *Med. Sci. Sports Exerc.* 14:276-80.

Ulmer, H.V. 1986. Perceived exertion as a part of a feedback system and its interaction with tactical behavior in endurance sports. In *Perception of exertion in physical work,* ed. G. Borg and D. Ottoson, 317-26. London: Macmillan.

Van Den Burg, M., and R. Ceci. 1986. A comparison of a psychophysical estimation and a production method in a laboratory and a field condition. In *Perception of exertion in physical work,* ed. G. Borg and D. Ottoson, 35-46. London: Macmillan.

Van Herwaarden, C.L., R.A. Binkhorst, J.F. Fennis, and A. Van 'T Laar. 1979. Effects of propranolol and metroprolol on haemodynamic and respiratory indices and on perceived exertion during exercise in hypertensive patients. *Br. Heart J.* 41:99-105.

Wasserman, K., B.J. Whipp, S.N. Koyl, and W.L. Beaver. 1973. Anaerobic threshold and respiratory gas exchange during exercise. *J. Appl. Physiol.* 35:236-43.

12

CHAPTER

Global Perspectives and Future Directions

Previous chapters have considered the evolution of theoretical and empirical models that explain the psychophysiological basis of exertional perceptions. It is recognized that when examined separately none of the models is sufficiently comprehensive to account for all the inputs (i.e., physiological, psychological, and performance) that shape the perceptual milieu during dynamic exercise. A global model that expresses the gestalt of this milieu is needed. Such a model recognizes that exertional perceptions represent an intricate grouping of information derived from physiological mediators, psychological factors, and performance settings. The following is an attempt to model the mechanism whereby the preceding factors function interactively to set the intensity of exertional perceptions during dynamic exercise.

Mediating Inputs

Physiological Mediators

Exertional perceptions reflect the mediating influence of respiratory-metabolic, peripheral, and nonspecific physiological processes. These physiological mediators have been examined extensively in previous chapters. In order to provide a physiological framework for a global perceptual model, examples of the three types of mediators are reviewed here. Respiratory-metabolic mediators take the form of responses such as minute volume ventilation, respiratory rate, and the relative oxygen uptake. As such, they are primarily perceived through mechanisms that control changes in ventilatory drive secondary to oxidative metabolism and carbon dioxide excretion. Peripheral mediators arise from the active limbs and involve exercise-induced changes in blood pH, plasma glucose pools, and regional blood flow. Nonspecific physiological mediators influence exertional perceptions through generalized systemic processes such as increased catecholamine secretion and elevated skin temperature. Under many exercise conditions, the most intense perceptual signal arises from the peripheral mediators, while the respiratory-metabolic and nonspecific physiological responses provide a potentiating influence that fine-tunes the conscious expression of the perceptual response.

Psychological Mediators

Psychological mediators of perceived exertion are classified as either *dispositional* or *situational*. This classification reflects the setting-dependent influence of psychological processes in shaping perceptual responsiveness during exercise. That is, dispositional factors are enduring traits that mediate perceptual signals in a consistent and predictable manner during most performance settings. Examples of dispositional psychological mediators are stimulus intensity modulation, locus of control, sex-role orientation, cognitive style, self-efficacy, and personality. The perceptual mediating influence of situational psychological factors is specific to a given time and performance setting, altering the exertional response under one condition and not another. Examples of situational mediators are performance duration, outcome expectation, self-presentation, and attentional focus.

The various dispositional and situational psychological factors either directly mediate the intensity of exertional perceptions in a manner analogous to physiological mediators or else function as components of a perceptual-cognitive reference filter that systematically modulates the intensity of the exertional signal according to individual differences in personality, mood state, and symptomatic responses.

Performance Milieu

The intensity of exertional perceptions during dynamic exercise is influenced by two unique properties of the performance milieu.[1] In the first instance, specific features of the performance setting are incorporated into the global interpretation of the exertional experience, subsequently modulating perceptual intensity. Examples are (1) competitive advantage (i.e., score), (2) position of competitors in relation to completion of the event, (3) comparative difficulty of the competitive venue, (4) awareness of sweating and temperature-induced changes in skin color, (5) environmental factors (e.g., terrain, ambient temperature, weather conditions),

---

[1]The influence of the performance milieu in mediating exertional perceptions has not been considered extensively in previous chapters. Therefore, this section gives comparatively more attention to those performance factors that modulate perceptual intensity during physical exertion. In this way, the various physiological, psychological, and performance inputs that shape global perceptual responsiveness can be weighted according to their respective importance.

(6) audience composition (i.e., supportive or oppositional), (7) history of competition with opponent, (8) comparative importance of the competitive event, and (9) support from coaches and teammates. These performance-related factors function in a manner similar to physiological and psychological mediators in shaping the global perceptual experience during dynamic exercise.

In the second case, the various components of the performance setting are monitored to determine the appropriateness of a prearranged perceptual set point that regulates exercise intensity and race strategy. In this context, Noble et al. (1986) point out that perceptions are a link between internal neurophysiological functions and external performance environments. An exercise stimulus is sensed, and interpretations subsequently are made regarding the quality and quantity of the external environment. In an applied context, internalized perceptual responses are evaluated so that decisions can be made about performance intensity and race strategy. For example, an endurance athlete consciously matches sensory signals that are linked to internal neurophysiological events with the demands of the competitive setting. Race pace is subsequently adjusted to achieve optimal performance.

Perhaps the most elaborate example of the interaction between the perceptual and performance domains is described by Ulmer (1986) using a feedback loop. The loop is by definition self-adjusting, simultaneously accommodating changes in both the perceptual experience and the competitive strategy to optimize performance outcomes. At the center of the feedback loop is a perceptual set point. Adjusting performance intensity to produce exertional perceptions that match the set point assures an optimal tactical arrangement for competition. The tactical arrangement depends on the time or distance to be performed and positions of competitors relative to race completion. During competition, the perceptual set point regulates performance intensity in accordance with the tactical arrangement. When the perceptual set point is accurately produced by adjusting race pace, energy expenditure is optimal and competitive outcomes are maximized.

Adjustment of the tactical arrangement (i.e., race pace) to produce the perceptual set point uses a feedback loop that receives and evaluates signals from respiratory-metabolic and peripheral physiological mediators. The feedback loop instantaneously samples and transmits information regarding the degree of physiological and subjective strain induced by the performance. Based on this perceptual feedback, decisions are made concerning the appropriateness of the preset tactical arrangement and the athlete's physiological capacity to continue the performance without inducing fatigue. Performance-related information that is transmitted within the loop indicates when the prearranged level of exertion is too intense (i.e., the set point is too high), thus inducing early onset of fatigue and contributing to a poor performance. In such a case, the perceptual set point is lowered, causing a corresponding adjustment in the tactical arrangement. Race pace is in turn changed in order to produce the level of exertion consistent with the revised set point. Precise matching of the performance intensity with the perceptual set point is learned through training and actual competition. Therefore, what the individual perceives he or she is doing to a large extent actually determines the performance outcome (Morgan 1973).

Components of the Global Model

By its nature, a global model that attempts to identify and explain the totality of those factors that shape exertional perceptions must be sufficiently robust to account for a wide variety of physiological, psychological, and performance variables. The intent of the model is to demonstrate the totality of these combined inputs, expressing exertional perceptions as a gestalt of the individual's internal and external environments. To appreciate the exertional milieu as a gestalt, it is necessary to distinguish between perception and sensation. Sensation is typically viewed in a comparatively restricted context involving direct stimulation of sense organs. As such, a true sensation—that is, hearing, seeing, touching, tasting, and smelling—can only involve impressions for which an end organ exists. Perception, on the other hand, involves an awareness of objects and data that are in part mediated directly by sensory organs and are also in part influenced by more obtuse internal and external stimuli. From a functional standpoint, perception is more global in its conscious expression and reaction to a stimulus than is sensation. As such, perception involves both pure sensation and an array of factors for which there are no direct links with sensory end organs. These factors involve elements of the psychological and performance domains as well as selected physiological processes.

The global model presented here attempts to explain the exertional milieu during dynamic exercise using perception as opposed to sensation as its organizing conceptual framework. In this way the perceptual signal can be viewed as a gestalt involving an array of information, some of which is directly linked to sense organs and some of which is not. Figure 12.1 presents a global model of perceived exertion. The model is a fourth-generation conceptualization that was derived from previous explanatory models presented by Noble et al. (1986) and Robertson et al. (1986). The intent of the model is to explain the flow of neurosensory information from physical stimulus to perceptual response. Perceptual responsiveness is explained in a sequential pattern by interpreting the model from left to right. Physiological responses to an exercise stimulus serve as the initial mediators in setting the intensity of the perceptual signal. These signal mediators act individually or collectively to alter tension-producing properties of skeletal muscle. An exercise-induced increase in peripheral or respiratory muscle tension is accomplished by greater discharge of feedforward commands from the motor cortex. A copy of these commands is sent by corollary pathways to the sensory cortex, where they are interpreted as perceptual signals of exertion. The final mediating step occurs when the signal arising from the sensory cortex is matched with the contents of the perceptual-cognitive reference filter. It is this filter that fine-tunes the perceptual signal, modulating its intensity in accordance with the

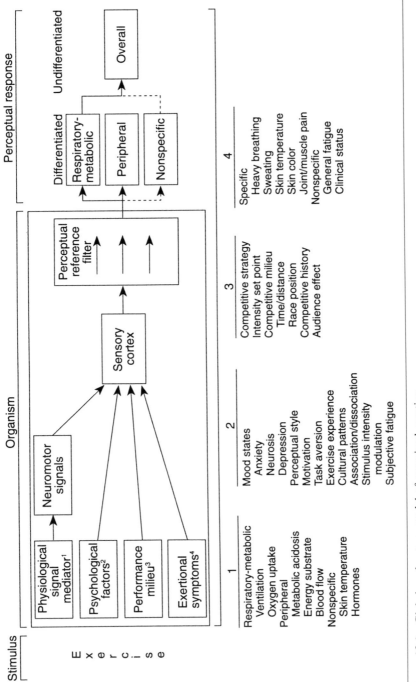

Figure 12.1 Global explanatory model of perceived exertion.
Adapted from Noble et al. 1986; Robertson et al. 1986.

299

matrix of past and present events that determine an individual's perceptual style. The actual expression of the perceptual response occurs as either a differentiated or undifferentiated report. Differentiated exertional reports are linked to specific perceptual signals arising from the active limbs (i.e., peripheral mediators) and the respiratory system (i.e., respiratory-metabolic mediators). The undifferentiated response for the overall body is an integration of the differentiated signals arising from involved body regions.

Future Directions

The following section conceptualizes a number of research and clinical initiatives that we feel will expand the knowledge base in the study of perceived exertion. These initiatives are listed here as "first-pass" ideas that may stimulate future scientific investigation in the field.

Perceptually Based Exercise Prescription

Research is needed to develop or validate

- estimation-production prescriptive procedures according to unique features and requirements of clinical, sport, pedagogical, occupational or military, and recreational settings;
- cross-modal estimation-production procedures that employ exertional perceptions to prescribe and regulate exercise intensity during circuit training (i.e., prescription of training intensity for cycling, rowing, stepping, and arm cranking) using perceptual responses from a graded treadmill test;
- estimation-production procedures that prescribe exercise intensity according to the RPE equivalent of the lactate or ventilatory threshold; and
- the relation between perceptual preference and metabolic efficiency in prescribing and regulating exercise intensity within the context of (1) normal daily physical activity, (2) structured regimens for therapeutic and sport training, and (3) a range of environmental conditions and activity modes.

Perceptually Based Graded Exercise Testing

Research is needed to develop or validate

- submaximal laboratory tests and field-based performance tests using perceived exertion as the criterion variable with applications for both clinically normal and diseased population subsets;
- a simple walk-run field test format for use with young children and older adults;

- a perceptually modified Sjostrand submaximal cycle protocol that (1) is technically simple to administer, (2) is low cost, and (3) predicts maximal aerobic power; and
- specificity and sensitivity of perceptually based laboratory and field tests for the assessment of physiological or clinical adaptations to exercise training.

Scaling Methods

Research is needed to develop or validate

- a standardized perceived exertion category scale for use by males and females of all ages and clinical status and in multicultural settings;
- verbal scale descriptors in a variety of languages using semantic differential analysis;
- a psychophysically optimal number of perceptual scale categories for use with a wide range of population subsets; and
- visual or pictorial scale descriptors of perceptual intensity for use with young children.

Psychological Mediators

Research is needed to develop or validate

- dispositional and situational psychological factors that (1) *directly* mediate perceptual intensity (e.g., personality) and (2) *indirectly* influence sensory responsiveness by operating as a component of a perceptual-cognitive reference filter (e.g., style of sensory augmentation or reduction); and
- theoretical and empirical models that explain how psychological mediators function in consort with physiological and performance factors in shaping a global perceptual response during exercise.

Physiological and Neuromuscular Mediators

Research is needed to develop or validate

- the perceptual influence of (1) energy substrate pools (i.e., blood glucose and muscle glycogen), (2) metabolic hormones (i.e., insulin, glucagon), (3) nonspecific systemic factors (e.g., catecholamines, beta-endorphins, and cortisol);
- the comparative importance of core and skin temperature in mediating perceptual intensity for a wide range of thermal conditions and relative metabolic rates in both men and women;

- the influence of muscle fiber type on perceptual responses, with specific reference to relative metabolic rate, energy substrate depletion, and type of training in men and women; and
- the comparative importance of neuromuscular feedback in fine-tuning the intensity of perceptual signals arising from peripheral and respiratory skeletal muscle.

Exertional Symptoms

Research is needed to develop or validate

- mechanisms whereby such exercise-related symptoms as fatigue, pain, exhaustion, discomfort or comfort, and pleasure interact with psychological and physiological factors to mediate the intensity of perceived exertion.

Differentiated Perceptual Responses

Research is needed to develop or validate

- differential signal strength and mode of sensory integration of exertional perceptions arising from peripheral and respiratory skeletal muscle, with specific attention to exercise mode, relative and absolute metabolic rate, and performance duration.

Individual Differences

Future experimental research and subsequent clinical applications involving perceptions of physical exertion should take into account the potential systematic influence of a wide range of individual differences. Examples include differences in gender, age, physical fitness, clinical status, cultural background, sport or athletic experience, and physical activity preference. Accounting for individual differences in sensory processes during exercise will increase the potential for pedagogical, sport, and therapeutic applications of perceptions of physical exertion.

Summary

This chapter presents a global model that explains the totality of the perceptual experience during physical exertion. This global conceptualization is effectively a fourth-generation model that has evolved from earlier theoretical and empirical models that described both physiological and psychological inputs to the exertional milieu during dynamic exercise. The organizational scheme of the global model depicts the exertional experience as a highly integrated perceptual gestalt that reflects inputs from physiological, psychological, and performance factors. In the final section, a brief summary of research initiatives that will facilitate future pedagogical, sport, and clinical applications of perceived exertion is presented.

References

Morgan, W.P. 1973. Psychological factors influencing perceived exertion. *Med. Sci. Sports* 5:97-103.

Noble, B.J., W.J. Kraemer, J.G. Allen, J.S. Plank, and L.A. Woodard. 1986. The integration of physiological cues in effort perception: Stimulus strength vs. relative contribution. In *The perception of exertion in physical work,* ed. G. Borg and D. Ottoson, 83-96. London: Macmillan.

Robertson, R.J., J.E. Falkel, A.L. Drash, A.M. Swank, K.F. Metz, S.A. Spungen, and J.R. LeBoeuf. 1986. Effect of blood pH on peripheral and central signals of perceived exertion. *Med. Sci. Sports Exerc.* 18:114-22.

Ulmer, H.V. 1986. Perceived exertion as a part of a feedback system and its interaction with tactical behavior in endurance sports. In *The perception of exertion in physical work,* ed. G. Borg and D. Ottoson, 317-26. London: Macmillan.

Credits

Figure 2.2   Adapted from S.S. Stevens, 1957, "On the psychophysical law," *Psychological Review* 64: 153-181.

Figure 3.1   Reprinted, by permission, from G. Borg, 1961, "Interindividual scaling and perception of muscular force," *Kungliga Fysiografiska Sallskapets I Lund Forhandlingar* 31(12): 120.

Figure 3.2   Adapted, by permission, from G. Borg, 1961, "Perceived exertion in relation to physical work load and pulse rate," *Kungliga Fysiografiska Sallskapets I Lund Forhandlingar* 37(11): 110.

Figure 3.3   Reprinted, by permission, from G. Borg, 1971, The perception of physical performance. In *Frontiers of fitness*, edited by R.J. Shephard (Springfield, IL: Charles C Thomas), 287.

Figure 3.4   Reprinted from C.M. Maresh and B.J. Noble, 1984, Utilization of perceived exertion ratings during exercise testing and training. In *Cardiac rehabilitation: Exercise testing and prescription*, edited by L.K. Hall, 157.

Figure 3.7   Reprinted, by permission, from G. Borg, 1971, The perception of physical performance. In *Frontiers of fitness*, edited by R.J. Shephard (Springfield, IL: Charles C. Thomas), 288.

Figure 3.8   Reprinted, by permission, from G. Borg, 1973, "A note on a category scale with ratio properties for estimating perceived exertion," *Reports from the Institute of Applied Psychology*: 4.

Figure 3.9   Reprinted, by permission, from G. Borg, 1982, A category scale with ratio properties for intermodal and interindividual comparisons. In *Psychophysical judgment and the process of perception*, edited by H-G Geissler and P. Petzold (Germany: VEB Deutscher Verlag der Wissenschaften), 31.

Figure 3.11   Adapted, by permission, from J.C. Hogan and E.A. Fleishman, 1979, "An index of the physical effort required in human task performance," *Journal of Applied Psychology* 64(2): 199.

Figure 3.13   Adapted, by permission, from A.P. Gagge, J.A.J. Stolwijk, and J.D. Hardy, 1967, "Comfort and thermal sensations and associated physiological responses at various ambient temperatures," *Environmental Research* 1, and from American College of Sports Medicine, 1986, *Guidelines for exercise testing and exercise prescription*.

Figure 4.1   Adapted, by permission, from P.C. Weiser, R.A. Kinsman, and D.A. Stamper, 1973, "Task specific symptomatology changes resulting from prolonged submaximal bicycle riding," *Medicine and Science in Sports* 5: 79-85.

Figure 4.2   Reprinted, by permission, from P.C. Weiser and D.A. Stamper, 1977, Psychophysiological interactions leading to increased effort, leg fatigue, and respiratory distress during prolonged, strenuous bicycle riding. In *Physical work and effort*, edited by G. Borg (New York: Pergamon Press), 402.

Table 5.1   Reprinted, by permission, from B.J. Noble et al., 1973, "Perceptual responses to exercise: A multiple regression study," *Medicine and Science in Sports* 5: 104-109.

Figure 5.1 Reprinted, by permission, from R.J. Robertson, 1982, "Central signals of perceived exertion during dynamic exercise," *Medicine and Science in Sports and Exercise* 14: 390-396.

Figure 5.2 Reprinted, by permission, from R.J. Robertson and K.F. Metz, 1986, Ventilatory precursors for central signals of perceived exertion. In *The perception of exertion in physical work*, edited by G. Borg and D. Ottoson (London: Macmillan Press), 111-121.

Figure 5.3 Reprinted, by permission, from R.J. Robertson, 1982, "Central signals of perceived exertion during dynamic exercise," *Medicine and Science in Sports and Exercise* 14: 390-396.

Figure 5.4 Reprinted, by permission, from R.J. Robertson, 1982, "Central signals of perceived exertion during dynamic exercise," *Medicine and Science in Sports and Exercise* 14: 390-396.

Figure 5.5 Reprinted, by permission, from K.B. Pandolf, 1977, Psychological and physiological factors influencing perceived exertion. In *Physical work and effort*, edited by G. Borg (New York: Pergamon Press), 371-384.

Figure 5.6 Reprinted, by permission, from R.J. Robertson, 1982, "Central signals of perceived exertion during dynamic exercise," *Medicine and Science in Sports and Exercise* 14: 390-396.

Figure 6.1 Reprinted, by permission, from R.J. Robertson et al., 1986, "Effect of blood pH on peripheral and central signals of perceived exertion," *Medicine and Science in Sports and Exercise* 18: 114-122.

Figure 6.2 Reprinted, by permission, from R.J. Robertson et al., 1986, "Effect of blood pH on peripheral and central signals of perceived exertion," *Medicine and Science in Sports and Exercise* 18: 114-122.

Figure 6.3 Reprinted, by permission, from R.J. Robertson et al., 1992, "Abatement of exertional perceptions following high intensity exercise: Physiological mediators," *Medicine and Science in Sports and Exercise* 24: 346-353.

Figure 6.4 Reprinted, by permission, from G. Borg, P. Hassmen, and M. Lagerstrom, 1987, "Perceived exertion related to heart rate and blood lactate during arm and leg exercise," *European Journal of Applied Physiology* 56: 679-685.

Figure 6.5 Reprinted, by permission, from H. Löllgen, T. Graham, and G. Sjogaard, 1980, "Muscle metabolites, force, and perceived exertion bicycling at varying pedal rates, *Medicine and Science in Sports and Exercise* 12: 345-351.

Figure 6.6 Reprinted, by permission, from B. Noble et al., 1983, "A category-ratio perceived exertion scale: Relationship to blood and muscle lactates and heart rate," *Medicine and Science in Sports and Exercise* 15: 523-529.

Figure 6.7 Reprinted, by permission, from R.J. Robertson et al., 1988, "Effect of simulated altitude erythrocythemia in women on hemoglobin flow rate during exercise," *Journal of Applied Physiology* 64: 1674-1679.

Figure 6.8 Reprinted, by permission, from G. Borg, P. Hassmen and M. Lagerstrom, 1987, "Perceived exertion related to heart rate and blood lactate during arm and leg exercise," *European Journal of Applied Physiology* 56: 679-685.

Figure 6.9 Reprinted, by permission, from R.J. Robertson et al., 1990, "Blood glucose extraction as a mediator of perceived exertion during prolonged exercise," *European Journal of Applied Physiology* 61: 100-105.

Figure 6.10   Reprinted, by permission, from R.J. Robertson et al., 1990, "Blood glucose extraction as a mediator of perceived exertion during prolonged exercise," *European Journal of Applied Physiology* 61: 100-105.

Figure 6.11   Reproduced with permission of the authors and publisher from: Skrinar, G.S., Ingram, S.P., & Pandolf, K.B. Effect of endurance training on perceived exertion and stress hormones in women. *Perceptual and Motor Skills*, 1983, 57, 1239-1250. © Perceptual and Motor Skills 1983.

Figure 6.12   Reprinted, by permission, from J.M. Pivarnik and L.C. Senay, 1986, "Effect of endurance training and heat acclimation on perceived exertion during exercise," *Journal of Cardiopulmonary Rehabilitation* 6: 499-504.

Figure 7.1   Reprinted, by permission, from E. Cafarelli, 1982, "Peripheral contributions to the perception of effort," *Medicine and Science in Sports and Exercise* 14: 382-389.

Figure 7.2   Reprinted, by permission, from E. Cafarelli, 1982, "Peripheral contributions to the perception of effort," *Medicine and Science in Sports and Exercise* 14: 382-389.

Figure 7.4   Reprinted, by permission, from J.R. Coast, R.H. Cox, and H.G. Welch, 1986, "Optimal pedalling rate in prolonged bouts of cycle ergometry," *Medicine and Science in Sports and Exercise* 18: 225-230.

Figure 7.5   Reprinted, by permission, from A. El-Manshawi and K.J. Killian, 1986, "Breathlessness during exercise with and without resistive loading," *Journal of Applied Physiology* 61: 896-905.

Figure 8.1   Reprinted, by permission, from H. Leventhal and O. Everhart, 1979, Emotion, pain and physical illness. In *Emotions in personality and psychopathology*, edited by C.E. Izard (New York: Plenum).

Figure 8.3   Reprinted, by permission, from G. Borg and D. Ottoson, 1986, *Perception of exertion in physical work* (London: Macmillan Press Ltd.).

Figure 8.5   Reprinted, by permission, from W.J. Rejeski, 1981, "The perception of exertion: A social psychophysiological integration," *Journal of Sport Psychology* 3(4): 316.

Table 10.1   Reprinted, by permission, from American College of Sports Medicine, 1991, *Guidelines for Exercise Testing and Prescription* (Philadelphia: Lea & Febiger).

Figure 10.1   From Herbert A. DeVries and Terry J. Housh, *Physiology of Exercise for Physical Education, Athletics and Exercise Science*, 5th ed. Copyright © 1994 Wm. C. Brown Communications, Inc. Reprinted by permission of Times Mirror Higher Education Group, Inc., Dubuque, Iowa. All Rights Reserved.

Figure 10.2   Reprinted, by permission, from M.L. Pollock, J.H. Wilmore, and S.M. Fox, 1984, *Exercise in health and disease: Evaluation and prescription for prevention and rehabilitation* (Philadelphia: W.B. Saunders).

Figure 10.3   Reprinted, by permission, from B.J. Noble, 1973, "Perceived exertion during walking and running-II," *Medicine and Science in Sports* 5(2): 116-120.

Figure 10.5   Reprinted, by permission, from R.J. Robertson, F.L. Goss, and K.F. Metz, Ratings of perceived exertion (RPE) in cardiac rehabilitation: Application and validation. In *Proceedings of the Vth world congress on cardiac rehabilitation*, edited by J.P. Broustet (England: Intercept Ltd.), 151-159.

Figure 10.6   Reprinted, by permission, from R.J. Robertson, F.L. Goss, and K.F. Metz, Ratings of perceived exertion (RPE) in cardiac rehabilitation: Application and validation. In *Proceddings of the Vth world congress on cardiac rehabilitation*, edited by J.P. Broustet (England: Intercept Ltd.), 151-159.

Figure 10.7 Reprinted, by permission, from G. Borg, 1982, "Ratings of perceived exertion and heart rates during short-term cycle exercise and their use in a cycling strength test," *International Journal of Sports Medicine* 3: 153-158.

Figure 10.8 Reprinted, by permission, from C.R. Davies and A.J. Sargeant, 1979, "The effects of atropine and practolol on the perception of exertion during treadmill exercise," *Ergonomics* 22: 1141-1146.

Figure 10.10 Reprinted, by permission, from H. Linderholm, 1986, Perceived exertion during exercise in the discrimination between circulatory and pulmonary disorders. In *Perception of exercise in physical work*, edited by G. Borg and D. Ottoson (London: Macmillan Press), 199-206.

Figure 10.11 Reprinted, by permission, from G. Borg, A. Holmgren and I. Lindblad, 1980, "Perception of chest pain during physical work in a group of patients with angina pectoris," *Reports from the Institute of Applied Psychology* 81:8.

Figure 10.12 Reprinted, by permission, from J. Karlsson et al., 1984, "Angina pectoris and blood lactate concentration during graded exercise," *International Journal of Sports Medicine* 5: 348-351.

Figure 11.2 Reprinted, by permission, from M.L. Pollock, J.H. Wilmore, and S.M. Fox, 1984, *Exercise in health and disease: Evaluation and prescription for prevention and rehabilitation* (Philadelphia: W.B. Saunders).

Figure 11.3 Reprinted, by permission, from M.C. Guttman et al., 1981, "Perceived exertion-heart rate relationship during exercise testing and training in cardiac patients," *Journal of Cardiac Rehabilitation* 1: 52-59.

Figure 11.4 Reprinted, by permission, from M. Van Den Burg and R. Ceci, 1986, A comparison of a psychophysical estimation and a production method in a laboratory and a field condition. In *Perception of exertion in physical work*, edited by G. Borg and D. Ottoson (London: Macmillan Press), 35-46.

Figure 11.6 Reprinted, by permission, from C.M. Maresh and B.J. Noble, 1984, Utilization of perceived exertion ratings during exercise testing and training. In *Cardiac rehabilitation: Exercise testing and prescription*, edited by L.K. Hall (New York: Spectrum Publications), 155-173.

Figure 11.7 Reprinted, by permission, from G. Borg, 1985, *An introduction to Borg's RPE scale* (Ithaka, NY: Mouvement Publications).

Figure 11.8 Reprinted, by permission, from C.M. Bayles et al, 1990, "Perceptual regulation of prescribed exercise," *Journal of Cardiopulmonary Rehabilitation* 10: 25-31.

Figure 11.9 Reprinted, by permission, from R.J. Robertson et al., 1990, "Cross-modal exercise prescription at absolute and relative oxygen uptake using perceived exertion," *Medicine and Science in Sports and Exercise* 27 (5): 656.

Figure 11.10 Reprinted, by permission, from R.J. Robertson et al., 1990, "Cross-modal exercise prescription at absolute and relative oxygen uptake using perceived exertion," *Medicine and Science in Sports and Exercise* 27 (5): 656.

Figure 11.11 Reprinted, by permission, from B.J. Noble et al., 1973, "Perceived exertion during walking and running-II," *Medicine and Science in Sports* 5: 116-120.

Figure 11.12 Reprinted, by permission, from M.C. Gutmann et al., 1981, "Perceived exertion-heart rate relationship during exercise testing and training in cardiac patients," *Journal of Cardiopulmonary Rehabilitation* 1: 52-59.

Figure 11.13 Reprinted, by permission, from G. Borg, A. Holmgren and I. Lindblad, 1980, "Perception of chest pain during physical work in a group of patients with angina pectoris," *Reports from the Institute of Applied Psychology* 81: 8.

Index

About the Authors

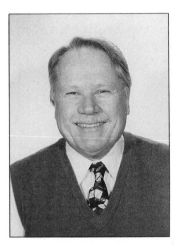

Bruce J. Noble, PhD, is professor of exercise physiology at Purdue University. He has done research in the field of perceived exertion since 1967 and has published widely on the subject, including his previous book, *Physiology of Exercise and Sport*. Noble served as doctoral advisor to coauthor Robert J. Robertson, as well as to Kent Pandolf and Enzo Cafarelli, all major figures in perceived exertion research for the past two decades.

In 1970 and 1973 Noble was visiting professor at the Institute of Applied Psychology in Stockholm, Sweden, where he worked with Gunnar Borg, eminent researcher in the field of perceived exertion and father of modern scaling methods. Noble was also an invited lecturer at the International Symposium on Perceived Exertion in Stockholm in 1980 and distinguished visiting professor at the University of North Carolina–Greensboro in 1988.

Noble has been a professor at the universities of Pittsburgh, Wyoming, and Illinois and a member of the board of directors for the American College of Sports Medicine, the American Alliance for Health, Physical Education, Recreation and Dance (AAHPERD), and the American Heart Association. He also served as President of AAHPERD'S Research Consortium.

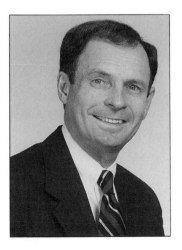

Robert J. Robertson, PhD, is Professor of Health and Physical Education at the University of Pittsburgh. He earned his PhD in Health and Physical Education/Exercise Physiology from the University of Pittsburgh in 1973 and has extensive teaching, research, and writing experience in the field of perceived exertion. Robertson has served as Director of the Human Energy Research Laboratory at the University of Pittsburgh and the Physical Fitness Research Laboratory at the University of Nebraska at Lincoln. Over the years, he has made numerous presentations on perceived exertion at international symposia.

In 1982 Robertson authored an influential article, "Central Signals of Perceived Exertion During Dynamic Exercise," which synthesized what was then known about the respiratory-metabolic mediators of exertional perceptions. Published in *Medicine and Science in Sports and Exercise*, the paper remains an important reference.

Robertson is a Fellow of the American College of Sports Medicine and a member of the American Association of Cardiovascular and Pulmonary Rehabilitation. He received the Professional Honor Award from the Pennsylvania Association for Health, Physical Education, Recreation and Dance in 1985.